INTRODUCTION TO QUALITY AND SAFETY EDUCATION FOR NURSES

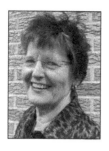

Patricia Kelly, MSN, RN, earned a diploma in nursing from St. Margaret Hospital School of Nursing, Hammond, Indiana; a baccalaureate in nursing from DePaul University in Chicago, Illinois; and a master's degree in nursing from Loyola University in Chicago, Illinois. She is professor emeritus, Purdue University Calumet, Hammond, Indiana. She has worked as a staff nurse, school nurse, and nurse educator. Patricia has traveled extensively in the United States, Canada, and Puerto Rico, teaching conferences for The Joint Commission, Resource Applications, Pediatric Concepts, and Kaplan, Inc. She currently teaches nationwide National Council Licensure Examination for Registered Nurses® (NCLEX-RN®) review courses for Evolve Testing & Remediation/Health Education Systems, Inc. (HESI), Houston, Texas. Patricia currently is a nursing volunteer at the Old Irving Park Community Clinic in Chicago, a free clinic for patients without health care insurance.

Patricia was director of Quality Improvement at the University of Chicago Hospitals and Clinics. She has taught at Wesley-Passavant School of Nursing and Chicago State University. Patricia was program director of the Associate Degree Nursing Program and Faculty at Purdue University Calumet. Patricia has taught Fundamentals of Nursing, Adult Nursing, Nursing Leadership and Management, Nursing Issues, Nursing Trends, Quality Improvement, and Legal Aspects of Nursing. She is a member of Sigma Theta Tau, the American Nurses Association, and the Emergency Nurses Association. She is listed in Who's Who in American Nursing, Notable American Women, and the International Who's Who of Professional and Business Women.

Patricia has served on the Board of Directors of Tri-City Mental Health Center, St. Anthony's Home, and the Mosby Quality Connection. She is the editor of *Nursing Leadership and Management*, now in its third edition; *Essentials of Nursing Leadership and Management* (with Janice Tazbir, coeditor), now in its third edition; and *Nursing Delegation, Setting Priorities, and Making Patient Care Assignments* (with Maureen Marthaler, coeditor) second edition. She contributed a chapter, "Preparing the Undergraduate Student and Faculty to Use Quality Improvement in Practice," to *Improving Quality*, second edition, by Claire Gavin Meisenheimer. She also contributed a chapter on obstructive lung disease to *Medical Surgical Nursing* by Rick Daniels. She has published several articles and has served as a national disaster volunteer for the American Red Cross. She has also been a health care team member on health care relief trips to Nicaragua.

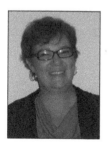

Beth A. Vottero, PhD, RN, CNE, earned a baccalaureate degree in liberal studies with a focus in business management from the University of Maine at Presque Isle; a baccalaureate degree in nursing from Valparaiso University; a master's degree in nursing from University of Phoenix; and a PhD in nursing education from Capella University. Previously, Beth taught undergraduate nursing at Purdue University North Central and taught in the graduate nursing program at Bethel College. Beth currently is an assistant professor of nursing at Purdue University Calumet, teaching graduate courses in informatics and in the Nurse Executive program. At the undergraduate level, she teaches Quality and Safety for Professional Nursing Practice, Informatics, and facilitates evidence-based quality-improvement student Capstone projects.

Beth's background includes over 18 years as a staff and charge nurse. After completing her doctorate, Beth coordinated and led a successful Magnet redesignation for Indiana University Health La Porte Hospital in La Porte, Indiana. She brought a desire to instill quality concepts to academia where she co-created a course at Purdue University Calumet focused on quality and safety in health care. Beth is a research associate with the Indiana Center for Evidence-Based Practice in Hammond, Indiana, a Joanna Briggs Institute (JBI) Collaborating Center. Through this association, she has completed a systematic review that was translated into a Best Practice Information Sheet for the JBI, assisted in developing an Evidence-Based Practice Fellowship program at Purdue University Calumet, and presented at the International JBI Conference in Chicago, Illinois.

Beth has published chapters such as "Systems for Evidence-Based Practice" in Hopp and Rittenmeyer's *Introduction to Evidence-Based Practice: A Practical Guide for Nurses*; "E-learning

Assessment" in Bristol and Zerwekh's *Essentials of E-Learning for Nurse Educators*; and has developed case studies for Zerwekh and Zerwekh's *Nursing Today: Transitions and Trends*. She has presented on topics concerning informatics at the undergraduate and graduate levels; developing a quality and safety course at the 2013 Quality and Safety Education for Nurses Conference in Atlanta, Georgia; and was the keynote speaker on the social obligation for evidence-based practice at the 2011 Evidence-Based Nursing Practice Conference in Hammond, Indiana. As a funded researcher through Purdue University, Beth has studied factors affecting medication errors in the clinical setting. Currently, she is completing a study on the effects of interruptions on medication error rates.

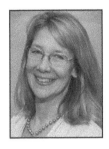 **Carolyn A. Christie-McAuliffe, PhD, FNP,** obtained her diploma in nursing from Crouse-Irving Memorial Hospital School of Nursing, Syracuse, New York; a baccalaureate and master's degree in nursing from the State University of New York, Health Science Center at Syracuse, Syracuse, New York; and a PhD in nursing from Binghamton University, Binghamton, New York. Her clinical experience has included staff nursing, home health care, oncology care, and private practice. She has functioned as an administrator primarily in clinical research and taught at the undergraduate and graduate nursing levels at Crouse-Irving Memorial Hospital School of Nursing, Syracuse, New York; The College of Notre Dame of Maryland, Baltimore, Maryland; State University of New York (SUNY) Institute of Technology, Utica, New York; and Keuka College, Keuka Park, New York. She has implemented multiple evidence-based practice and quality assurance programs and served as a compliance officer and Institutional Review Board chair at SUNY Institute of Technology. Carolyn's research interest and efforts have focused on primary prevention. The majority of her publications and speaking engagements have centered on topics of research, evidence-based practice, and leadership.

Currently Carolyn is an associate professor of nursing at Keuka College and co-principal investigator of a National Institutes of Health (NIH)/National Center for Complementary and Alternative Medicine (NCCAM) R01 grant through the University of Rochester on preventing chemotherapy-induced nausea. In addition, Carolyn is in independent practice as a nurse practitioner in Syracuse, providing primary care.

INTRODUCTION TO QUALITY AND SAFETY EDUCATION FOR NURSES
CORE COMPETENCIES

Patricia Kelly, MSN, RN
Beth A. Vottero, PhD, RN, CNE
Carolyn A. Christie-McAuliffe, PhD, FNP
Editors

SPRINGER PUBLISHING COMPANY
NEW YORK

Springer Publishing Company, LLC
11 West 42nd Street
New York, NY 10036
www.springerpub.com

Acquisitions Editor: Joseph Morita
Composition: Newgen Imaging

ISBN: 978-0-8261-2183-7
e-book ISBN: 978-0-8261-2184-4
Instructors' PowerPoint Material: 978-0-8261-2607-8

Instructors may request supplements by e-mailing textbook@springerpub.com

15 16 17 / 5 4

The author and the publisher of this Work have made every effort to use sources believed to be reliable to provide information that is accurate and compatible with the standards generally accepted at the time of publication. Because medical science is continually advancing, our knowledge base continues to expand. Therefore, as new information becomes available, changes in procedures become necessary. We recommend that the reader always consult current research and specific institutional policies before performing any clinical procedure. The author and publisher shall not be liable for any special, consequential, or exemplary damages resulting, in whole or in part, from the readers' use of, or reliance on, the information contained in this book. The publisher has no responsibility for the persistence or accuracy of URLs for external or third-party Internet websites referred to in this publication and does not guarantee that any content on such websites is, or will remain, accurate or appropriate.

Library of Congress Cataloging-in-Publication Data

Introduction to quality and safety education for nurses : core competencies / [edited by] Patricia Kelly, Beth A. Vottero, Carolyn Christie-McAuliffe.
  p. ; cm.
Includes bibliographical references and index.
  ISBN 978-0-8261-2183-7 (alk. paper) — ISBN 978-0-8261-2184-4 (e-book)
  I. Kelly, Patricia, 1941- editor of compilation. II. Vottero, Beth, editor of compilation. III. Christie-McAuliffe, Carolyn, editor of compilation.
  [DNLM: 1. Nursing—standards—United States. 2. Quality of Health Care—United States. 3. Patient Safety—United States. 4. Safety Management—United States. WY 16 AA1]
  RT73
  610.73071'1—dc23

2013040388

Printed in the United States of America by Courier.

This book is dedicated by Patricia Kelly to her loving dad and mom,
Ed and Jean Kelly; to her dear partner, support, and best friend,
Ron Vana; to her super sisters, Tessie Kelly Dybel and Kathy Kelly Milch;
to her dear aunts and uncles, Aunt Pat and Uncle Bill Kelly
and Aunt Verna and Uncle Archie Payne; to her nieces, Natalie Dybel Bevil,
Melissa Milch Arredondo, and Stacey Milch Monks; to her nephew, John Milch;
to her grandnephew, Brock Bevil, and grandniece, Reese Bevil;
and to her nephews-in-law, Tracy Bevil, Peter Arredondo,
and Derek Monks.

Beth Vottero would like to thank her support, her rock, and her hero...her
ever-patient husband Dino. Thanks also go to her son Tom (Army Strong),
Mitchell (umpire extraordinaire), Micah, and Trisha; to her ever-loving parents
Tom and Judy, Ray and Dolly; to her fashionista sister and her husband,
Becky and Shannon; and to her dog Ben, who sat on a chair and stared at her for
hours while she worked. To her super-fantastic, unbelievably incredible
coworkers; you know who you are and how much your support means to me.

Carolyn A. Christie-McAuliffe would like to thank her incredible husband
and best friend, Chris, as well as her two precious sons who provide
inspiration and unending support; thanks also to her parents
and siblings, colleagues and friends and, most of all,
thank you to her patients who motivate her to continually
seek better ways to provide safe and efficacious care.

CONTENTS

UNIT III. QUALITY IMPROVEMENT

UNIT IV. SUPPORTS FOR PATIENT SAFETY AND QUALITY OF CARE

UNIT V. ENSURING FUTURE FIDELITY IN PATIENT SAFETY AND QUALITY: THE EVOLVING ROLE OF THE REGISTERED NURSE

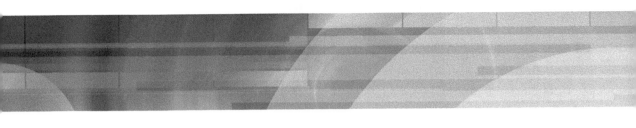

CONTRIBUTORS

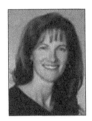

Gerry Altmiller, EdD, APRN, ACNS-BC
Associate Professor
CNS Track Director
Chair Faculty Search
    Committee
La Salle University
School of Nursing and Health
    Sciences
Philadelphia, Pennsylvania

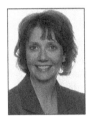

Anne K. Anderson, DNP, MHSA, RN, CPHQ, NEA-BC
Director
Patient Care Services and
    Magnet Quality Leader
Central DuPage Hospital
Winfield, Illinois

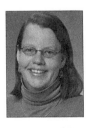

Gail Armstrong, DNP, ACNS-BC, CNE
Associate Professor
University of Colorado College
    of Nursing
Aurora, Colorado

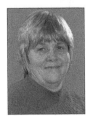

Pauline Arnold, MSN MSA RN HACP
Chief Nursing and Quality
    Officer
VP Clinical Operations
Indiana University Health La
    Porte Hospital
La Porte, Indiana

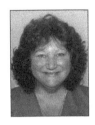

Esther Bankert, PhD, RN
Consultant in Nursing Education
Remsen, New York
Adjunct Professor of Nursing
New England Institute of
    Technology
East Greenwich, Rhode Island
Provost and Dean Emerita
State University of New York
    Institute of Technology
Utica, New York

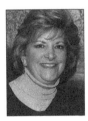

Amy J. Barton, PhD, RN, FAAN
Associate Dean for Clinical and
    Community Affairs
Professor, Daniel and Janet
    Mordecai Endowed Chair in
    Rural Health Nursing
University of Colorado College
    of Nursing
Aurora, Colorado

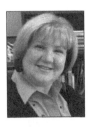

Michelle E. Block, PhD, RN
Associate Professor
    of Nursing
School of Nursing
Purdue University Calumet
Hammond, Indiana

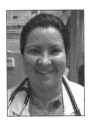

Lindsay Bonaventura, MS, RN, FNP-BC
Family Nurse Practitioner
Chesterton, Indiana

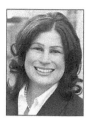

Ashley Currier, MSN, RN, NE-BC
Director of Operations-Process
   Improvement
Northwestern Memorial
   Physicians Group
Chicago, Illinois

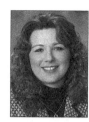

Andrea Lazarek-LaQuay, MS, RN
Vice President of Strategic
   Innovation
Visiting Nurse Association of
   Central New York
Syracuse, New York

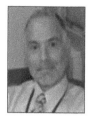

Anthony L. D'Eramo, MSN, RN, CPHQ
ISO Consultant, Region 1
VHA ISO Consultation
   Division, Office of Quality,
   Safety, and Value
Coventry, Rhode Island
Providence VA Medical Center
Providence, Rhode Island

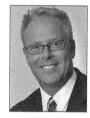

Jerry A. Mansfield, PhD, RN
Chief Nursing Officer
University Hospital and the
   Richard M. Ross Heart
   Hospital
The Ohio State University
   Wexner Medical Center
Columbus, Ohio

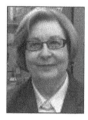

Mary Gillaspy, MLS, MS
Manager, Health Learning
   Centers, Retired
Northwestern Memorial
   Hospital
Woodland Park, Colorado

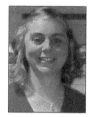

Karen L. McCrea, DNP, FNP-C
Assistant Professor
School of Nursing and Health
   Studies
Georgetown University
Washington, DC

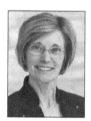

Corinne Haviley, RN, MS, PhD
Associate Chief Nursing
   Officer
Outpatient, Behavioral Health,
   and Emergency Services
Central DuPage Hospital
Winfield, Illinois

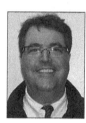

Peter D. Mills, PhD, MS
Director
VA National Center for Patient
   Safety Field Office
White River Junction, Vermont
Adjunct Associate Professor
   of Psychiatry, Dartmouth
   Medical School
Hanover, New Hampshire

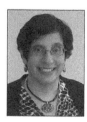

Joanne M. Joseph, PhD
Professor of Psychology
SUNY Institute of Technology
Utica, New York
Director of Assessment
   and Coordinator for the
   Center for Service-Based
   Learning and Community
   Engagement
Clinton, New York

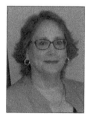

Joanne Belviso Puckett, EdM, RN
Organizational Excellence
   Coach
VA New England Healthcare
   System (VISN 1)
Hanover, New Hampshire

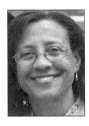

Francia I. Reed, MS, RN, FNP-C
Nurse Executive, Lt Col, New York Air National Guard
Clinical Assistant Professor and Coordinator
Masters in Nursing Education Program
State University of New York, Institute of Technology
Utica, New York

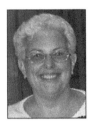

Christine Rovinski-Wagner, ARNP, MSN
Accreditation/Performance Improvement Coordinator
VA Medical Center
White River Junction, Vermont

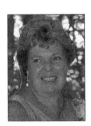

Kathleen Fischer Sellers, PhD, RN
Professor and Chair, Department of Nursing
Alfred State College
Alfred, New York

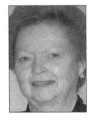

Donna L. Silsbee, PhD, RHIA, CTR, CCS
Associate Professor and Coordinator, Health Information Management/ Health Services Management
State University of New York Institute of Technology
Utica, New York

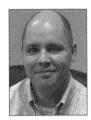

J. Scott Thomson, MLIS, AHIP
Library Director, Boxer Library
Rosalind Franklin University of Medicine and Science
North Chicago, Illinois

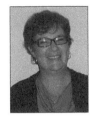

Beth A. Vottero, PhD, RN, CNE
Assistant Professor of Nursing
Purdue University Calumet
College of Nursing
Research Associate
Indiana Center for Evidence-Based Nursing Practice
Joanna Briggs Collaborating Center
Hammond, Indiana

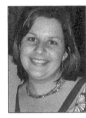

Cibele C. Webb, MSN Ed., RN
Adjunct Professor
Bethel College School of Nursing
Mishawaka, Indiana

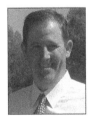

Patrick M. Webb, MD
Beacon Health System
Medical Group, Family Practice
La Porte, Indiana

FOREWORD

More than a decade ago, the Institute of Medicine initiated a call to action challenging health care providers to adopt competencies to improve the quality and safety of health care. Like-minded nursing trailblazers, who were focused on health care improvement, heeded that call. Through vigilance and a generous grant from the Robert Wood Johnson Foundation (RWJF), the Quality and Safety Education for Nurses (QSEN) collaboration began. The collaboration developed competencies reflecting a nursing identity where knowledge, skills, and attitudes support actions that emphasize patient-centered care, collaboration with other members of the health care team, evidence-based practice, quality improvement, safety, and the integrated use of informatics. The initial RWJF grant funded 15 pilot schools to join with the original founders and develop strategies and tools to support quality and safety education. What began as a small group of dedicated individuals grew into a network of innovative educators and practitioners with a single vision: to transform the professional identity of nurses by changing basic education for nurses. QSEN's vision was to position nurses to create a safer health care system. The authors of this book share that vision.

The QSEN competencies have become the underpinning of practice at all levels of nursing education. Moving away from task-oriented instruction, nursing education has become focused on the development of attributes that direct a nurse not only to focus on how to provide safe and effective care, but also to continuously strive to improve the quality and efficiency of that care. It is now imperative that upon entering the workforce, nurses immediately take the lead in terms of their ability to ensure a safe environment for patients and effect change for continuous quality improvement.

As a QSEN consultant, and with many years working to incorporate the QSEN competencies into classroom and clinical experiences for nursing students, I have learned that quality and safety are not new ideas, although the skills needed to ensure quality and safety in our rapidly advancing, technologically challenging, and culturally diverse world are new. Principles that guide nursing work can be traced back to Florence Nightingale, and enacting those principles in our sophisticated health care system has become complex. Students need guidance to become effective caregivers, proficient communicators, contributing team members, and staunch patient advocates.

Students need a clear road map for developing their professional nursing identity. This book is that road map.

Introduction to Quality and Safety Education for Nurses: Core Competencies provides a comprehensive overview of essential knowledge, skills, and attitudes that support quality and safety competencies in nursing practice. It contains many practical examples from real-life experiences. Each chapter includes interviews with experts in their respective health care field to provide an interprofessional team perspective. Interviewees include pharmacists, nurses, lawyers, physicians, librarians, quality improvement nurses, radiology technologists, nurse practitioners, hospital board members, and patients. Discussion questions and case studies are designed to facilitate application of interprofessional collaboration.

The textbook is written by nurse educators, nurse researchers, librarians, nurse administrators, nurse case managers, physicians, nurse quality improvement practitioners, nurse practitioners, nurse entrepreneurs, and others whose work in quality improvement and safety education has been nationally recognized. Contributors to this text come from all over the United States, including Colorado, Illinois, Indiana, New Hampshire, New Jersey, New York, Ohio, Pennsylvania, Rhode Island, Vermont, and Washington, DC, emphasizing a diverse and broad view of quality and safety. Chapter contributors include members from the original 15 pilot schools of the QSEN collaboration. Many contributors have developed teaching strategies that are shared internationally through the QSEN website and have presented at the annual QSEN National Forum. Their collective expertise provides a solid foundation for students working to develop a professional nursing identity grounded in high-quality practice.

Faculty will find that this text is an excellent resource to support their efforts to prepare future nurses for the demands of current practice in health care. Health care organizations expect quality-minded practitioners, and each chapter addresses pertinent quality-focused topics of nursing practice. Nurses need to understand quality metrics and data and be able to utilize them to effect change that leads to improved care for patients. While it has always been identified that quality and safety are important aspects of nursing care, research now provides us with evidence that quality and safety practices ensure safe, high-quality, consistent patient outcomes. That research translates into evidence-based practice. New quality measures and benchmarking are emerging. Current accreditation standards for educational institutions dictate stringent expectations for the new health care workforce. Quality and safety competencies have been incorporated into the essentials of baccalaureate education, and are becoming a condition of nursing licensure through the Transition to Practice Program developed by the National Council of the State Boards of Nursing. Students recognize their individual responsibility to provide high-quality, safe care. This textbook will provide the resources needed for students to frame their professional nursing identity and build a strong foundation for their current and future nursing practice.

Gerry Altmiller, EdD, APRN, ACNS-BC
Associate Professor, La Salle University, Philadelphia, Pennsylvania
QSEN Consultant and QSEN Advisory Board Member

FOREWORD

*H*ealth care providers and consumers of care demand excellence. When that is not achieved, and less than optimal outcomes are realized, the competence of individual providers pushes to the forefront of discussions, complaints, and root cause investigations. Assuming or judging individual competence is complicated, particularly when other causes, such as organizational factors, are disregarded or not appreciated. In too many instances, particularly when care does not meet our expectations or an adverse event occurs, the key factors indicate troubles with the competency of not just one but many.

With the increasing complexity of health care and patient needs, there is a demand for qualified and competent health care providers for high-quality, safe patient care. The attainment of nursing quality and safety competencies begins during coursework and clinical preparation, is developed in practice, and is refined with experience. While we may agree that all health care providers need to demonstrate specific competencies in practice, we struggle with the definition, context, attainment, importance, and demonstration of competencies within various health care environments. A common understanding of the definitions, standards, and domains of competencies is essential and antecedent to potential associations with understanding and improving organizational, professional, and patient outcomes.

Each day, nurses fulfill many different expectations in different contexts with changing demands and multiple challenges. To do so, nurses apply and adapt their competencies as part of their professional practice performance. The application and adaptation of one's competencies are influenced by many factors, including attitudes, motives, and perceptions. Notwithstanding, perceptions of functioning competencies or levels of competencies may be intertwined with the performance of other nurses and health care providers. As such, there are challenges in measuring competencies and understanding the confluence of competencies across health care teams. It may be that differences in scope of practice among the professions do not necessarily indicate discipline-specific competencies. Instead, competencies are interdependent and practice specific.

Core competencies for quality and patient safety have been defined by the Quality and Safety Education for Nurses (QSEN) initiative, funded by the Robert Wood Johnson

Foundation, to prepare the future nursing workforce with necessary knowledge, skills, and attitudes to be actively engaged in improving the quality and safety of health care. The approach in this book is based on QSEN and is structured to ensure that students will obtain the recommended competencies and knowledge necessary to provide care that is both high quality and safe in practice. Patricia Kelly, Beth A. Vottero, and Carolyn A. Christie-McAuliffe bring the QSEN core competencies together in an introductory book to improve student preparation. It is a book that will be an essential tool on our journey to realize the quality and safety of care we all demand.

Ronda G. Hughes, PhD, MHS, RN, CLNC, FAAN
Associate Professor, Nursing, Marquette University, Milwaukee, Wisconsin
Member, Institute of Medicine Committee on Credentialing Research in Nursing
Editor, *Patient Safety and Quality: An Evidence-Based Handbook for Nurses*
Agency for Healthcare Research and Quality

PREFACE

The 1994 Institute of Medicine (IOM) report, *America's Health in Transition: Protecting and Improving Quality*, highlighted the seriousness and pervasiveness of health care error rates and their effect on patient outcomes and morbidity and mortality rates. Then, in 2000, the IOM released the report, *To Err Is Human: Building a Safer Health System*. This IOM report instantly received national attention from policy makers, health care providers, and consumers. The IOM report stated, "At least 44,000 people, and perhaps as many as 98,000 people, die in hospitals each year as a result of medical errors that could have been prevented." This IOM report caused major ripples throughout the health care system and highlighted the need to change how health care is delivered.

The 2001 release of the IOM report, *Crossing the Quality Chasm: A New Health System for the 21st Century*, spotlighted general problems in health care in an attempt to close the gap between what is known to provide quality health care and what is actually occurring in practice. The IOM report defined six aims for health care: Health care should be safe, effective, patient-centered, timely, efficient, and equitable. The IOM report also identified 10 rules for care delivery redesign, available at http://www.nap.edu/openbook.php?record_id=10027&page=6. This IOM report spawned a series of IOM reports on priority health care areas, for example, public health; biomedical and health research; diseases; quality and patient safety; health services, coverage, and access; select populations and health disparities; food and nutrition; veterans' health; health care workforce; environmental health; global health; substance abuse and mental health; women's health; aging; and education. The IOM report, *The Future of Nursing: Leading Change, Advancing Health* (2011), recommended that nurses practice to the full extent of their education, improve nursing education, provide nursing leadership positions in health care redesign, and improve data collection for workplace planning and policy making. These IOM reports called for changes in how health care organizations provide safe, quality patient care services. Currently, the IOM and many others, including clinicians, health care organizations, employers, consumers, foundations, research agencies, government agencies, and quality organizations, are working to create a more patient-centered, 21st-century health care system.

A primary movement for change in nursing academia toward the inclusion of more educational information on safe, effective, patient-centered, timely, efficient, and equitable patient care has been the Quality and Safety Education for Nurses (QSEN) initiative. QSEN followed the IOM lead and stated that changes in health care needed to focus on the development of nursing competencies in patient-centered care, teamwork and collaboration, quality improvement, evidence-based practice, and informatics. Because of nurses' unique position to protect patient safety, safety was added as a sixth competency. The QSEN initiative convened a national panel of experts to identify the core knowledge, skills, and attitudes (KSAs) required for each of the six competencies. Information about the KSAs is available at http://qsen.org.

Another significant movement for health care change has been the Agency for Healthcare Research and Quality (AHRQ). This agency, with funding from the Robert Wood Johnson Foundation, published *Patient Safety and Quality: An Evidence-Based Handbook for Nurses* (2008), edited by Ronda G. Hughes, to provide all nurses with evidence-based techniques and interventions to improve patient outcomes.

WHY THIS BOOK, *INTRODUCTION TO QUALITY AND SAFETY EDUCATION FOR NURSES: CORE COMPETENCIES?*

The idea for this book was born when two of the editors, Patricia Kelly and Dr. Beth A. Vottero attended the 2011 QSEN conference in Milwaukee, Wisconsin. Patricia and Beth, from the Chicago area, invited Dr. Carolyn A. Christie-McAuliffe, from New York, to join them as the third editor to facilitate the development of a broad look at quality and safety. The three coeditors experienced the rapid evolution of quality and safety information in their clinical and academic practices and they identified the need for nursing students to receive an understanding of quality and safety in their basic nursing preparation. The coeditors believed in the need to organize existing information about quality and safety into one basic, easily understood textbook.

The purpose of this book is to provide a comprehensive overview of essential KSAs about quality and safety competencies in nursing practice. Many practical examples from real-life experiences are discussed. Exposing nursing students to key concepts related to the QSEN areas of quality, safety, patient-centered care, teamwork and collaboration, evidence-based practice, and informatics helps students build a foundation for their current and future nursing practice.

The contributors to this text include nurse educators, nurse faculty, nurse researchers, librarians, nurse administrators, nurse case managers, physicians, nurse quality improvement practitioners, nurse practitioners, nurse entrepreneurs, psychologists, and others. These contributors are from all over the United States, emphasizing a broad view of quality and safety. There are contributors from Colorado, Illinois, Indiana, New Hampshire, New Jersey, New York, Ohio, Pennsylvania, Rhode Island, Vermont, and Washington, DC.

Each chapter includes interviews with experts in their respective health care field to provide an interprofessional team perspective. Interviewees include pharmacists, nurses, lawyers, physicians, librarians, quality improvement nurses, radiology technologists, nurse practitioners, hospital board members, patients, and others.

Appendix A lists key IOM reports that have influenced changes in health care today. Additional IOM reports, updated June 2013, are found at http://www.iom .edu/~/media/Files/About%20the%20IOM/IOMPublicationList63013.pdf.

An important feature of this book is the listing of QSEN competencies and the associated KSAs found in Appendix B. Appendix B also identifies the chapter in which the QSEN competency's KSA information can be found in the text. This will help both students and faculty plan for the development of KSA competency in students.

Appendix C identifies additional critical thinking exercises with answers designed to build competency in the six QSEN competencies.

Appendix D contains answers and rationale for each of the chapter Review Questions.

Appendix E contains answers to the chapter Review Activities.

ORGANIZATION

Introduction to Quality and Safety Education for Nurses: Core Competencies consists of 13 chapters organized into five units. Each unit provides nursing students and beginning nurses with a background and foundational knowledge of quality and safety in today's health care environment.

- Unit I, "Introduction to Quality and Safety Education for Nurses: Core Competencies," covers a broad overview of the importance of quality and safety for health care professionals from a national and organizational perspective. The three chapters in this unit include "Overview of Patient Safety and Quality of Care," "Quality and Safety Education for Nurses," and "Quality and Safety in High-Reliability Organizations."
- Unit II introduces concepts of patient safety, interprofessional teamwork and collaboration, and patient-centered care. There are three chapters in this unit, one chapter on each of the three concepts.
- Unit III focuses on quality improvement. There are three chapters: "Essentials of Quality Improvement," "Benchmarking Quality Performance," and the "Tools of Quality Improvement."
- Unit IV, "Supports for Patient Safety and Quality of Care," includes three chapters: "Informatics," "Basic Literature Search Strategies," and "Evidence-Based Practice."
- Unit V has one chapter, "The Future Role of the Registered Nurse in Patient Safety and Quality."

CHAPTER FEATURES

Several chapter features are used throughout the text to provide the reader with a consistent format for learning. Chapter features include:

- Photos, tables, and figures to enhance student understanding
- Health care or nursing quotes related to chapter content
- Objectives that state the chapter's learning goals
- Opening Scenario, a mini entry-level clinical situation that relates to the chapter, with two or three critical thinking questions
- Key Concepts, a listing of the primary understandings the reader is to take from the chapter
- Key Terms, a listing of important new terms defined in the chapter
- Review Questions, several multiple-choice and alternate-style National Council Licensure Examination for Registered Nurses (NCLEX-RN®) questions (answers to Review Questions are in Appendix D)
- Review Activities, to help students apply chapter content to patient care situations (answers to Review Activities are in Appendix E)
- Exploring the Web activities
- References
- Suggested Reading

Special elements are sprinkled throughout the chapters to enhance student learning and encourage critical thinking and application of the knowledge presented. These include:

- Evidence from the literature with a synopsis of key findings from nursing and health care literature.

- Real-World Interviews with health care leaders and managers, including nursing staff, clinicians, administrators, risk managers, faculty, nurses, physicians, patients, nursing assistive personnel, lawyers, pharmacists, hospital administrators, and others.
- Critical Thinking exercises regarding a safety or quality-related issue (answers to Critical Thinking exercises are at the end of each chapter).
- Case Studies to provide the nursing student with a patient care situation calling for critical thinking to solve an open-ended problem (answers to Case Study questions can be found at the end of each chapter).

Highlights of the Text

- A strong foundation for evidence-based health care with attention to high-quality, safe care is emphasized throughout the text.
- Chapters include new information from national, federal, and state health care and nursing organizations.
  - Teamwork and interprofessional collaboration is stressed throughout the text.
  - The six QSEN competencies with their KSAs are highlighted in the chapters and in Appendix B.
  - There are extensive critical thinking activities and case studies throughout the chapters and Appendix C contains additional critical thinking activities with answers.

INSTRUCTOR RESOURCES

1. Suggested answers to the text's Critical Thinking exercises, Review Questions, Review Activities, and Case Studies, as well as a guided discussion of each chapter's Opening Scenario, are included in the text's chapters and appendices.
2. Lecture slides in PowerPoint for each chapter serve as guides for presentation in the classroom. **These can be obtained for qualified instructors by e-mailing Springer Publishing Company at textbook@springerpub.com.**

Patricia Kelly
Beth A. Vottero
Carolyn A. Christie-McAuliffe

REFERENCES

Agency for Healthcare Research and Quality (AHRQ). (2008). *Patient safety and quality: An evidence-based handbook for nurses*. AHRQ Publication No. 08–0043. Rockville, MD: Author. Retrieved from http://www.ahrq.gov/professionals/clinicians-providers/resources/nursing/resources/nurseshdbk/index.html

Institute of Medicine (IOM). (1994). *America's health in transition: Protecting and improving quality*. Washington, DC: National Academy of Sciences. Retrieved from http://www.nap.edu/openbook.php?record_id=9147&page=R1

Institute of Medicine (IOM). (2000). *To err is human: Building a safer health system*. Washington, DC: National Academy of Sciences. Retrieved from http://www.nap.edu/openbook.php?record_id=9728&page=R1

Institute of Medicine (IOM). (2001). *Crossing the quality chasm: A new health system for the 21st century*. Washington, DC: National Academy of Sciences. Retrieved from http://www.nap.edu/openbook.php?booksearch=1&term=crossing%20the%20quality%20chasm%20a%20new%20health%20system%20for%20the%2021st%20century%20(&record_id=10027

Institute of Medicine (IOM). (2010). *The future of nursing: Leading change, advancing health*. Retrieved from http://www.iom.edu/Reports/2010/The-future-of-nursing-leading-change-advancing-health.aspx

ACKNOWLEDGMENTS

A book such as this requires much effort and the coordination of many persons. Pat, Beth, and Carolyn would like to thank all of the contributing authors for their time and effort in sharing their knowledge gained through years of experience in both clinical and academic settings. All of the contributing authors worked within tight time frames to share their expertise. Thanks also to Jane Woodruff for her computer support and Jane A. Walker, PhD, RN, for her networking support.

We would like to acknowledge and sincerely thank the Springer Publishing Company team who worked to make this book a reality. Joseph Morita, senior acquisitions editor, and Chris Teja, assistant editor, are great people who worked hard to bring this book to publication.

OVERVIEW OF PATIENT SAFETY AND QUALITY OF CARE

Corinne Haviley, Anne K. Anderson, and Ashley Currier

To know one's strengths, to know how to improve them, and to know what one cannot do are the keys to continuous learning. (Peter Drucker, 2004)

Upon completion of this chapter, the reader should be able to

1. Define patient safety and quality of care
2. Identify forces influencing health care safety and quality including the role of national health care accreditation organizations
3. Discuss core measures, sentinel events, and never events
4. Discuss health care in industrialized countries
5. Describe the costs of health care salaries, medications, technology, and malpractice in the United States
6. Discuss variation in health care delivery
7. Describe the American Nurses Credentialing Center (ANCC) Magnet™ Recognition Program
8. Discuss the Baldrige Awards
9. Identify the Institute of Medicine (IOM) report, *The Future of Nursing: Leading Change, Advancing Health*
10. Discuss the role of nurses at the "sharp" end of health care
11. Discuss efforts to increase health care transparency, improve public reporting of health care, and reduce unwarranted variation in health care safety and quality
12. Identify the Patient Protection and Affordable Care Act
13. Identify ethical and legal responsibilities of the professional nurse related to Quality and Safety Education for Nurses (QSEN) including knowledge, skills, and attitudes (KSAs) related to patient-centered care, teamwork and collaboration, evidence-based practice (EBP), quality improvement (QI), safety, and informatics

*Y*ou have completed an orientation to patient care delivery on a medicine inpatient unit.

- What elements of quality care would you look for on the unit to better understand the patient care that the staff is delivering?
- What type of questions might you ask the staff related to their QI work?
- What type of quality concerns do the patients have?

*P*atient safety and quality of care are very important topics because they touch every patient and family experience within health care. Ensuring that patients are safe and that they receive high-quality care is at the top of the health care provider's mind. Understanding safety and quality is very complex. Multiple providers deliver patient care and they depend on and complement each other to support safe, high-quality patient care.

This chapter provides information about patient safety and quality of care. It defines safety and quality. Then, forces influencing health care safety and quality including the role of national health care accreditation organizations, **core measures**, sentinel events, and never events are discussed. The chapter discusses health care in industrialized countries and the costs of health care salaries, medications, technology, and malpractice in the United States. Variation in health care delivery, the ANCC Magnet Recognition Program and the Baldrige Award are explored. The chapter then identifies the IOM report *The Future of Nursing: Leading Change, Advancing Health* and discusses the role of nurses at the "sharp" end of health care. Efforts to increase health care transparency, improve public reporting of health care, and reduce unwarranted variation in health care safety and quality are explored and the Patient Protection and Affordable Care Act is discussed. Finally, ethical and legal responsibilities of the professional nurse related to QSEN including KSAs related to patient-centered care, teamwork and collaboration, EBP, QI, safety, and informatics are explored.

PATIENT SAFETY AND QUALITY OF CARE

Patient safety and quality are key concepts that have been studied, defined, and redefined over time. QSEN, a Robert Wood Johnson Foundation project that addresses the challenge of preparing future nurses with the KSAs necessary to continuously improve the quality and safety of the health care systems in which they work, suggests that **safety** is the process of minimizing risk of harm to patients and providers through both system effectiveness and individual performance (QSEN, 2012b). The Joint Commission, a prominent health care regulatory agency further expands the definition of safety as "the degree to which the risk of an intervention, for example, use of a drug, or a procedure, and risk in the care environment are reduced for a patient and other persons, including health care practitioners. Safety risks may arise from the performance of tasks, from the structure of the physical environment, or from situations beyond the organization's control, such as weather" (The Joint Commission, 2011, p. GL-34).

Health care quality is "the degree to which care, treatment, or services for individuals and populations increases the likelihood of desired health or behavioral health outcomes; considerations include the appropriateness, efficacy, efficiency, timeliness, accessibility and continuity of care, the safety of the care environment and the individual's personal values, practices and beliefs" (The Joint Commission, 2011b, p. GL-31). Patients' quality concerns are often related to health care access, safety, outcomes, and respect (Table 1.1; Healthcare Financial Management Association's [HFMA's] Value Project, 2011).

TABLE 1.1 PATIENT'S QUALITY CONCERNS

Access	Make my care available and affordable
Safety	Do not hurt me
Outcomes	Make me better
Respect	Respect me as a person, not a case

Source: HFMA's Value Project (2011).

Quality has been further discussed by the Agency for Healthcare Research and Quality (AHRQ, 2011) as follows:

- "Doing the right thing (getting the health care services you need)
- At the right time (when you need them)
- In the right way (using the appropriate test or procedure)
- To achieve the best possible results" (AHRQ, 2011)

Importance of Patient Safety and Quality of Care

Why are we so prescriptive in defining safety and quality? Think about patients as consumers. Patients should be able to have access to care, be respected, and receive health care that is directed toward meeting individual needs based on evidence-based research. Patients expect to receive safe, high-quality treatment and care without negative outcomes, for example, harm from medication administration, infection passed from a caregiver to a patient, surgical procedure done on the wrong body part. Patients should receive treatment in a timely enough fashion to save their life. Patients do not want to be a part of any of the mishaps named above. Yet it does happen within our health care system.

Error-Free Care and Lack of Evidence

The U.S. health system has not provided consistent error-free care to all patients. In addition, many health care treatments are not based upon scientific evidence partially because health care providers such as nurses and doctors find it difficult to keep up with the pace of development of new knowledge, scientific findings, and new technology development (Leape, 2008).

Patients often have multiple chronic conditions that interplay, such that caregivers are often not just treating one acute illness or problem. They are treating multiple illnesses or problems in one patient. Coordinating this care has become increasingly more difficult. The process for handing off patients from one provider to another provider is often slowed down, delaying care delivery because of the time-consuming efforts required to treat the whole patient and not just one problem (Leape, 2008). It is not that we have uncaring individuals, inadequate training, or uncommitted people providing care within our health care system. Rather, our health care work processes have not always been able to support the complex care needed by our patients.

Landmark Safety and Quality Stories

Two stories related to safety and quality care have publically rocked the United States and have sent shock waves through our health care system. The first story occurred in 1994. A 39-year-old patient with breast cancer, Betsy Lehman, died from an overdose of chemotherapy at a highly prestigious academic institution. Betsy was the wife of a cancer researcher affiliated with Dana Farber Institute in Boston, Massachusetts, and lost her life at the very same hospital where her husband worked. She received four times the dose of Cytoxan ordered for her treatment. The nurses and pharmacists reportedly misinterpreted a physician's order to give 6,520 mg of the drug daily for 4 days. The physician's intent was to give a total dose of 6,520 mg over 4 consecutive days (Kenney, 2008).

The second story occurred in 2001. Josie King, a 17-month-old girl, was admitted to Johns Hopkins Hospital, Baltimore, Maryland, after she had turned on the hot water in a bath tub and climbed into scalding water at her home. After 2 weeks of treatment, Josie began to show signs of improvement. Sorrel King, Josie's mother, was at her bedside most of the time and wanted to partner with the staff to help her child recover. Josie began to have unexplained symptoms, for example, her eyes rolling upwards and being lethargic to the point of listlessness. At that point, a decision was made to hold the patient's methadone injections for pain, which seemed to be contributing to her symptoms. Mrs. King did not trust the nurse who was caring for her daughter in spite of reassurance from other staff. Later that same nurse administered an additional dose of methadone in error. Josie subsequently went into cardiac arrest and died from a narcotic overdose and dehydration (Josie King Foundation, 2002). After Josie's death, Mrs. King, worked endlessly to publicly share this horrific story. Mrs. King's passion has led to the requirement for all The Joint Commission–accredited hospitals in the United States to have rapid response teams to provide care for patients with deteriorating conditions.

The stories of Betsy Lehman and Josie King, like many others, have touched the hearts of caregivers nationwide and have helped us to learn from our mistakes. They were pivotal in igniting a call to action to improve patient safety. As health care providers, we have taken a strong look in the mirror trying to understand how we can make improvements so that no one will be harmed in any way. Even though these stories happened several years ago, we are still not where we want to be in confidently providing care of the highest safety and quality and without error.

REAL-WORLD INTERVIEW

Every nurse wants and intends to deliver safe, accurate, healing care to every patient. When an error does occur, it can be personally and professionally devastating, even if there is little or no harm to the patient. We know that the nurse can be a "second victim" of health care error, struggling with self-doubt and fear, even shame, often in silence.

The overwhelming majority of health care errors occur as a result of poor systems design, poor handoffs and communication, wrong assumptions, and from the explosion of technology, drugs, and devices that are challenging to master. Many errors are related to poor teamwork and a steep power gradient that makes it difficult for a junior member of the team to speak up. Health care errors cause serious harm to the person we are most committed to help, our patient. As a nurse, you can reduce your patients' vulnerability to harm by thinking critically about the health care systems within which you work and investing energy and commitment in your clinical team. Strong health care organizations welcome your thoughtful attention to opportunities for improvement.

Cynthia Barnard, MBA, MSJS, CPHQ
Director, Quality Strategies, Northwestern Memorial Hospital, Chicago, Illinois

FORCES INFLUENCING HEALTH CARE SAFETY AND QUALITY

A provocative IOM *To Err Is Human* publication in 1999 became the impetus for propelling the safety and quality movement forward. This IOM report proclaimed alarming data, including the finding that there were up to 98,000 preventable deaths yearly; but as important, the cause was defective processes, not defective people (Leape, 2008).

Another IOM report, *Crossing the Quality Chasm: A New Health System for the 21st Century* (National Research Council, 2001), zoomed in on the need to collect and analyze data related to the cause and effect of health care errors, reducing dependence on our ability to recall and increasing our need to standardize approaches to routine care. These IOM reports and subsequent reports were the forces behind the health care QI revolution involving the government, consumers, providers, and the health care industry. This revolution led health care to reduce errors in clinical practice through a comprehensive strategy. Since 1994, there have been 164 IOM reports developed and published under the heading of Quality and Safety (Institute of Medicine of the National Academy of Sciences, 2012).

National Health Care Accreditation Organizations

There are many national health care accreditation organizations (Table 1.2). The Joint Commission is one of the most highly visible not-for-profit organizations in the United States. The Joint Commission accredits more than 19,000 health care organizations and programs in the nation. An **accredited hospital** is one that demonstrates that the hospital meets the minimal standards for quality developed by The Joint Commission or another accrediting agency; this includes monitoring of standards such as infection control standards, medication management standards, emergency management standards, and so on, as well as measurement of core accountability measures, safe practice measures, and process improvement.

Cost of Accreditation

Meeting The Joint Commission accreditation requirements has significant monetary compensation implications because hospitals must to be accredited to be reimbursed

---

TABLE 1.2 HEALTH CARE ACCREDITATION ORGANIZATIONS

Centers for Medicare and Medicaid Services (CMS) (http://www.cms.gov)

The Joint Commission (www.jointcommission.org)

Healthcare Facilities Accreditation Program (HFAP) (www.hfap.org)

Det Norske Veritas Healthcare Inc. (DNVHC, Inc.) (http://www.dnvusa.com/industry/healthcare/index.asp)

The American Osteopathic Association (AOA; http://www.osteopathic.org)

Commission on Accreditation of Rehabilitation Facilities (CARF; http://www.carf.org/home)

Community Health Accreditation Program (CHAP; www.chapinc.org)

The Accreditation Commission for Health Care Inc. (ACHA; www.achc.org)

Utilization Review Accreditation Commission (URAC; www.urac.org)

The Exemplary Provider Program of the Compliance Team (www.exemplaryprovider,com)

The Healthcare Quality Association on Accreditation (HQAA; www.hqaa.org)

for patient care covered by Medicare and Medicaid. The Medicare and Medicaid patient population is often a sizable proportion of patients treated in hospitals. The average fee for a hospital's full accreditation survey in 2010 was $46,000 (The Joint Commission International, 2011a).

Core Measures of Quality

Core measures are standardized performance indicators that allow for comparison of quality measures between organizations. Currently, hospitals are required to collect and transmit data to The Joint Commission on 45 core measures. Core measures for a patient with an acute myocardial infarction include such measures as

- Aspirin on patient arrival
- Statin prescribed at discharge
- Beta blocker prescribed at discharge (The Joint Commission, 2012a)

A listing of the top hospital performers on 45 core accountability measures, 2012, for heart attack, heart failure, pneumonia, surgical care, children's asthma care, inpatient psychiatric services, venous thromboembolism, and stroke care is available at The Joint Commission (2012b). Since the inception of The Joint Commission Core Measure data tracking requirements, remarkable improvements in core measures have been realized often due to interprofessional efforts that are coordinated rather than each profession working alone in individual silos (The Joint Commission, 2012b).

REAL-WORLD INTERVIEW

Inherent in our roles as registered nurses (RNs) is a commitment to quality and safety in our delivery of patient care. As the largest group of health care providers, RNs are on the "front line" of care delivery and are acutely aware of what works and what does not work. Over time, however the constant work-around by staff to get the patient/family what they need can be "opportunities" for error. Going around systems and policies may seem the right thing to do, in the moment, but in the long run may set up the nurse and/or system for a near miss or even more serious—a sentinel event. Standing by as a silent member of an interprofessional team can mean the difference between patient safety and harm. Nursing's call to action and the responsibility held by our professional licensure asks us to take a more active role.

Solutions to our health care delivery system to promote quality and safety are best handled with the interprofessional team. Recognizing that patients' needs are complex, with shorter lengths of stays in hospitals, high rates of readmissions and multiple chronic conditions, all elevate the need for greater surveillance by the RN. The eyes, ears, and hands of the nurse are tools to discern quality and safety concerns—but the work of the nurse is enhanced when others join the process (e.g., pharmacists, dietitians, respiratory therapists, etc.). Getting to know your fellow clinical providers and joining in dialogue of how to promote safety

(continued)

and quality in the work setting puts the patient in an environment with care we would ask be given to a loved one.

Jerry A. Mansfield, PhD, RN
Chief Nursing Officer, Ambulatory Services—Health System
The Ohio State University Medical Center Columbus, Ohio

Sentinel Events

A **sentinel event** is an unexpected occurrence involving death or serious physical or psychological injury, or the risk thereof (The Joint Commission, 2012c). Sentinel events are carefully reviewed for quality problems when they occur. From 2004 to 2011, there were 4,909 sentinel events reported to The Joint Commission. They included

• Wrong-Patient, Wrong-Site, Wrong-Procedure	734 sentinel events
• Delay In Treatment	604 sentinel events
• Operative/Postoperative Complication	570 sentinel events
• Retention of Foreign Body (since 2005)	546 sentinel events
• Suicide	518 sentinel events
• Medication Error	310 sentinel events
• Criminal Event	211 sentinel events
• Perinatal Death/Injury	185 sentinel events
• Medical Equipment Related	151 sentinel events

From The Joint Commission (2011).

HEALTH CARE COSTS IN INDUSTRIALIZED COUNTRIES

There has been mounting pressure as a result of a U.S. economic downturn to manage the rising costs of health care while ensuring that value and choice are maintained. **Value for health care organizations** is defined as quality divided by cost (Porter, 2010). Choices are made at a number of levels within a health system such as whether to seek care, what types of care to seek and when, which health care providers to see, what benefits to prioritize in selecting a health plan, and which health plan to join. Health care value increases when health care outcomes demonstrate improvement and health care costs are reduced.

Note that health care spending per capita in the United States is close to double compared to five other industrialized countries, namely, Canada, Germany, France, Australia, and the United Kingdom (Figure 1.1). This is after adjusting the per capita spending rates to international dollars to account for purchasing power parity (PPP). In a 2007 study comparing six health care quality indicators, health care access, quality care, efficiency, equity, healthy lives, and health expenditures per capita, the United States ranked last in contrast with the five countries mentioned earlier (Davis et al., 2007). At the present time, health care costs continue to rise and there is considerable strain on the U.S. national income while at the same time there is significant consumer dissatisfaction with health care.

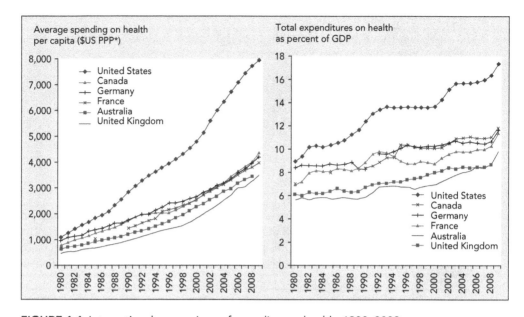

FIGURE 1.1 International comparison of spending on health, 1980–2009.

Source: University of California Atlas of Global Inequality (2012) and The Commonwealth Fund (2011).

Note the international health care comparisons in Table 1.3. European health care systems use price controls, negotiated physician fees, and hospital budgets with limits on expenditures and use of new technology. They keep annual cost increases within the 3% to 4% range (United States = 7%), have better health outcomes than we do in many areas, and achieve all of this at significantly less cost (Callahan, 2008).

REAL-WORLD INTERVIEW

Staff nurses should be aware of the way hospitals look at quality measures and how they use these to make decisions. Typically hospitals make decisions based on a series of strategic goals. These strategic goals are usually grouped into:

1. Quality and safety
2. Financial performance
3. Patient satisfaction/experience
4. Strategic growth
5. Workforce

When hospitals make decisions about programs they look at each of these five strategic goal groups to make sure goals are being met. Hospitals would not make a decision based on financial performance if it would negatively impact quality and safety.

(continued)

To track progress on decisions and to point out opportunities to improve, hospitals use dashboards. Each department has target measures and goals to obtain. Variation from these targets are tracked. If we are off target, we put in place a plan to get back on track. We are always mindful to not negatively impact any one of the five strategic goal areas. The things we measure can also be determined by regulatory agencies such as The Joint Commission, the Department of Public Health, or by government agencies such as Medicare. For example, core measures are measured to comply with The Joint Commission regulations.

Staff nurses should be aware of their hospitals goals and metrics for decision making. If the hospital is not posting these in a common area, the staff nurse should ask his or her supervisor to see the dashboards.

An example of a common measure on hospital dashboards is length of stay (LOS). LOS is important from a financial performance, patient satisfaction, and quality perspective. Payments to hospitals are typically paid per discharge and adding days to the patients stay results in higher cost. Additionally, patients are more satisfied if they can recover at home and have the same quality outcomes if we are careful to give good discharge instructions and home care.

Ann McMackin, MS
Health Care Consultant, Belmont, Massachusetts

Life Expectancy and Health Care Spending

Though health care organizations strive to deliver high levels of quality, along with safe and effective care, they are challenged to do so at low cost. The United States spends more on health care than most other countries in the world yet life expectancy falls short in comparison to many other countries. Note that life expectancy in the five countries mentioned earlier, Canada, Germany, France, Australia, and the United Kingdom, is higher than life expectancy in the United States, yet the United States spends significantly more for health care (Figure 1.2).

HEALTH CARE SALARY, MEDICATION, MEDICAL TECHNOLOGY, AND MALPRACTICE COSTS IN THE UNITED STATES

Several categories of health care costs, for example, health care workers' salaries, add to the cost of health care in the United States. Table 1.4 illustrates several different health care workers' salaries.

Medication Cost

The cost of medications has also been an area of concern for Americans. Differences in medication costs are not reported as frequently as other expenses. Here are a few examples of the cost of medications in the United States, United Kingdom, and Canada (Table 1.5). U.S. medication costs are three to six times greater than many other countries (Motheral, 2011). U.S. pharmaceutical companies justify these high U.S. costs to support drug trials and research.

TABLE 1.3 INTERNATIONAL HEALTH CARE COMPARISONS

COUNTRY	WHO RANK	SPENDING PER PERSON PER YEAR	YEARS OF LIFE EXPECTANCY	ADULTS WHO REPORT GOOD HEALTH	TYPE OF SYSTEM	ADULTS NOT HAPPY WITH SYSTEM
France	11	$3,926 80% government	80.9	80%	Universal coverage in employment-based system with supplemental private insurance available.	N/A
Japan	10	$2,908 83% government	82.1	39%	Universal care for all. Half the population has insurance through employers. Other half in national insurance program.	N/A
United Kingdom	18	$3,065 87% government	78.7	74%	Universal care for all. Also funded through patient co-pays and a small amount of private, supplemental insurance.	15%
Germany	25	$3,628 77% government	78.9	73%	World's oldest universal health care system with both national and private insurance.	27%
Canada	30	$3,678 70% government	80.3	88%	Government-sponsored and –funded	12%
United States	37	$6,347 45% government	78.1	89%	Employer–employee-insurance based with government coverage for some children, elderly, disabled, poor, veterans, and government employees.	34%

Sources: World Health Organization (WHO), Organization for Economic Development and Cooperation, International Development Research Centre, Commonwealth Fund, University of Michigan, University of Maine, Henry J. Kaiser Family Foundation, National Center for Policy Analysis, reported in, A World of Options on Health Care Reform (2009).

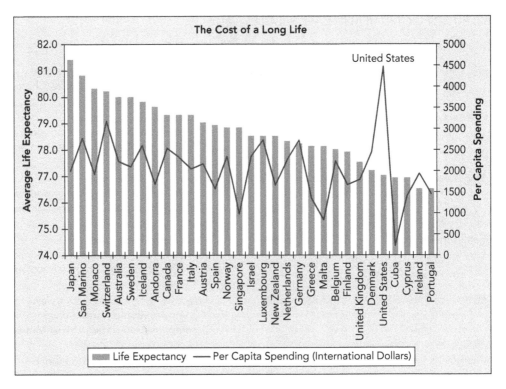

FIGURE 1.2 Average life expectancy and per capita spending.
Source: University of California Atlas of Global Inequality (2012).

Medical Technology

Medical technology costs are also worthy of concern. There has been an increase in the use of this technology. It is estimated that 40% to 50% of annual health care cost increases are associated with the development of new technologies or the increased use of existing ones. Health care economists suggest that the control of technology is the most important factor in bringing costs down (The Hastings Center, 2012).

Technology can be used to record, review, and collaborate with other team members on test and procedure results, progress notes, patient history, medications, and potential surgery. It can be used to initiate referrals and make work lists, for example, a list of today's patients, orders, and test results. Technology also offers current and future clinical decision support and the use of clinical alerts to avoid medication errors or warn of panic levels of laboratory results. It can offer evidence-based guideline support with suggested orders and illustrations of problem-based documentation. Technology can provide health maintenance reminders; it can capture patient outcome data; generate a patient's problem list; and analyze variability in patient care costs, outcomes and treatment patterns.

Also note the use of robotic devices now available in hospitals that are willing to pay for the equipment. Laparoscopic surgery done with the use of robotics is linked to decreased length of hospital stays as compared to conventional surgery. These devices are reported to have been responsible for a reduction in postoperative pain, scarring, infections, and blood transfusions. Robots cost an average of $1.3 million in addition

TABLE 1.4 SELECTED HEALTH CARE SALARIES

ROLE	SALARY	SOURCE
CEO, Kaiser	$1,965,682 average	http://www.kaiserhealthnews.org/Stories/2011/September/28/Chart-CEO-Pay-Packages.aspx
Anesthesiologist	$372,750 median	http://cejka.force.com/PhysicianCompensation#compdata; AMGA Physician Compensation Survey excerpt
General surgeon	$367,315 median	http://cejka.force.com/PhysicianCompensation#compdata; AMGA Physician Compensation Survey excerpt
Family medicine MD	$208,658 median	http://cejka.force.com/PhysicianCompensation#compdata; AMGA Physician Compensation Survey excerpt
Dentist	$167,389 median	http://www.cejkasearch.com/view-compensation-data/mid-level-compensation-data/; AMGA Mid-Level Compensation Data 2009
Pharmacist	$112,160 mean	May 2011 National Occupational Employment and Wage Estimates United States. Retrieved from http://www.bls.gov/oes/current/oes_nat.htm#29–0000
Dietitian and nutritionist	$55,460 mean	May 2011 National Occupational Employment and Wage Estimates United States. Retrieved from http://www.bls.gov/oes/current/oes_nat.htm#29–0000
Nurse practitioner	$86,410 median	http://www.cejkasearch.com/view-compensation-data/mid-level-compensation-data/; AMGA Mid-Level Compensation Data 2009
Registered nurse	$67,720 mean	United States Department of Labor, Bureau of Labor Statistics. (2011). *May 2010 national occupational employment and wage estimates United States.* Retrieved from http://www.bls.gov/oes/current/oes_nat.htm#29–0000
Licensed practical nurse	$41,360 mean	United States Department of Labor, Bureau of Labor Statistics. (2011). *May 2010 national occupational employment and wage estimates United States.* Retrieved from http://www.bls.gov/oes/current/oes_nat.htm#29–0000
Nursing aide	$25,420 annual mean wage	United States Department of Labor, Bureau of Labor Statistics. (2011). *May 2010 national occupational employment and wage estimates United States.* Retrieved from http://www.bls.gov/oes/current/oes_nat.htm#31–0000

TABLE 1.5 COST OF SELECTED MEDICATIONS IN THE UNITED STATES, UNITED KINGDOM, AND CANADA

MEDICATION	U.S. COST	UK COST	CANADA COST
Plavix	$152	$57	$76
Lipitor	$129	Less than $40	Less than $40

Adapted from Motheral (2011).

TABLE 1.6 TECHNOLOGY COSTS

TECHNOLOGY	COST
Implantable pacemaker	$4,218
Knee implant—femoral	$2,601
Drug-eluting stent	$1,414
Computerized tomography (CT) scanner	$1,081,200
MRI	$1,674,332
Bed, electric	$14,712
Portable ultrasound system	$35,112

Adapted from Modern Healthcare (2012).

to several hundred thousand dollars of annual maintenance fees (Feder, 2008). It has been reported that the number of robot-assisted procedures throughout the world has increased by approximately three times since 2007. The number of da Vinci robotic systems (the premier robotic technology) that were installed in U.S. hospitals grew by approximately 75% between 2007 and 2009 (Barbash & Glied, 2010). Note other technology costs found in hospitals today in Table 1.6. It is important to use technology in cost-effective ways to improve quality and safety.

Malpractice

Malpractice in the United States currently runs at about $55.6 billion a year, $45.6 billion of which is spent on defensive medicine practiced by physicians seeking to stay clear of lawsuits. Note that $55.6 billion comprises 2.4% of the nation's total health care expenditure (Mello, Chandra, Gawande, & Studdert, 2010).

Reimbursement and Insurance

Health care organizations are partially reimbursed for patient health care costs through health care insurance, including Medicare, Medicaid, and private insurance such as Blue Cross Blue Shield, Aetna, and so on. When patients do not have insurance, they are required to pay "out of pocket" for health care services, which means that they are personally responsible for payment. In an effort to contain costs, one government payer source, the Centers for Medicare and Medicaid Services (CMS) has developed criteria to measure and pay hospitals related to patient care in the past several years. Hospitals are obligated to publicly report specific measures on patients who use

TABLE 1.7 SELECTED NEVER EVENTS

- Patient suicide
- Sexual assault on a patient
- Abduction of a patient of any age
- Patient death associated with a fall
- Infant discharged to the wrong person
- Surgery performed on the wrong body part
- Patient death/serious disability associated with the use of restraints/bedrails

Adapted from Serious Reportable Events (2012).

Medicare and Medicaid services. These specific measures include mortality, readmission rates, and patient satisfaction responses, along with quality measurement data for common health problems and diseases. These measures are reported on the CMS information website, Health Care Compare (http://www.hospitalcompare.hhs.gov). Hospitals that do not participate can receive an annual reduction of 2% in patient care reimbursement (Chassim, Loeb, Schmaltz, & Wachter, 2011).

Never Events

Hospital reimbursement has recently been eliminated for certain never events. **Never events** are health care situations that arise that are serious, often preventable, and not expected to occur in a hospital, such as a patient acquiring a new Stage IV pressure ulcer (Table 1.7). Safety and quality activities must be directed toward the prevention of these never events.

EVIDENCE FROM THE LITERATURE

Citation

Neuspiel, D. R., Stubbs, E. H., & Liggin, L. (2011). Improving reporting of outpatient pediatric medical errors. *Pediatrics, 128*(6), e1608–e1613.

Discussion

Error reporting systems have not been effective historically in getting staff to report errors. Error reporting systems are often seen as punitive. This article discusses a study involving an academic pediatric practice that implemented a nonpunitive error reporting system to promote patient safety. They developed an interprofessional team in a large pediatric ambulatory clinic to develop an error reporting system that staff would be more inclined to use. This interprofessional team implemented a voluntary, anonymous, nonpunitive, error reporting system. All practitioners were educated and encouraged to report adverse events and near misses. The team was trained in root cause analysis and system review. An **error** was defined as "any event in a patient's medical care that did not go

(continued)

as intended and either harmed or could have harmed the patient" (Plews-Ogan, Nadkarni, Forren et al., 2004). Errors were reported anonymously on forms and bins to collect information were located in several areas. Suggestions for preventing the errors were also requested.

Information was reviewed monthly by the team. A rapid redesign methodology was used to improve health care processes. Interventions were implemented after root cause analysis. Progress was tracked for over a period of time and monthly summaries of reported errors were distributed to staff. Data was displayed by frequency of error reports per month and was compared with the number of patient visits per month using a statistical control chart.

The project demonstrated an improvement in error reporting. In a 12-month period before the project was started, five errors were reported using the traditional system. During the first 30 months of the project, 216 errors were reported. RNs reported 42% of the errors, physicians 28%, mid-level providers 7%, and the remaining errors were reported from a variety of sources. The data reviewed allowed for staff to better understand the most commonly occurring errors.

The significant increase in reporting may have resulted from many factors, that is, education, efforts to overcome a culture of blame, a dedicated safety team, data sharing, anonymous reporting, and feedback to staff. Endorsement by leadership also contributed to the increase in reporting.

Implications for Practice

It is important to have reliable error reporting systems if efforts to improve care are to be successful. A nonpunitive error reporting environment that supports staff as they work to reduce errors, report them accurately, and improve quality care is critical.

UNWARRANTED VARIATION IN HEALTH CARE SAFETY AND QUALITY

Over the last several years, a number of studies have focused on variability in the quality of health care and among health care organizations (Jha, Perlin, Kizer, & Dudley, 2003; McHugh, Kang, & Hasnain-Wynia, 2009; Popescu, Nallamothu, Vaughan-Sarrazin, & Cram, 2008; Wener, Goldman, & Dudley, 2008; Wennberg & Fischer, 2006). **Unwarranted variation** is variation in use of medical care that cannot be explained on the basis of illness, medical evidence, or patient preferences. Over the years, Wennberg, as reported by McCue (2003) has categorized four types of variation:

- Variations from the underuse of effective treatment or intervention that has been shown in clinical studies to improve health status or quality of life, for example, the use of beta blockers post–myocardial infarction
- Variations in outcomes attributable to the quality of care, for example, increased mortality following surgery
- Variations from the misuse of preference-sensitive treatments, for example, hysterectomy versus hormone treatment
- Variations from the overuse of supply-sensitive services, for example, supplies that are overused because they are easily available to patients and health care practitioners, for example, medications and various technologies

According to Wennberg, health care prices are typically stable, especially in U.S. programs such as Medicare. As a result, having an oversupply of a given type of health care provider or service does not reduce the price, it just increases the likelihood of that service or treatment being provided (McCue, 2003). There is variability in health care delivery in various areas of the United States, variability provided by different health care practitioners and agencies, and variability in services available to different socioeconomic groups. Nurses and other members of the health care team must work to improve health care safety and quality and reduce variability.

Variation in Cost

Financial data is being released from the CMS (2013) that show significant variation across the country and within communities in what health care providers charge for common services. These financial data include information comparing the charges for the 100 most common inpatient services and 30 common outpatient services. Providers determine what they will charge for items and services provided to patients and these charges are the amount the providers bill for an item or service.

HEALTH CARE REFORM LEGISLATION

Health care reform legislation is affecting health care reimbursement and is forecasted to have lasting results through 2029. Health care reform is estimated to increase insurance coverage to 32 million additional people, currently uninsured, costing over $940 billion in the next 10 years (www.cnn.com; CNN Politics, 2010).

In this health care reform environment, health care organizations face risks such as decreased reimbursement from government and private health care insurance payers, resulting in low or negative operating margins; loss of accreditation due to increasing quality standards; and an increased threat that patients will seek health care services from other health care organizations (Goetz, Janney, & Ramsey, 2011). Under health care reform, a very real impetus for quality for a health care organization occurs when patients are empowered to choose a health care facility based on quality performance. Organizations that fail to demonstrate quality care delivery as compared to their peers risk the loss of their health care customers. This leads to the loss of health care revenue and may ultimately lead to the demise of an organization's existence. The gravity of this pressure for organizations is yet another reason why high-quality care has taken precedence in the complex health environment. As organizations place optimizing value at the top of their priority lists, the quality bar will continue to rise. Organizations must continue on a path of quality and cost improvement (Porter, 2010). This path will ensure safe care for patients and high quality for organizations.

The Patient Protection and Affordable Care Act (ACA)

In 2010, the president of the United States, Barack Obama, signed into law the ACA to transform health care and provide safer, high-quality, and more accessible care. This health care legislation is affecting health care reimbursement and is forecasted to have lasting results through 2029. It is estimated to increase insurance coverage to 32 million additional people, currently uninsured, costing over $940 billion in the next 10 years (www.cnn.com; CNN Politics, 2010). The new law is discussed at http://www.

healthcare.gov/law/features/rights/bill-of-rights/index.html (The Patient Protection and Affordable Care Act, 2010; CNN Politics, 2010). The full text of this Act is available at http://www.gpo.gov/fdsys/pkg/BILLS-111hr3590enr/pdf/BILLS-111hr3590enr. pdf.

HEALTH CARE TRANSPARENCY

Patients and families trust that the hospital and health care team will take care of them when they are ill. Providers have a duty of trust to patients. Health care transparency allows for consumers to review providers on cost and quality. **Health care transparency** has been defined by the IOM (2001) as making available to the public, in a reliable and understandable manner, information on the health care system's quality, efficiency, and consumer experience with care, which includes price and quality data, so as to influence the behavior of patients, providers, payers, and others to achieve better outcomes (quality and cost of care). According to the American College of Physicians, major domains of health care transparency include sharing information with the patient about:

- Clinical quality and safety
- Resource use
- Efficiency
- Patient experience of care
- Professionalism
- Health care system/facility recognition and accreditations for meeting national standards
- Financial relationship of physicians and other health care professionals, and
- Industry and health insurance company processes (American College of Physicians, 2010)

Much has changed in health care transparency in the last decade. In the past, hospitals and providers did not always disclose errors to patients. Patients who were the victims of errors had to pursue a more litigious solution. This resulted in many malpractice cases. More recently, the external forces of change related to quality and patient safety have demanded that providers report errors and pursue a culture of transparency. "Professional and organization policies and procedures, risk management and performance improvement initiatives demand prompt reporting" (Wolf & Hughes, 2009).

The University of Michigan Health System Transparency Policy

The University of Michigan Health System has developed a transparency policy of apologizing and having an open discussion when clinical care does not go as planned. Good communication, full disclosure, and learning from experience have been critical in reducing the number of malpractice claims pending against it, slashing its malpractice expenses, dramatically dropping the amount paid out in judgments or settlements, and cutting the time it takes to handle a claim. In July 2001, this health system had over 260 presuit claims and lawsuits pending. It currently has just over 100. Its average legal expense per case is down by more than 50% since 1997 (University of Michigan Health System, 2012).

EVIDENCE FROM THE LITERATURE

Citation

Peredino, D. A (2011). *Overhauling America's health care machine.* Upper Saddle River, NJ: FT Press.

Discussion

The physician author of this text discusses the need for the following five elements in America's health care system.

- Universal health care coverage
- Retention of a private market for additional health care services
- Providers must be able to price their services freely
- The price of all health care goods and services must be transparent, fully disclosed, and easily available
- The system must ration health care overtly, rather than covertly

Implications for Practice

Each of these five elements deserves discussion along with a review of what other developed countries are doing to achieve quality outcomes and cost. The U.S. health care system needs improvement.

PUBLIC REPORTING OF QUALITY

Consumers now have the opportunity to research how their hospital is performing or if their physician or nurse has had any malpractice issues. Quality outcome measures that are felt to be meaningful and measurable are publicly reported. Even patient opinions about their hospital experience are available (Minch, 2012, p. 5). Patient's perceptions are increasingly being sought about their communication with nurses and doctors, responsiveness of hospital staff, pain management, communication about medicines, and cleanliness and quietness of the hospital environment, for example, the Hospital Consumer Assessment of Healthcare Providers and Systems (HCAHPS) survey (HCAHPS: Patients' Perspectives of Care Survey, 2012).

Consumers can search the Internet and find website information on hospitals and providers at various sites (Table 1.8).

Health care transparency allows for patients to make informed decisions on where they want to receive care. The ease of accessibility of information on quality care for patients and families may positively or negatively impact whom patients choose for health care services. Thus, providing quality health care is currently at the top of most organization's missions. Health care transparency can improve care. Using data to compare results allows hospitals and providers to benchmark themselves. Identifying high-performing organizations allow for others to adapt successful protocols and practices and control costs. QI organizations such as the Institute

TABLE 1.8 HEALTH CARE WEBSITES

SPONSORING ORGANIZATION	HEALTH CARE WEBSITE
Centers for Medicare and Medicaid Services (CMS)	www.hospitalcompare.hhs.gov
Centers for Medicare and Medicaid Services, Health Care Costs	http://www.cms.gov/Research-Statistics-Data-and-Systems/Statistics-Trends-and-Reports/Medicare-Provider-Charge-Data/index.html
The Commonwealth Fund, Why not the Best?	http://www.whynotthebest.org
The Joint Commission Quality Check	http://www.qualitycheck.org/consumer/searchQCR.aspx
Health Grades	www.healthgrades.com
U.S. News and World Report	http://health.usnews.com/best-hospitals/rankings
United Health Foundation	http://www.americashealthrankings.org
World Health Organization	http://www.who.int
The Leapfrog Group Hospital Safety Score program	http://hospitalsafetyscore.org
Consumer Reports	http://www.consumerreports.org/hospitalratings, and, http://www.consumerreports.org/cro/magazine/2012/08/how-safe-is-your-hospital/index.htm
Improving Healthcare for the Common Good (IPRO)	http://www.ipro.org/index/compare-hospitals

for Healthcare Improvement (IHI) are dedicated to the sharing of information to improve health care processes and patient safety. The IHI website (www.IHI.org) includes white papers, evidence-based protocols, blogs, improvement stories, and other tools to promote the sharing of information to improve safety and ultimately patient outcomes.

The Patient Self-Determination Act (PSDA)

The PSDA was passed by the U.S. Congress in 1990. "The PSDA requires many Medicare and Medicaid providers (hospitals, nursing homes, hospice programs, home health agencies, and health maintenance organizations [HMOs]) to give adult individuals, at the time of inpatient admission or enrollment, certain information about their rights under state laws governing advance directives, including:

- The right to participate in and direct their own health care decisions
- The right to accept or refuse medical or surgical treatment
- The right to prepare an advance directive
- Information on the provider's policies that govern the utilization of these rights

PSDA also prohibits institutions from discriminating against a patient who does not have an advance directive" (Ascension Health, 2012).

Critical Thinking 1.1

Go to www.dartmouth-hitchcock.org; click "Quality Reports"; click "Dartmouth-Hitchcock Medical Center (DHMC) Quality Reports"; click ""Reports A to Z." Click on a health care condition of your choice. Note what you see there. Then, search for "Health care charges." Click on " Surgeries, Procedures, and Medical Conditions."

1. What did you see there?
2. Does this type of cost transparency have the ability to improve quality care? (Note also, http://www.cms.gov/Research-Statistics-Data-and-Systems/Statistics-Trends-and-Reports/Medicare-Provider-Charge-Data/index.html)
3. Note the information comparing charges for the 100 most common inpatient services and 30 common outpatient services at the CMS site. Were you surprised at this information?

BALDRIGE AWARD

The Baldrige Health Care Criteria for Performance Excellence have been used by many health care organizations to improve quality. Baldrige identifies criteria to improve organizational:

- Leadership
- Strategic planning
- Customer focus
- Measurement, analysis, and knowledge management
- Workforce focus
- Operations focus
- Results (The National Institute of Standards and Technology [NIST], 2013–2014)

Many organizations have received the Baldrige Award based upon achievement of their best in class performance, role model organization, and best management practices, principles, and strategies.

THE FUTURE OF NURSING: LEADING CHANGE, ADVANCING HEALTH

A 2010 IOM report *The Future of Nursing: Leading Change, Advancing Health,* is a blueprint for nursing action that focuses on eight main recommendations (Table 1.9). This IOM report aims to allow quality health care to reach diverse populations and fosters a health care system that promotes wellness and disease prevention; improves health outcomes; provides professional, compassionate care; and empowers the profession of nursing to make modifications in nursing practice to achieve the eight recommendations and influence health care so that it is safe, quality driven, and effective.

TABLE 1.9 EIGHT IOM RECOMMENDATIONS FOR THE FUTURE OF NURSING

- Remove scope of practice barriers
- Expand opportunities for nurses to lead collaborative improvement
- Implement nurse residency programs
- Increase the proportion of nurses with a baccalaureate degree to 80% by 2010
- Double the number of nurses with a doctorate by 2020
- Ensure that nurses engage in lifelong learning
- Prepare and enable nurses to lead change to advance health
- Build an infrastructure for collection and analysis of health workforce data

Source: Institute of Medicine (IOM) (2010).

EVIDENCE FROM THE LITERATURE

Citation

Headrick, L. A., Barton, A. J., Ogrinc, G., Strang, C., Aboumatar, H. J., Aud, M. A.,…Patterson, J. E. (2012). Results of an effort to integrate quality and safety into medical and nursing school curricula and foster joint learning. *Health Affairs, 31*(12), 2669–2680.

Discussion

Improvements in health care are slow, in part because doctors and nurses lack skills in quality improvement, patient safety, and interprofessional teamwork.

This article reports on the Retooling for Quality and Safety initiative of the Josiah Macy Jr. Foundation and the IHI, which sought to integrate quality improvement and patient safety into medical and nursing school curricula. In one academic year, 2009 to 2010, the initiative supported new learning activities (87% of which were interprofessional, involving both medical and nursing students) in classrooms, simulation centers, and clinical care settings that involved 1,374 student encounters at six universities. The work generated insights, described in this article, into which learning goals require interprofessional education; how to create clinically based improvement learning for all students; and how to demonstrate the effects on students' behavior, organizational practice, and benefits to patients. A commonly encountered limiting factor for the programs was the lack of a critical mass of clinically based faculty members who were ready to teach about the improvement of care.

Implications for Practice

Interprofessional medical and nursing education is necessary to improve future patient care. The pace for improving this education must improve.

Critical Thinking 1.2

You are a student nurse and have just introduced yourself to a patient. In response to your introduction, the patient asks you, "How do I know that the nurses are qualified to give safe, high-quality care to me?"

1. How will you answer this patient?
2. How can you begin to assure patient-centered care that improves health care access, safety, outcomes, and respect for this patient?

NURSES AT THE SHARP END OF HEALTH CARE

Nurses at the "sharp" end of health care are able to provide perspective on barriers and challenges to providing effective and efficient care that those further away from the bedside may not see (Hughes, 2008). The term, **sharp end**, has been used to identify the important and significant direct contact role that nurses at the bedside, closest to clinical activities, play in recognizing the need for and potential impact of practice change. Nurses may see the sharp-end effects on patients and others first when the right care is not provided. The profession of nursing has a unique opportunity to bridge gaps internally and externally and to standardize and elevate the expectations for effective and efficient practice (Goetz et al., 2011).

Nurses at the bedside play a vital role in bringing clinical expertise and firsthand experience to the tables of discussion for organizational improvements. Nurses must step up, speak out, and take action to improve the way care is delivered across the health care continuum. Being an active part of the solution to safety and quality challenges is what organizations and patients require of nurses today.

Nurses must practice with a spirit of inquiry, consistently evaluating the way care is delivered to ensure that it is evidence based. QI projects that marry clinical need with organizational and national agendas provide the greatest opportunity for support that leads the way to lasting positive outcomes (Stillwell, Fineout-Overholt, Mazurek-Melnyk, & Williamson, 2010).

CASE STUDY 1.1

You were part of the interprofessional team that developed guidelines for the prevention of intravascular catheter-related infections, using information from the CMS website, http://partnershipforpatients.cms.gov/p4p_resources/1presources.html. You are now caring for a 72-year-old male who requires an urgent insertion of a central line catheter at the bedside. It is 3 a.m. The doctor on call is Dr. Smith. You are dreading the procedure, because Dr. Smith can be difficult and often condescending in her tone to nurses. Dr. Smith arrives from home to insert the central line. Fortunately, she seems to be in a decent mood and preparation for the central line insertion is going well. However, immediately before inserting the

(continued)

catheter, you note that Dr. Smith contaminates her glove on the bedside rail. She briefly pauses, and then returns to the insertion.

1. *What do you do?*
2. *What authority do you have to speak out against Dr. Smith's decision to proceed with a contaminated glove?*
3. *How can quality and safety for the patient be provided if nurses and other health care team members do not speak up when patient safety is in jeopardy?*

EVIDENCE FROM THE LITERATURE

Citation

Kydona, C. K., Malamis, G., Giasnetsova, T., Tsiora, V., & Gritsi-Gerogianni, N. (2010). The level of teamwork as an index of quality in ICU performance. *Hippokratia, 14*(2), 94–97.

Discussion

The benefits of improved interprofessional collaboration in health care are well documented in the literature including fewer errors and shorter delays and thus enhanced effectiveness and maximized patient safety. Given that the first step in improving teamwork involves uncovering individual team member's attitudes, this study was planned to investigate the level of interprofessional collaboration as part of organizational culture in the environment of intensive care unit (ICU) in Hippokratio Hospital. All the medical and nursing ICU personnel was included in the study as well as that of other cooperating clinical departments and labs of Hippokratio hospital. For the purpose of the study a questionnaire was adopted and was given to 250 individuals, 196 of whom responded (response rate 78.4%). The results were that responders, in general, valued teamwork as crucial for the performance of the ICU. However, the study revealed a relative low consensus regarding the level of teamwork within each unit and inadequate collaboration between certain departments and ICU. Most of the responders stated they were willing to share responsibility but unwilling to share decision making or accept questioning of their actions. Low consensus was also observed regarding the composition of the team. Certain differences were detected across departments as well as between physicians and nurses. The study concluded that although the benefits of teamwork are well understood, realization of effective cooperation seems to be far from interprofessional practice. Teaching of teamwork skills and team concepts should become part of medical and nursing education if a substantial improvement in the quality of health care services is desired.

Implications for Practice

Education in interprofessional nursing and medical teamwork is a priority for the future. Patient care quality and safety is dependent on this.

THE ANCC MAGNET RECOGNITION PROGRAM

The ANCC Magnet Recognition Program focuses health care organizations on achieving superior performance that is measured by the achievement of outcomes and is often referred to as the ultimate credential for high-quality nursing worldwide. The Magnet Recognition Program evaluates sources of evidence that creates the foundational infrastructure for excellence, while its focus on results fosters a culture of quality and innovation (Table 1.10).

ETHICAL AND LEGAL RESPONSIBILITY OF THE PROFESSIONAL NURSE

In the current high-pressure push for health care safety and quality, health care providers are especially challenged to practice both ethically and legally and do the right thing. Every nurse must understand important, basic, ethical, and legal principles when determining what the "correct" action is to take. The American Nurses Association (ANA) developed the Code of Ethics for Nurses as a guide for carrying out nursing responsibilities in a manner consistent with quality in nursing care and the ethical obligations of the profession. All practicing nurses should be aware of the ANA Code of Ethics, which can be found at http://www.nursingworld.org/codeofethics.

TABLE 1.10 MAGNET SOURCES OF EVIDENCE

SOURCE OF EVIDENCE	HIGHLIGHTS
Transformational leadership	• Uses visionary, influential, knowledgeable, and strong professional leadership practice. • Leads people where they need to be in order to meet the demands of the future.
Structural empowerment	• Provides superior quality health care structures and processes that permit the health care practice environment to demonstrate the organization's mission, vision, and values. • Empowers employees who seek strong partnerships internally and externally to deliver the best patient care and achieve exceptional outcomes.
Exemplary professional practice	• Highlights superior nursing skills and behavior that are delivered through professional practice and care delivery models that facilitate superior application of the nursing role and allow for achievement of extraordinary results with patients, families, communities, and the interprofessional team. • Includes the application of new knowledge and evidence that commands respect and admiration.
New knowledge, innovation, and improvements	• Highlights high-quality health care organizations that are redesigned and redefined to contribute to quality health care and to the nursing profession. • Fosters a culture of inquiry and making improvements, innovations, and new knowledge a must.
Empirical quality results	• Demonstrates superior organizational clinical outcomes related to nursing; workforce outcomes; patient and consumer outcomes; and organizational outcomes. • Establishes quantitative benchmarks or report cards.

Prepared with information from American Nurses Credentialing Center (2012).

Ethical and Legal Responsibilities and QSEN

QSEN suggests that nurses can make a difference in ensuring safety and quality for patients. QSEN states that nurses should incorporate KSAs regarding six key elements into nursing practice. These six elements are

- Patient-centered care
- Teamwork and collaboration
- EBP
- QI
- Safety
- Informatics (http://qsen.org/about-qsen/project-overview)

Patient-centered care occurs when nurses and interprofessional team members show respect for patients' individual needs, preferences, and values. For example, they work to ensure optimal patient access to high-quality, safe health care outcomes. Patient-centered nurses and interprofessional team members demonstrate respect and caring for patients, dress professionally, and achieve good patient satisfaction scores. They give patients friendly explanations of their care and the need for any delays; they work to manage any patient pain or discomfort; and they acknowledge patient requests for hand washing, asepsis measures, and privacy.

Patient-centered nurses on interprofessional teams collaborate and work to resolve any patient complaints. For example, patient-centered nurses on interprofessional teams are respectful, show appreciation to others, and are friendly and approachable. They say hello/thanks/goodbye, demonstrate politeness, network and work with the team, the boss, and others, do their job, and avoid leaving work for the next shift. Interprofessional team members do not act unprofessional, miss deadlines, promise what they can't deliver, write unprofessional emails that others can see, participate in sexual harassment, gossip, or tell off-color jokes.

Interprofessional team members are discreet; avoid complaining, arguing, and interrupting; and provide good backup for the team. They are the team members whom others love to work with. Interprofessional team members don't take up the boss's and others' time needlessly. They anticipate patient care orders and maintain good patient flow in busy patient care areas; they work with others, go the extra mile, and help other team members find missing labs, take vitals, and so on. Interprofessional team members question orders that do not make sense and make suggestions to the RN/MD team if something is omitted from patient care. They communicate clearly in patient report handoffs to ensure quality and safety.

Interprofessional team members incorporate EBP into their daily work and use consistent hand washing and bundled patient care approaches based on evidence to reduce infections. They always try to improve quality and safety by managing patient care by the facts, collecting data, and looking for ways to make a positive patient care difference based upon real statistics and numbers. Interprofessional team players minimize the risk of patient harm by following established standardized work processes such as checking two patient identifiers and completing medication reconciliation, and so on. Interprofessional team members use informatics to its fullest in a cost-effective manner and use technology systems to support patient information and make it accessible to caregivers and patients (QSEN, 2012a).

Note selected implications of QSEN for the ethical and legal responsibilities of the nurse (Table 1.11).

CASE STUDY 1.2

The risk manager at a community hospital had been reviewing occurrence report data trends over the last quarter. There appeared to be an increasing trend of patients who were not appropriate candidates for an MRI due to the patients having implanted metal devices. The lead MRI technologist is very concerned that these patients were not being correctly screened by the nurses on the unit.

The risk manager pulled together a team of staff from the nursing, medical, and MRI departments. After reviewing the MRI screening process, it was discovered that a new scheduling system that had been put in place in the radiology department was so efficient in getting inpatients an MRI appointment, the unit nurses did not have time to complete an MRI patient screening after the doctor had ordered it. A new MRI screening process was immediately implemented. The MRI order would now not be placed by the unit secretary until the RN communicated that the MRI patient screening was completed. Note that the problem reported by MRI staff led to the work process change. This protected patients from a potential injury.

1. *Why is it important that patients with implants be identified on the unit by the nurse rather than later by the MRI technologist?*
2. *How did the risk management process of reviewing the MRI screening process help with this patient safety issue?*

TABLE 1.11 SELECTED IMPLICATIONS OF QSEN FOR NURSING ETHICAL AND LEGAL RESPONSIBILITIES

QUALITY AND SAFETY EDUCATION ELEMENT	LEGAL IMPLICATIONS	ETHICAL IMPLICATIONS
Patient-centered care	• Develop policy to guide the practice of transparency, for example, work with risk management and the interprofessional team to inform the patient and family what happened, why, when, what you are doing to fix it, and assure that it does not happen again. • Prevent errors. • Monitor health care system for errors, develop error prevention systems, and take action.	• Offer all patients respect and access to care. • Respect patients' rights to make all health care decisions. • Communicate health care risks to patients. • Make decisions based on helping, not harming, the patient. • Respect the patient's religious and other beliefs. • Monitor patient outcomes. See http://pcori.org • Monitor patient satisfaction with the HCAHPS (Hospital Consumer Assessment of Healthcare Providers and Systems) tool at http://www.hcahpsonline.org/surveyinstrument.aspx

(continued)

TABLE 1.11 SELECTED IMPLICATIONS OF QSEN FOR NURSING ETHICAL AND LEGAL RESPONSIBILITIES (*continued*)

QUALITY AND SAFETY EDUCATION ELEMENT	LEGAL IMPLICATIONS	ETHICAL IMPLICATIONS
		• Take action on any problems identified from monitoring patient outcomes and patient satisfaction scores.
Teamwork and collaboration	• Develop rapport and communicate clearly with the interprofessional team. • Collaborate to improve patient report handoffs and achieve high-quality, safe outcomes. • Take action to assure prompt responses of the responsible licensed caregiver to critical test results and values.	• Verify verbal and telephone orders or reporting of critical test results by having the person receiving the information "read-back" the complete order or test result.
Evidence-based practice (EBP)	• Manage as sentinel events all identified cases of unanticipated patient deaths or major permanent loss of patient function from a health care–associated infection. • Review the literature regularly and maintain EBP.	• Reduce the risk of health care-associated infections. • Comply with current World Health Organization (WHO) hand hygiene guidelines or Centers for Disease Control and Prevention (CDC) hand hygiene guidelines.
Quality improvement	• Monitor patient outcome standards. • Develop standardized approaches to identify patients at risk for suicide or change in condition. • Develop an error prevention mindset to avoid quality problems. • Become a high-reliability organization (see Chapter 3).	• Reduce the risk of patient harm resulting from falls. • Implement a fall reduction program including an evaluation of the effectiveness of the program.
Safety	• Annually review a list of look-alike/sound-alike drugs used by the organization and take action to prevent errors involving the interchange of these drugs. • Use at least two patient identifiers when providing care, treatment, or services. • Develop a culture of safety (see Chapter 4).	• Define and communicate the means for patients and their families to report concerns about safety and encourage them to do so.
Informatics	• Follow legal guidelines in adopting new technology. • Value the contributions of standardization and reliability to safety using technology. • Explore the cost-effectiveness and quality of new informatics technology.	• Consider ethics when adopting new technology. • Value technologies that support clinical decision making, error prevention, and care coordination. • Review resources at http://www.nlm.nih.gov/hsrinfo/informatics.html

PROFESSIONAL HEALTH CARE ORGANIZATIONS

Professional organizations such as the ANA, http://www.nursingworld.org; the American Medical Association, http://www.ama-assn.org; and the American Hospital Association, http://www.aha.org, have produced position statements to assist hospitals and health care practitioners in focusing on the move to health care safety and quality. Position statements can be found at the websites on a variety of important topics, that is, culture, nurse staffing hours, patient safety, environmental safety, social causes, payment systems, education levels, and so on. Position statements provide strategies and guidance to health care professionals regarding the forces of change. Professional organizations and their lobbyists also advocate for health care legislation and health care worker's rights such as safe work environments.

Health care quality and safety is an interprofessional and complex process. It is clear that no one is alone in the pursuit of quality patient care outcomes and safety measures. Nurses and the interprofessional team depend upon each other to provide optimum care to each patient while appreciating the important health care systems that lead to safe and appropriate care delivery. There is much to learn about quality and safety within our health care system. Nurses are well-positioned to have a voice in the overall care that patients receive. The future of health care and all the health care professions is dependent upon the decisions that we make today.

KEY CONCEPTS

- Patient safety and quality of care have been defined and studied over time and have become increasing regulated by the government and regulatory agencies.
- There are several national health care accreditation organizations that strive to ensure health care safety and quality.
- Health care salaries, medications, technology, and malpractice all contribute to the high cost of health care in the United States.
- The cost of health care in the United States is higher than most industrial countries; yet select quality outcomes do not demonstrate that the United States has health care advantages over other countries.
- Health care reimbursement is increasingly being scrutinized by health care payer sources such as Medicare, Medicaid, and insurance companies.
- The U.S. health system does not provide consistent error-free care to all patients.
- The ANCC Magnet Recognition Program focuses health care organizations on achieving superior performance.
- The Baldrige Award provides recognition to organizations that perform at exceptionally high levels.
- Nurses at the bedside and thus at the "sharp" end of health care have a very valuable role in influencing EBP decisions that can influence safety and quality.

- There are increased efforts to reduce unwarranted variation in health care delivery.
- The intent of the Patient Protection and Affordable Care Act is to improve quality and safety for patients.
- There are several national efforts to improve transparency and public reporting of health care quality and cost.
- The interprofessional team has an obligation to report health care practice errors and provide health care transparency to patients.
- Professional standards provide a level of protection to the public for safety and quality and help guide the nurses' professional actions.
- The IOM *Future of Nursing* report has identified nursing directions for the future.
- QSEN develops KSAs in patient-centered care, teamwork and collaboration, EBP, QI, safety, and informatics.
- Ethical and legal responsibilities of the professional nurse related to QSEN are important in patient care.

KEY TERMS

Accredited hospital

Core measures

Error

Health care quality

Health care transparency

Never events

Safety

Sentinel event

Sharp end

Unwarranted variation

Value for health care organizations

DISCUSSION OF OPENING SCENARIO

1. What elements of quality care would you look for on the unit to better understand the patient care that the staff is delivering?

    The elements of quality care you would look for on the unit to better understand the patient care that the staff is delivering include evidence that elements of quality unit structures and work processes have been put in place to achieve quality patient outcomes. Often units display results of their quality measures in their break rooms or conference rooms so that all can be reminded that patient safety is being safeguarded with QI activities. Many units have developed a quality dashboard that provides important quality data such as clinical outcomes, work flow processes, financial measures, and other quality achievements. This quality dashboard provides a snap shot of the unit's progress.

2. What type of questions might you ask the staff related to their QI work?

    You might want to ask the charge nurse, nurse manager, and nursing staff what QI projects the staff and they are working on and where they are in the process. It is interesting and helpful to ask why the staff chose the QI issues that they are focusing on. Often there has been a patient safety or quality issue that gives insight into a quality challenge or problem that has been bothersome to the point of keeping staff up at night worrying about a work process problem that has not been resolved or needs to be fixed.

3. What type of quality concerns do the patients have?

    Patients may have questions related to their need for quality health care access, safety, respect, and quality outcomes.

CRITICAL THINKING ANSWERS

Critical Thinking 1.1

1. What did you see there?

    The Dartmouth website has much information about cost and other elements of quality that can be openly shared with patients and used to improve the quality of health care in this country.

2. Does this type of cost transparency have the ability to improve quality care? (Note also, http://www.cms.gov/Research-Statistics-Data-and-Systems/Statistics-Trends-and-Reports/Medicare-Provider-Charge-Data/index.html)

    This type of cost transparency shares information about price and quality with patients. Both the Dartmouth website and the CMS website have much information that can be viewed by patients and used to improve the quality of health care in this country.

3. Note the information comparing charges for the 100 most common inpatient services and 30 common outpatient services at the CMS site. Were you surprised at this information?

    The CMS website has much information comparing charges for the 100 most common inpatient services and 30 common outpatient services that can be viewed by patients. Many of these charges are very surprising. It is a helpful thing for nurses to be aware of health care costs.

Critical Thinking 1.2

1. How will you answer this patient?

    Nurses are required to complete nursing education from an accredited college or university. Additionally, they are required to pass a state licensure exam that confirms that they possess essential nursing knowledge. Nurses often are also required to complete a competency validation process within their health care organization, which demonstrates the nurse's ability to apply their knowledge and technical skills to specific situations. Many nurses obtain specialty certifications in their area of practice, for example, Advanced Cardiac Life Support (ACLS), Trauma Nurse Specialist (TNS), and so on. Finally, many nurses return to school and seek advanced education, for example, master of science in nursing (MSN), nurse practitioner, and PhD.

2. How can you begin to ensure patient-centered care that improves health care access, safety, outcomes, and respect for this patient?

    You can begin to ensure health care access, safety, outcomes, and respect for this patient by becoming more aware of the health care environment, speaking up for improved health care, and working to be the best, most qualified nurse you can be.

CASE STUDY ANSWERS

Case Study 1.1

1. What do you do?

    The nurse should notify Dr. Smith that her glove is contaminated and tell her that she will get her a new glove. The procedure stops until the sterile field is ensured.

2. What authority do you have to speak out against Dr. Smith's decision to proceed with a contaminated glove?

An RN has a professional state license and individual professional accountability to advocate and protect the patient's interest. It is the job of the nurse to ensure the patient is safe.

3. How can quality and safety for the patient be provided if nurses and other health care team members do not speak up when patient safety is in jeopardy?

If nurses and other health care team members do not speak up when patient safety is in jeopardy, patient safety cannot be ensured. The health care team must hold each other accountable for delivery of care and all care decisions. We all need to work as a team with the focus on what is best for the patient. If Dr. Smith does not respond appropriately, the nurse should discuss the situation with her charge nurse or nurse manager to ensure patient safety and quality.

CASE STUDY 1.2

1. Why is it important that patients with implants be identified on the unit by the nurse rather than later by the MRI technologist?

It is important that patients with implants be identified on the unit by the nurse rather than later by the MRI technologist as the assessment of the patient by the nurse on the unit is the first safety check. Safety systems have redundancy in them. A two-step process is safest. Missing the implant device on the floor puts the patient at greater risk for a dangerous error to occur. If the MRI technician did not check for the implant device or assumed the nurse had checked for it, the patient could be hurt.

2. How did the risk management process of reviewing the MRI screening process help with this patient safety issue?

The risk management process of reviewing the MRI screening process helped with this patient safety issue as the patient care unit staff may not have realized that there was a problem with patients being sent down for MRI without assessment. The error could have continued on for quite a while and patients could be hurt. By aggregating the patient data from the MRI screening process and noting trends, the MRI problem was picked up.

REVIEW QUESTIONS

Please see Appendix D for answers to Review Questions.

1. A group of emergency room nurses are asked to develop an action plan to improve the time before patients who presented with chest pain received an electrocardiogram (EKG). Which of the following would *not* be helpful when working on a QI effort like this?

   A. Identify an interprofessional group of individuals to help review current performance.
   B. Compare current hospital data results to benchmark comparison information reported on a national website.
   C. Post current hospital performance data results openly to staff in the nursing lounge.
   D. Identify whose fault it is that results are not very good.

2. As a staff nurse you are interested in making QIs in the overall care of patients with heart failure. Where would be most helpful to you as you start to look for data and information to help you get started with these improvements?

    A. Explore IHI website (www.IHI.org), which includes white papers, evidence-based protocols, blogs, and improvement stories for patients with heart failure.
    B. Review the National Cancer Institute's website, which includes facts and statistics related to cancer care, resources, and latest research developments.
    C. Review drug companies' websites to see if there are any new medications available to treat heart failure.
    D. Google "heart failure" to see if you can get access to the latest treatment options for this patient population.

3. An 87-year-old patient was admitted to an acute care hospital. The patient was in a severe automobile vehicle accident. He is unconscious in intensive care and on a ventilator. On Day 3 of the patient's hospitalization, the patient experiences a cardiac arrest and a code blue is called. The code blue lasts for an hour. The patient's heart rhythm is restored. When the family is notified of the event, the wife is very upset. She stated she had provided the hospital with the patient's advance directive, which clearly stated the patient should not be resuscitated. You are the nurse talking to the wife. What do you do?

    A. Apologize, but state that the patient was a full code, which means he must be resuscitated.
    B. Apologize, and assure the wife that you will be contacting the attending physician and your nurse manager that the problem occurred. The risk management department will probably review this case.
    C. Notify the wife that the advance directive is not legal or binding and that the wife needed to tell them specifically that the patient did not want to be resuscitated.
    D. Try to focus on the positive, that her 87-year-old husband is still alive.

4. A patient asks a nurse what it means to have a hospital accredited by The Joint Commission. Which one of the following is not a Joint Commission quality compliance requirement?

    A. Billing models
    B. Core measures
    C. Safe practice measures
    D. Process improvement efforts

5. A coworker has read a recent report on the U.S. economy and asks a nurse to explain where the U.S. stands in comparison to other Westernized counties. The coworker heard that the U.S. spends more per capita than most Westernized countries. Which of the following is of national concern?

    A. U.S. life expectancy is lower than most Westernized countries.
    B. U.S. life expectancy rate is higher than most Westernized countries.
    C. U.S. life expectancy rate is the same as most Westernized countries.
    D. U.S. life expectancy data is not available for review.

6. A patient read that hospitals are not getting reimbursed by CMS for certain never events and asks a nurse to explain. Which one of the following is an example of a never event?

   A. Absence of a hospice unit within the hospital
   B. Emergency department admissions over 1,000 per month
   C. Nursing stations located at the end of the hall versus in the middle of the patient care unit
   D. Stage IV hospital-acquired pressure ulcer

7. What is a common cause of errors within health care settings?

   A. Uncaring professionals
   B. Incompetent caregivers
   C. Communication problems between caregivers
   D. Phones not connecting to the nurse's station

8. QSEN has developed multiple quality and safety elements to guide nursing practice. Identify which of these are considered a part of the six key elements.

   A. QI, teamwork and collaboration, and EBP
   B. Fact finding, mission statements, and strategic planning
   C. Stakeholder feedback, budget reconciliation, and strategic planning
   D. Financial reporting, wait time measurements, and time delays in getting treatments

9. You are the nurse caring for a patient who was recently told he has heart failure. The patient will be relocating next week to a different state. The patient has a primary care provider in his new state and intends to follow up as instructed upon discharge. However, he would like to identify an acute care hospital in his new state that is adept in caring for heart failure patients in the event that he needs to be admitted. The patient asks for your recommendation. All of the suggestions below may give him good information. What would be your *best* suggestion to the patient so that he may make a well-informed, objective decision?

   A. Tell the patient that hospitals publicly report their quality data associated with caring for heart failure patients on a website and instruct him where he can retrieve this information.
   B. Tell him to ask members in the community or family and friends where they have had good experiences.
   C. Tell him to ask his primary care provider for a recommendation.
   D. Tell him to visit the websites of hospitals in the community where he is moving.

10. You are an administrator working in an urban health system. You have been charged to lead the efforts of redesigning the patient care delivery model. This model is intended to best represent the patient expectations. As such, in developing the model you recognize the importance of taking into account the patient's quality concerns. Which answer best represents the top patient quality concerns as described by the HFMA Value Project (2011).

    A. Access: Make care available and affordable. Safety: Don't hurt me. Outcomes: Make me better. Respect: Respect me as a person, not a case.
    B. Access: Make care available and affordable. Safety: Don't hurt me. Quality: Provide high-quality care. Respect: Respect me as a person, not a case.

    C. Safety: Don't hurt me. Outcomes: Make me better. Value: Deliver care at a reasonable price. Inclusion: Include my loved ones in any care plans.

    D. Safety: Don't hurt me. Quality: Provide high-quality care. Value: Deliver care at a reasonable price. Respect: Respect me as a person, not a case.

REVIEW ACTIVITIES

Please see Appendix E for answers to Review Activities.

1. Look around your agency. Do you see any evidence of QI activities? What do they reveal about your agency?
2. What kinds of activities do you see on your unit to support patient safety? Who is involved in the activities?
3. Go to the QSEN Institute website, http://qsen.org. Click on Competencies, Pre Licensure. Also, click on Teaching Strategies. What did you find at these sites?

EXPLORING THE WEB

1. QSEN Institute—http://qsen.org
2. Partner in Health—http://partnerhealth.com
3. Partnership for Patients—http://partnershipforpatients.cms.gov
4. The Leapfrog Group—http://www.leapfroggroup.org
5. Health Grades—http://www.ahrq.gov/consumer/guidetoq/guidetoq9.htm
6. IOM, *Future of Nursing*—http://www.iom.edu/~/media/Files/Report%20Files/2010/The Future-of-Nursing/Future%20of%20Nursing%202010%20Recommendations.pdf
7. Fair Health—http://www.fairhealthconsumer.org

REFERENCES

Agency for Health Care Research and Quality (AHRQ). (2011). *Moving forward with quality improvement*. Retrieved from http:/www.ahrq.gov/consumer/guidetoq/guidetoq9.htm

American College of Physicians. (2010). *Healthcare transparency—Focus on price and clinical performance information*. Retrieved January 4, 2014 from http://www.acponline.org/advocacy/current_policy_papers/assets/transparency.pdf

American Nurses Credentialing Center (ANCC). (2012). Retrieved from http://www.nursecredentialing. org/MagnetModel.aspx

American Nurses Credentialing Center (ANCC). (2012). *Sources of evidence*. Retrieved from http:// www.nursecredentialing.org/Magnet/ProgramOverview

Ascension Health. (2012). *Health care ethics, issues and concepts*. Retrieved from http://www.ascensionhealth.org/index.php?option=com_content&view=article&id=188&Itemid=172

A World of Options on Health Care Reform. (2009). *International health care comparison*; compiled by Jason Brudereck. Retrieved from http://readingeagle.com/mobile/article.aspx?id=152758

Barbash, G. I., & Glied, S. A. (2010). New technology and health care costs: The case of robotas-sisted surgery. *The New England Journal of Medicine, 363*(8), 701–704.

Callahan, D. (2008). Health care costs and Med. Tech. In M. Crowley (Ed.), *From birth to death and bench to clinic: The Hastings center bioethics briefing book for journalists, policymakers, and campaigns* (pp. 79–82). Garrison, NY: The Hastings Center. Retrieved from http://www.thehastingscenter.org/Publications/BriefingBook/Detail.aspx?id=2178

Centers for Medicare & Medicaid Services. (2012). *Hospital Consumer Assessment of Healthcare Providers and Systems (HCAHPS)*. Retrieved from http://www.cms.gov/Medicare/Quality-Initiatives-Patient-Assessment-Instruments/HospitalQualityInits/HospitalHCAHPS.html

Centers for Medicare & Medicaid Services (CMS). (2013). *Medicare provider charge data*. Retrieved from http://www.cms.gov/Research-Statistics-Data-and-Systems/Statistics-Trends-and-Reports/Medicare-Provider-Charge-Data/index.html

Chassim, M., Loeb, J., Schmaltz, St., & Wachter, R. (2011). Accountability measures-using measurement to promote quality improvement. *The New England Journal of Medicine, 343*(7), 683–688.

CNN Politics. (2010). *Where does healthcare reform stand?* Retrieved August 2012, from: http://articles.cnn.com/2010–03-18/politics/health.care.latest_1_health-care-bill-cbo-report-new-cbo-estimates?_s=PM:POLITICS

The Commonwealth Fund. (2011). *Why not the best? Results from the national scorecard on U.S. health system performance, 2011*. Retrieved from http://www.commonwealthfund.org/Publications/Fund-Reports/2011/Oct/Why-Not-the-Best-2011.aspx?page=all

Davis, K., Schoen, S., Schoenbaum, M., Doty, M., Homgren, A., Kriss, J., & Shea, K. (2007, May). *Mirror, mirror on the wall, an international update on the comparative performance of American health care*. The Commonwealth Fund Report. Retrieved from http://www.common-wealthfund.org/Publications/Fund-Reports/2007/May/Mirror--Mirror-on-the-Wall--An-International-Update-on-the-Comparative-Performance-of-American-Healt.aspx

Drucker, P. (2004). *The daily Drucker*. New York, NY: Harper Business.

Feder, B. J. (2008, May 4). *Prepping robots to perform surgery*. The New York Times. Retrieved from http://www.nytimes.com/2008/05/04/business/04moll.html?_r=0

Goetz, K., Janney, M., & Ramsey, K. (2011). When nursing takes ownership of financial outcomes:achieving exceptional financial performance through leadership, strategy, and execution.*Nursing Economics, 29*(4), 173–182.

The Hastings Center. (2012). *Health care costs and medical technology*. Retrieved from http://www.thehastingscenter.org/Publications/BriefingBook/Detail.aspx?id=2178

Headrick, L. A., Barton, A. J., Ogrinc, G., Strang, C., Aboumatar, H. J., Aud, M. A.,…Patterson, J. E. (2012). Results of an effort to integrate quality and safety into medical and nursing school curricula and foster joint learning. *Health Affairs, 31*(12), 2669–2680.

Healthcare Financial Management Association's (HFMA) Value Project. (2011). *Value in health care: Current state and future directions*. HealthcareFinancial Management Association. Retrieved from http://www.aramarkhealthcare.com/RelatedFiles/1157_value-report_w3.pdf

Hughes, R. G. (Ed.) (2008). *Patient safety and quality: An evidence-based handbook for nurses*. (Prepared with support from the Robert Wood Johnson Foundation). AHRQ Publication No. 08–0043. Rockville, MD: Agency for Healthcare Research and Quality.

Institute of Medicine (IOM). (2001). *To err is human: building a safer health system*. Retrieved from http://www.nap.edu/catalog/9728.html

Institute of Medicine (IOM). (2010). *The future of nursing: Leading, changing advancing health*. Retrieved from http://iom.edu/Reports/2010/The-Future-of-Nursing-Leading-Change-Advancing-Health.aspx

Institute of Medicine of the National Academy of Sciences. (2012). *About reports*. Retrieved from http://www.iom.edu/Reports.aspx?Topic1={DE49DD61–623A-438F-932B-6921-E7BE9F6A}& page=17

Jha, A., Perlin, J., Kizer, K., & Dudley, A. (2003). Effect of the transformation of the veterans' affairs health care system on the quality of care. *The New England Journal of Medicine, 348*(22), 2218–2227.

Josie King Foundation. (2002). *What happened, Sorrel King's speech to the 2002 IHI conference*. Retrieved from http://www.josieking.org

Kenney, C. (2008). *The best practice: How the new quality movement is transforming health care*. New York, NY: Public Affairs.

Kydona, C. K., Malamis, G., Giasnetsova, T., Tsiora, V., & Gritsi-Gerogianni, N. (2010). The level of teamwork as an index of quality in ICU performance. *Hippokratia, 14*(2), 94–97.

Leape, L. (2008). Scope of problem and history of patient safety. *Obstetrics and Gynecology Clinics of North America, 35*, 1–10.

McCue, M. T. (2003). Clamping down on variation. *Managed Health Care Executive.* Retrieved from http://managedhealthcareexecutive.modernmedicine.com/mhe/article/articleDetail.jsp?id=46508&sk=&date=&&pageID=1

McHugh, M., Kang, R., & Hasnain-Wynia, R. (2009). Understanding the safety net: Inpatient quality of care varies based on how one defines safety-net hospitals. *Medical Care Research and Review,66*(5), 590–605.

Mello, M. M., Chandra, A., Gawande, A. A., & Studdert, D. M. (2010). National costs of the medical liability system. *Health Affairs, 29*(9), 1569–1577.

Minch, F. M. (2012, May). *Thoughts on transparency and a few final words.* Tennessee Medicine (p. 5).

Modern Healthcare. (2012). *The modern healthcare/ECRI Institute Technology price index.* Retrieved from http://www.modernhealthcare.com/section/technology-price-index#

Motheral, B. (2011, February). *U.S. drug prices 3- to 6-fold greater than other countries.* RX Outcomes Advisor. Retrieved from http://rxoutcomesadviser.wordpress.com/2011/02/07/drug-prices/

National Quality Forum. (2008, October). *Serious reportable events.* Retrieved from http://www.qualityforum.org/Publications/2008/10/Serious_Reportable_Events.aspx

National Research Council. (2001). *Crossing the quality chasm: A new health system for the 21st century.* Washington, DC: The National Academies Press.

Neuspiel, D. R., Stubbs, E. H., & Liggin, L. (2011). Improving reporting of outpatient pediatric medical errors. *Pediatrics, 128*(6), e1608–e1613.

The Patient Protection and Affordable Care Act. (2010). Retrieved January 4, 2014, from http://www.gpo.gov/fdsys/pkg/BILLS-111hr3590enr/pdf/BILLS-111hr3590enr.pdf

Peredino, D. A. (2011). *Overhauling America's health care machine.* Upper Saddle River, NJ: FT Press.

Plews-Ogan, M. L., Nadkarni, M. M., Forren, S., Leon, D., White, D., Marineau, D., ... Schectman, J. M. (2004). Patient safety in the ambulatory setting: A clinician-based approach. *Journal of General Internal Medicine, 19*(7), 719–727.

Popescu, I., Nallamothu, B., Vaughan-Sarrazin, M., & Cram, P. (2008). Do specialty cardiac hospitals have greater adherence to acute myocardial infarction and heart failure process measures? An empirical assessment using Medicare quality measures: Quality of care in cardiac specialty hospitals. *American Heart Journal, 156*, 155–159.

Porter, M. E. (2010). What is value in healthcare? *The New England Journal of Medicine, 363*, 2477–2481.

Quality and Safety Education for Nurses (QSEN). (2012a). *Quality and safety education for nurses: An introduction to the competencies and the knowledge, skills and attitudes.* Retrieved from http://www.qsen.org/search_strategies.php?id=148

Quality and Safety Education for Nurses (QSEN). (2012b). *Quality and safety education for nurses: Quality and safety competencies, quality safety definition.* Retrieved from http://www.qsen.org/definition.php?id=5

Serious Reportable Events. (2012). *The National Quality Forum.* Retrieved from http://www.qualityforum.org/Publications/2008/10/Serious_Reportable_Events.aspx

Stillwell, S., Fineout-Overholt, E., Mazurek-Melnyk, B., & Williamson, K. (2010). Asking the clinical question: A key step in evidence-based practice. *AJN, 10*(3), 58–61.

The Joint Commission International. (2011a). *Costs of accreditation.* Retrieved from http://www.jointcommissioninternational.org/Cost-of-accreditation

The Joint Commission. (2011b). *In the Joint Commission, the hospital accreditation standards manual 2011—Glossary* (pp. GL1–GL38). Oakbrook Terrace, IL: Joint Commission Resources.

The Joint Commission. (2012a). *Acute myocardial infarction core measure set.* Retrieved from http://www.jointcommission.org/assets/1/6/Acute%20Myocardial%20Infarction.pdf

The Joint Commission. (2012b). *Improving America's hospitals: The Joint Commission's Annual report on quality and safety. 2012 top performers on key quality measures.* Retrieved from http://www.jointcommission.org/assets/1/18/TJC_Annual_Report_2012.pdf

The Joint Commission. (2012c). *Sentinel events.* Retrieved from http://www.jointcommission.org/sentinel_event.aspx

University of California Atlas of Global Inequality. (2012). *Health care spending*. Retrieved from http://ucatlas.ucsc.edu/spend.php

University of Michigan Health System. (2012). *Medical malpractice and patient safety at UMHS*. Retrieved from http://www.med.umich.edu/news/newsroom/mm.htm#summary

U.S. Department of Commerce. The National Institute of Standards and Technology (NIST). *2013–2014 Health Care Baldrige Criteria for Performance Excellence*. Retrieved January 4, 2014, from http://www.nist.gov/baldrige/publications/criteria.cfm

Wennberg, J., & Fisher, E. (2006). *The care of patients with severe chronic illness: A report on theMedicare program by the Dartmouth Atlas Project*. Hanover, NH: Center for the Evaluative Clinical Sciences, Dartmouth Medical School.

Werner, R., Goldman, E., & Dudley, A. (2008). Comparison of change in quality care between safety-net and non-safety-net hospitals. *The Journal of the American Medical Association, 299*(18), 2180–2187.

Wolf, Z. R., & Hughes, R. G. (2009). Chapter 35 error reporting and disclosure. In R. G. Hughes (Ed.), *Patient safety and quality: An evidence-based handbook for nurses*. Retrieved from http://www.ncbi.nlm.nih.gov/books/NBK2652/

SUGGESTED READING

Aiken, L. H., Clarke, S. P., Sloane, D. M., Lake, E. T., & Cheney, T. (2008). Effects of hospital environment on patient mortality and nurse outcomes. *Journal of Nursing Administration, 38*(5), 223–229.

Eizenberg, M. M. (2010). Implementation of evidence-based nursing practice: nurses' personal and professional factors? *Journal of Advanced Nursing, 67*(1), 33–42.

Granner, T., Sendelback, S., Boland, L., & Koehn, K. (2011). Evidence-based nursing. Changing practice, one clinical question at a time. *Nursing Management, 42*(5), 14–17.

Makic, M. B., VonRueden, K., Rauen, C. A., & Chadwick, J. (2011). Evidence-based practice habits: Putting more sacred cows out to pasture. *Critical Care Nurse, 31*(2), 38–62.

Wennberg, J., & Gittelsohn, A. (1973). Small area variations in health care delivery. *Science, 182*(117), 1102–1108.

QUALITY AND SAFETY EDUCATION FOR NURSES

Gail Armstrong and Amy J. Barton

One goal of QSEN is to alter nursing's professional identity so that when we think of what it means to be a respected nurse, we think not only of caring, knowledge, honesty and integrity.... But also, that it means that we value, possess, and collectively support the development of quality and safety competencies. (Cronenwett, 2007)

Upon completion of this chapter, the reader should be able to

1. Review a brief history of the Quality and Safety Education for Nurses (QSEN) initiative in the United States
2. Discuss the various phases of development of the QSEN initiative
3. Identify the six QSEN competencies, which are: patient-centered care (PCC), quality improvement (QI), safety, teamwork and collaboration, evidence-based practice (EBP), and informatics
4. Identify the knowledge, skills, and attitudes (KSAs) associated with each of the six QSEN competencies
5. Identify QSEN competencies related to accreditation standards for nursing programs
6. Recognize resources available for further learning about QSEN competencies
7. Discuss special issues of nursing journals that have focused on QSEN

*A*n 86-year-old woman fell at home and suffered an intertrochanteric hip fracture. She will have a plate and screws surgically placed to stabilize the fracture. This patient has a past medical history of osteoporosis and atrial fibrillation. The patient takes Fosamax (alendronate sodium) 70 mg by mouth once a week and Coumadin (warfarin) 3 mg by mouth once a day. She proceeds to surgery without any member of the health care team checking her last dose of Coumadin or her international normalized ratio (INR) level. During surgery, the patient begins to bleed profusely and requires a transfusion of 5 units of packed red blood cells. The patient is transferred to the intensive care unit (ICU) for further monitoring. After this transfer, the interprofessional health care team gathers to review elements of this case.

- Which members of the interprofessional health care team should be present to review this case?
- How was patient safety and quality compromised in this case?
- Which processes of patient care might be reviewed to ensure that this type of error does not occur again?

*T*he national nursing initiative, QSEN, funded by the Robert Wood Johnson Foundation (RWJF), has trained over 1,000 nursing faculty in how to update quality and safety content in prelicensure nursing programs. QSEN offers rich faculty and student resources for the ongoing work of developing quality and safety. This chapter outlines a brief history of QSEN in the United States. It discusses the various phases of the QSEN initiative. The chapter then identifies six QSEN competencies, that is, PCC, QI, safety, teamwork and collaboration, EBP, and informatics and the KSAs associated with each of them. It then identifies how the QSEN KSAs are integrated into various phases of a nursing curriculum. It identifies QSEN competencies related to accreditation standards for nursing programs and recognizes resources available for further learning about QSEN competencies. Finally, the chapter discusses special issues of nursing journals that have focused on QSEN.

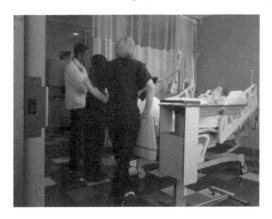

Interprofessional activities at the University of Colorado.

HISTORY OF QSEN IN THE UNITED STATES

To understand the history of the current emphasis on safety and quality in the United States and the background for QSEN, one must go back to 1999. Nurses practicing in 1999 remember the publication of *To Err Is Human* by the Institute of Medicine (IOM). Most startling to health care professionals, as well as the general public, was the revelation that each year 98,000 people die in hospitals as a result of medical errors that could have been prevented (IOM, 1999). *To Err Is Human* ushered in a new era of consciousness about quality and safety concerns in the U.S. health care system.

TABLE 2.1 INSTITUTE OF MEDICINE'S DEFINITIONS OF STEEEP

	IOM TERM	DEFINITION
S	Safe	Avoiding injuries to patients from the care that is intended to help them.
T	Timely	Reducing waits and sometimes harmful delays for both those who receive and those who give care.
E	Efficient	Avoiding waste, including waste of equipment, supplies, ideas, and energy.
E	Equitable	Providing care that does not vary in quality because of personal characteristics such as gender, ethnicity, geographic location, and socioeconomic status.
E	Effective	Providing services based on scientific knowledge to all who could benefit, and refraining from providing services to those not likely to benefit.
P	Patient-centered	Providing care that is respectful of and responsive to individual patient preferences, needs, and values, and ensuring that patient values guide all clinical decisions

Source: STEEEP Health Care Goals. Compiled with information from the IOM (2001).

For many years after the publication of *To Err Is Human*, the IOM focused its reports on suggesting health care system and professional responses to address the causes of the startling number of errors and preventable deaths in hospitals. Many health care clinicians are familiar with the 2001 IOM report, *Crossing the Quality Chasm*, where the attributes of safe, timely, efficient, equitable, effective, and PCC (the acronym STEEEP is often used as a mnemonic for these attributes) are offered as goals of care (Table 2.1).

QSEN: PHASES OF DEVELOPMENT

A group of nurse leaders, who had collaborated yearly since 1993 at an interprofessional conference with physicians and health care administrators, explored the impact of the 2003 IOM report, *Health Professions Education: A Bridge to Quality*. Engaging other national thought leaders in nursing, this influential group asked the question, "What teaching strategies will prepare nursing graduates with the necessary skills to continuously improve the quality and safety of the health care system in which they work?" Beginning in 2005, QSEN, Phase I was funded by the RWJF. Today, QSEN is a vibrant national initiative for nurses and nursing educators that offers resources for integrating IOM's recommendations into models of nursing education. See http://qsen.org.

The five competencies recommended by IOM for all health professions students (PCC, teamwork and collaboration, QI, EBP, and informatics) were closely examined by the nursing leaders. The goal was to identify competencies that would apply to all registered nurses (RNs). Due to nurses' unique position to protect patient safety, safety was added as a sixth competency. The QSEN core faculty outlined the KSAs appropriate for prelicensure education for each of the six competencies (Cronenwett et al.,

2007). These six competencies are the base of QSEN's foundation (PCC, QI, teamwork and collaboration, EBP, informatics, and safety).

Early QSEN data indicated that no nursing graduates were entering practice with updated knowledge about safe systems or knowledge from safety science. **Safety science** is an emerging content area that utilizes new theories and frameworks to describe how errors and near misses are recognized and reported, ways to manage the human factors that impact safe care delivery, and the competencies required for health professionals to provide safe care. Safety science has its roots in other high-performance industries (such as aviation) and is now being adapted to health care systems. Safety science not only focuses on considering personal responsibility and accountability in the delivery of safe care, but also considers how to direct efforts to make system changes to reduce the possibility of errors and increase patient safety. Nursing has historically focused on maintaining patient safety but now safety science calls for new KSAs to achieve practice changes identified in national reports from the IOM (Armstrong & Sherwood, 2012).

QSEN's Phase II work, also funded by RWJF, occurred between 2007 and 2009. Phase II focused on developing a QSEN Pilot School Learning Collaborative by accepting applications from all types of prelicensure programs across the country. Given the limited exposure to quality and safety education in the health professions to date, the QSEN faculty did not know how difficult it would be to integrate the teaching of the KSAs into all types of prelicensure nursing education programs. The goals of Phase II, the QSEN Pilot School Learning Collaborative, were for 15 schools to experiment with various teaching strategies to integrate the KSAs. Much of the work of Phase II pilot schools is now available on the QSEN website http://www.qsen.org.

QSEN's Phase III work, also funded by RWJF, occurred between 2009 and 2012. Three goals focused this work. They were to:

- Promote continued innovation in the development and evaluation of methods to elicit and assess student learning of KSAs of the six QSEN competencies and the widespread sharing of these innovations
- Develop the faculty expertise necessary to assist the learning and assessment of achievement of quality and safety competencies in all types of nursing programs
- Create mechanisms to sustain the will to change among all nursing education programs

This work included change in the content of nursing textbooks, accreditation and certification standards, licensure exams, and continued competence requirements. Through QSEN's Phase III work, more than 1,000 nurse educators were trained in how to integrate updated quality and safety concepts into their nursing education programs.

QSEN's Phase IV work began in 2012 with the announcement that the Tri-Council for Nursing, consisting of the American Association of Colleges of Nursing (AACN), National League for Nursing, American Nurses Association, and the American Organization of Nurse Executives (AONE) will lead a $4.3 million, 2-year initiative, funded by the RWJF, to advance state and regional strategies to create a more highly educated nursing workforce.

Understanding the KSAs: Integration Into Nursing Curricula

For practicing nurses, it is helpful to understand how nursing education is changing and to consider how QSEN KSAs are integrated into nursing curricula. Incorporating QSEN into a nursing curriculum requires not only an understanding of the six QSEN competency definitions of PCC, QI, teamwork and collaboration, EBP, informatics, and safety that are available on the QSEN website. Incorporating QSEN into a curriculum also requires a clear sense of how to effectively place the 162 KSA elements that operationalize those six QSEN competencies into a nursing curriculum. To provide guidance to faculty, a modified Delphi research strategy was used to gain consensus about where individual KSAs should be introduced in the nursing curriculum and where they should be emphasized (Barton, Armstrong, Preheim, Gelmon, & Andrus, 2009). Each of the KSAs were identified as appropriate for introduction and emphasis either in a beginning-level nursing course, an intermediate-level nursing course, or an advanced-level nursing course. A beginning-level nursing course is one of a student's first nursing education courses. An intermediate-level nursing course is taken in the middle of a student's nursing education program. And an advanced-level nursing course is taken by a student just before graduation. Table 2.2 provides a summary table of the Delphi results, indicating where KSAs from five of the six QSEN competencies should be introduced and where they should be emphasized in a prelicensure nursing curriculum. Most interesting of these Delphi results is the clear message that all six quality and safety competencies need to be introduced and emphasized throughout a prelicensure nursing student's education program.

THE SIX QSEN COMPETENCIES

Nursing students may assume that the six QSEN competencies have long been a part of the foundation of nursing education and practice; however, this is not the case (Preheim, Armstrong, & Barton, 2009). Students will likely work with many nursing preceptors who were not educated in the six QSEN competencies. The six QSEN competencies are updated quality and safety concepts that reflect current national quality and safety initiatives and reform in health care professions education. In the following section, a traditional explanation for each competency is contrasted with the QSEN-updated definition (Cronenwett et al., 2007).

PCC

The traditional concept of PCC involved the nurse in consistent listening to the patient and demonstrating respect and compassion. The new QSEN competency of PCC emphasizes recognition of the patient or designee as the source of control and full partner in providing compassionate and coordinated care based on respect for patient's preferences, values, and needs. Example KSAs for this PCC competency are:

- K—Integrate understanding of the multiple dimensions of PCC: Patient/family/community preferences and values; coordination and integration of care; information, communication, and education, physical comfort and emotional support; involvement of family and friends; transition and continuity.

TABLE 2.2 OVERVIEW OF DELPHI STUDY FINDINGS

QSEN COMPETENCY	BEGINNING INTRODUCTION	INTERMEDIATE INTRODUCTION	ADVANCED INTRODUCTION	BEGINNING EMPHASIS	INTERMEDIATE EMPHASIS	ADVANCED EMPHASIS
Patient-centered care	Knowledge, skill, and attitude competencies				Knowledge, skill and attitude competencies	
Teamwork and collaboration	Skill and attitude competencies	Knowledge and skill competencies			Attitude competencies	Knowledge and skill competencies
Evidence-based practice competencies	Knowledge and attitude competencies	Skill competencies			Knowledge and attitude competencies	Skill and attitude competencies
Safety competencies	Knowledge, skill, and attitude competencies			Attitude competencies	Knowledge, skill, and attitude competencies	Knowledge competencies
Informatics competencies	Skill and attitude competencies	Knowledge competencies			Skills competencies	Knowledge and attitude competencies
Quality improvement competencies	Attitude competencies	Skill and attitude competencies	Knowledge competencies		Attitude competencies	Knowledge, skill and attitude competencies

Compiled with information from Barton et al. (2009).

- S—Elicit patient values, preferences, and expressed needs as part of clinical interview, implementation of care plan, and evaluation of care.
- A—Value seeing health care situations through the patient's eyes (Cronenwett et al., 2007).

In the QSEN competency of PCC, the concept of patient as full partner is reflected in providing hygiene care, nutrition, and assisting with elimination for patients. The end point is not limited to skills associated with bathing, feeding, or toileting. Rather, it is important that new nurses learn that nursing skills are centered in the larger context of the patient's preferences and values. For example, when would a patient like to be bathed? How does he or she like to be fed? How often does he or she need to go to the bathroom? Are there aspects of self-care that a patient is capable of carrying out and that a patient would prefer to perform independently? Physical comfort and emotional support are one knowledge aspect of the larger PCC competence. An example of relevant reading that can provide the contemporary context for PCC is the report by the Picker Institute and the Commonwealth Fund (Shaller, 2007), *Patient-Centered Care: What Does It Take?* This report is accessible via QSEN's website (www.qsen.org) using "Related Links." Table 2.3 offers learning activities for PCC at the beginning, intermediate, and advanced levels of nursing education.

Critical Thinking 2.1

View the video in which Don Berwick shares his view of PCC: http://www.youtube.com/ watch?v=SSauhroFTpk

1. Why is "indignity" promulgated and tolerated within health care institutions?
2. How can families be more authentically included in a patient care experience?
3. Identify three concrete actions you can take to honor the concept of patient centeredness?

CASE STUDY 2.1

You are a nurse on a medical–surgical unit and have been asked to precept a new graduate nurse for a month. This new graduate nurse has had some new graduate training on another unit. Your job is to orient her to your medical–surgical unit's care. After working with her for 2 weeks, you notice a consistent approach in how she plans care with her patients. This new graduate nurse has developed a habit of developing a patient's plan of care based mainly on the physician's notes in the chart. She does not consider the patient's preferences, values, or needs in developing a plan of care.

1. *Which QSEN competency would help you in expanding this new graduate nurse's practice?*
2. *Which resources for this QSEN competency might help you in working with this new graduate nurse?*

TABLE 2.3 PATIENT-CENTERED CARE LEARNING ACTIVITIES

CURRICULUM LEVEL	LEARNING ACTIVITIES
Beginning level	Encourage students to interview a patient about his or her diagnosis. What does the diagnosis mean to him or her? How does the patient's perspective of the diagnosis differ from that of the health care team? Write up the patient's perspective, and share it with the patient. Ask the patient for feedback about accuracy and interpretation.
Intermediate level	Are there barriers in your practice environment to active involvement of families in patients' health care processes? Examine system barriers like limited visiting hours in the ICU or inability of family to be present in the perioperative setting. Are there policies that interfere with family involvement? What is the history of these policies?
Advanced level	Sometimes the nurse must initiate a conversation about patient-centered care. Use the following resource to identify effective strategies for such conversations: *Crucial Conversations: Tools for Talking When Stakes are High.* Patterson, Grenny, McMillan, and Switzler (2002).

Teamwork and Collaboration

The traditional concept of teamwork and collaboration has involved working side by side with other health care professionals while performing nursing skills. The updated QSEN competency emphasizes health care providers functioning effectively within nursing and interprofessional teams, fostering open communication, mutual respect, and shared decision making to achieve quality patient care. Examples of KSAs in this competency include:

- K—Describe scope of practice and roles of health care team members.
- S—Follow communication practices that minimize risk associated with handoff among providers and across transitions in care.
- A—Acknowledge own potential to contribute to effective team functioning (Cronenwett et al., 2007).

Students begin to value the nurse's role in planning care and the nurse's impact on patient outcomes when the nursing scope of practice is learned within the context of interprofessional teams. Teamwork is one of the core competencies (along with communication, roles and responsibilities, and ethics) that all health professions students should achieve (Interprofessional Education Collaborative Expert Panel, 2011). The nurse is often at the center of communication for the health care team and frequently facilitates important patient care transitions. For example, communication of the patient's changing status is vital to successful use of rapid response teams.

Rapid response teams are a group of individuals from a variety of disciplines (such as nursing, medicine, respiratory therapy) that use evidence-based interventions in the acute care setting to provide timely, focused care for patients experiencing rapid deterioration. The Institute for Healthcare Improvement's (IHI) *5 Million Lives* campaign facilitated widespread adoption of this team-based intervention (*The 5 Million Lives Campaign*, 2006). Details about rapid response teams can be explored at IHI's website, www.ihi.org. Table 2.4 offers learning activities that focus on the teamwork and collaboration competency at the beginning, intermediate, and advanced levels of nursing education.

Critical Thinking 2.2

Go to the QSEN website and search for the video on the Lewis Blackman story (http://www.qsen.org).

1. What are the factors specific to Lewis's clinical situation that eventually led to Lewis's death?
2. What interventions could have been engaged to prevent Lewis's death?
3. How will knowledge of the Lewis Blackman story affect your practice?

CASE STUDY 2.2

Gloria is a new graduate RN on a medical–surgical unit. She has been concerned lately about the incidence of decubitus ulcers on her unit. Gloria has built good rapport with other members of the health care team and she knows there are several strategies that must be employed by the team to effectively address this problem. When caring for John, a patient with postoperative spinal stenosis, Gloria is worried about a possible decubitus ulcer because of John's immobility and intake of high-dose steroids.

1. *How might Gloria build on her existing rapport with the interprofessional health care team to engage them in working to prevent John's decubitus ulcers?*
2. *How might Gloria use national standards and guidelines to address practice standards on her nursing unit?*
3. *When does an adverse patient outcome move from a quality and safety concern at the individual patient level to a concern of quality and safety at the unit or health care system level?*

TABLE 2.4 TEAMWORK AND COLLABORATION LEARNING ACTIVITIES

CURRICULUM LEVEL	LEARNING ACTIVITIES
Beginning level	Explore the tools recommended for health care teams in the TeamSTEPPS program. These tools can be found at http://teamstepps.ahrq.gov. Which TeamSTEPPs communication strategies would be helpful for patient care on your unit?
Intermediate level	Teamwork and collaboration are core elements of surgical care processes. The Institute for Healthcare Improvement (IHI) launched a national campaign to standardize aspects of perioperative teamwork and collaboration. Go to IHI's home page (www.ihi.org) and using the search box, type in "Surgical Care Improvement Project (SCIP)." Look at the elements of the SCIP project. What components of the SCIP campaign are present in your perioperative services?
Advanced level	Review the article below and examine the implications of these authors' findings on training health care teams. Note the impact of teamwork training on patient outcomes. The first author on this research article is a nurse (Neily et al., 2010).

EBP

The traditional concept of EBP has involved adhering to one facility's internal patient care policies. The QSEN competency of EBP emphasizes the integration of best current evidence with clinical expertise and patient/family preferences and values for delivery of optimal health care. Examples of KSAs for this competency include:

- K—Describe EBP to include components of research evidence, clinical expertise, and patient/family values.
- S—Base individualized care plans on patient values, clinical expertise, and evidence.
- A—Value the concept of EBP as integral to determining best clinical practice (Cronenwett et al., 2007).

Nursing skills are now often taught in the context of EBP. Recent nursing research highlights emerging best clinical practices related to patient care. Nursing texts now include evidence-based support to explain rationales for clinical practices. Table 2.5 offers learning activities at beginning, intermediate, and advanced levels of nursing education.

QI

A traditional concept of QI involves routinely updating nursing policies and procedures. The QSEN competency of QI recommends use of data to monitor the outcomes of patient care processes and the use of QI methods to design and test changes to

TABLE 2.5 EVIDENCE-BASED PRACTICE LEARNING ACTIVITIES

CURRICULUM LEVEL	LEARNING ACTIVITIES
Beginning level	There is an emerging body of research around barriers to nursing clinicians utilizing EBP in their practice. Read the following article: Leasure, Stirlen, and Thompson (2008). Do the authors' take-away points resonate with what you are seeing in practice around barriers to utilization of EBP?
Intermediate level	The following learning activity on the QSEN website allows teams of students to create EBP questions, evaluate the literature, and recommend changes to practice. All elements that are needed for this learning activity are provided: http://www.qsen.org/teachingstrategy.php?id=54
Advanced level	Nurses still struggle to get evidence into practice. An article, "Barriers and Facilitators to the Use of Evidence-Based Practice," by Scott and McSherry explains that for evidence-based nursing to occur, nurses need to be aware of what evidence-based nursing means, what constitutes evidence, how evidence-based nursing differs from evidence-based medicine and EBP, and what the process is to engage with and apply the evidence. The article examines the concept of evidence-based nursing and its application to clinical practice. Use the article as a basis for your of discussion of nursing's struggle to get evidence into practice (Scott & McSherry, 2009).

EBP, evidence-based practice; QSEN, Quality and Safety Education for Nurses.

continuously improve the quality and safety of health care systems. Example KSAs from this competency include:

- K—Recognize that nursing and other health professions students are parts of systems of care and care processes that affect outcomes for patients and families.
- S—Use tools (such as control charts and run charts) that are helpful for understanding variation.
- A—Appreciate continuous QI as essential in the daily work of all health professionals (Cronenwett et al., 2007).

Formal, systems-focused QI processes that engage a health care team, such as adverse events reporting, should be part of the early components of the nursing curriculum. Root cause analyses and resulting system changes are relevant to study in a clinical nursing course. As students progress through clinical courses, they will see many examples of nurses contributing to QI processes in the acute care setting. Nurses are well positioned to offer insights into how to improve patient care processes to improve patient outcomes. Table 2.6 offers learning activities at the beginning, intermediate, and advanced levels of nursing education.

In addition to learning about QI from a nursing perspective, engaging with other health professional students is an effective learning strategy. Students can learn about QI together in classroom, simulation, and clinical settings (Headrick et al., 2012). In fact, the IHI has established an "Open School" to distribute free online courses, provide experiential learning opportunities, as well as build community (http://www.ihi.org/offerings/ihiopenschool/Pages/default.aspx).

EVIDENCE FROM THE LITERATURE

Citation

Kovner, C. T., Brewer, C. S., Yingrengreung, S., & Fairchild, S. (2010). New nurses' views of quality improvement education. *Joint Commission Journal of Quality Improvement and Patient Safety, 36*(1), 29–35, AP1–AP5.

Discussion

QI skills are necessary to identify gaps between current care and best practices and to design, implement, test, and evaluate changes that are essential for RNs (registered nurses) to participate effectively in QI. Newly licensed RNs' positions as direct caregivers could have a negative impact on QI if these nurses lack sufficient knowledge, concepts, and tools required for QI. Data were examined from 436 respondents (69.4% response rate) to a 2008 eight-page mailed survey in a nationally representative panel survey of new nurses who graduated between August 1, 2004, and July 31, 2005. Overall, 159 (38.6%) of the new nurses thought that they were "poorly" or "very poorly" prepared about or had "never heard" of QI.

Implications for Practice

This study highlights new nurses' lack of preparation to participate in QI work. This is significant as bedside nurses have a significant role to play in QI. This study identifies the need to build QI concepts into all nursing curriculums.

TABLE 2.6 QUALITY IMPROVEMENT LEARNING ACTIVITIES

CURRICULUM LEVEL	LEARNING ACTIVITIES
Beginning level	Nurses are involved in QI work at every level in health care. A famous checklist, developed by Peter Pronovost, around central line insertion has standardized the practice of central line insertion and reduced central line-associated bloodstream infections. Read Atul Gawande's article on the development of this checklist, paying attention to the role of nurses in the checklist's implementation. (Gawande, 2007; http://www.newyorker.com/reporting/2007/12/10/071210fa_fact_gawande)
Intermediate level	The following case study illustrates the process of QI by having student teams review an adverse event and propose system solutions: Hall (2007); http://www.qsen.org/teachingstrategy.php?id=45
Advanced level	Partner with someone who works in the QI Department of your hospital. Shadow that person for 2 full days. Notice the focus of their work. Which patient outcomes is this department tracking? How is data gathered for these patient outcomes? What elements of nursing care are tracked for these patient outcomes? What insight can nurses provide about the patient care processes around these patient outcomes?

Safety

A traditional concept of safety focuses on giving attention to limited aspects of safe care, such as bed rails being used properly and ensuring that a patient does not fall out of bed during a nurse's shift. The QSEN updated competency of safety emphasizes broader concepts such as building a culture of safety and minimizing the risk of harm to patients through the implementation of both health care system effectiveness and high-quality individual performance. Examples of KSAs in the safety competency include:

- K—Examine human factors and other basic safety design principles as well as commonly used unsafe practices such as work-arounds and dangerous abbreviations.
- S—Demonstrate effective use of strategies to reduce the risk of harm to self or others.
- A—Value the contributions of standardization/reliability to safety (Cronenwett et al., 2007).

QSEN's definition of safety emphasizes team strategies to promote safe care in a health care system rather than focusing on blaming individuals for safety issues, for example, maintaining asepsis is a component of an individual nurse's practice and has multiple associated safety skills. Maintaining asepsis and reducing infections

---

REAL-WORLD INTERVIEW

The overall goal that I have for medical students is to consider safety and quality as a fundamental part of what they need to learn to be competent physicians. These content areas should not be an "add-on" or extra piece that they do when they have extra time to focus on a QI project. Instead, I teach safety and quality as core parts of both their professional duty and their own competencies. I want my medical students to include safe care and QI as part of their daily work. Part of making these goals achievable is to assure that students start to explore safety and quality concepts early in their medical education, and that they have authentic experiences in the clinical setting doing safety and quality work.

Dr. Wendy Madigosky, MD, MSPH
Director, Foundations of Doctoring Curriculum
Associate Professor, University of Colorado School of Medicine, Aurora, Colorado

---

CASE STUDY 2.3

You are a new nurse working in a busy operating room. You notice that in the past month, three patients being transferred from the same adult patient care unit in the hospital have not been given their preoperative (preop) antibiotics prior to transfer.

1. *What patient care processes might you address to attend to this recurring issue?*
2. *What data might you need?*
3. *Who would you invite to a meeting to address this patient care issue?*

TABLE 2.7 SAFETY LEARNING ACTIVITIES

CURRICULUM LEVEL	LEARNING ACTIVITIES
Beginning level	See http://www.jointcommission.org/2014_national_patient_safety_goals_slide_presentation for a free 2014 National Patient Safety Goals slide presentation.
Intermediate level	This article summarizes the system failures that led to a sentinel event with a newborn: Smetzer, J. L. (1998). Lesson from Colorado: Beyond blaming individuals. *Nursing Management, 29*(6), 49–51.
Advanced level	Note the Nine Patient Safety Solutions identified by The Joint Commission and the World Health Organization: The purpose of the nine patient safety solutions is to guide the redesign of patient care processes to prevent inevitable human errors from actually reaching patients. See http://www.who.int/mediacentre/news/releases/2007/pr22/en

in one's practice has direct implications for supporting patient outcomes related to various national safety goals in a health care system. The *National Patient Safety Goals* (The Joint Commission, 2012), *5 Million Lives Campaign* (IHI, 2012), and *Safe Practices for Better Healthcare* (National Quality Forum, 2009) all state common goals around decreasing nosocomial infection rates in the acute care setting. Table 2.7 offers learning activities at the beginning, intermediate, and advanced level of nursing education.

Informatics

A traditional concept of informatics involves focusing on timely and accurate documentation. The QSEN competency of informatics expands this definition and calls for using information and technology to communicate, manage knowledge, mitigate or reduce error, and support decision making. KSAs from this competency include:

- K—Explain why information and technology skills are essential for safe patient care.
- S—Apply technology and information management tools to support safe processes of care.
- A—Value technologies supporting decision making, error prevention, and care coordination (Cronenwett et al., 2007).

Documentation is an important skill in health care informatics. All members of a health care team contribute to an electronic health record that is used extensively to document shifting patient care priorities. A broader view of informatics emphasizes not only documenting patient care provided but also encourages the use of informatics in decision management, clinical alerts, and so on. Decision management in health care focuses on having the appropriate data available at points in the decision-making process to be able to make the best decision in a timely fashion. Data used in decision management may come from patient records, diagnostic results, providers' documentation, or EBPs. Table 2.8 offers learning activities at the beginning, intermediate, and advanced levels of nursing education.

TABLE 2.8 INFORMATICS LEARNING ACTIVITIES

CURRICULUM LEVEL	LEARNING ACTIVITIES
Beginning level	Many patients use Internet resources to become educated about their diagnosis. Use this QSEN learning activity to evaluate a health-related website that one of your patients may use. There is an evaluation form provided: http://qsen.org/website-evaluation-exercise
Intermediate level	The Commission on Systematic Interoperability has been charged with developing a strategy to make health care information increasingly accessible at various care points in the health care process. Use the following website: www.endingthedocumentgame.gov. Click on the "personal stories" link and read the narratives provided by patients, health care professionals, and nurses about the importance of timely access to patient data.
Advanced level	Consider the number of electronic health records (EHR) you have experienced during your nursing rotations. Answer the following questions: 1. How many EHR systems have you seen in your various clinical rotations? 2. What similarities have you seen among EHR systems? 3. Which EHR system seemed most "nurse friendly"? Identify what you mean by "nurse friendly." 4. What improvements do you think need to be made to existing EHR systems in the acute care setting to better support nursing care needs?

QSEN, Quality and Safety Education for Nurses.

NURSING EDUCATION ACCREDITATION STANDARDS AND QSEN COMPETENCIES

Nursing education accreditation standards are driven by rapid changes occurring in nursing practice. Recently, several national reports have focused on the need for updated quality and safety content in nursing education. A 2010 report by the Carnegie Foundation for the Advancement of Teaching National Nursing Education Study recommended a radical transformation of nursing education to effectively address the practice–education gap (Benner, Sutphen, Leonard, & Day, 2010). The report's authors emphasize that both didactic academic classroom teaching and clinical practice teaching models need to more fully reflect the current health care emphasis on QI and patient safety. An interprofessional report published by IOM in 2011, *The Future of Nursing: Leading Change, Advancing Health,* includes the key message that nurses need to be full partners with other health care team members to redesign health care in the United States. Quality and safety are two significant areas where interprofessional, collaborative efforts are needed to redesign U.S. health care systems. Accreditation standards for nursing programs have begun to clearly articulate the need for quality and safety content in prelicensure curricula. Standards from accrediting bodies for nursing programs, that is, the Accreditation Commission for Education in Nursing (ACEN), formerly the National League for Nursing Accrediting Commission (NLNAC) and the AACN are explicit about the necessity for the QSEN competencies in all nursing prelicensure curricula. Table 2.9 connects each of the AACN Essentials of Baccalaureate

TABLE 2.9 SELECTED AACN ESSENTIALS OF BACCALAUREATE EDUCATION AND QSEN COMPETENCIES

AACN ESSENTIALS OF BACCALAUREATE EDUCATION	QSEN COMPETENCY
II: Basic Organizational and Systems Leadership for Quality Care and Patient Safety	QI Safety
III: Scholarship for Evidence-Based Practice	Evidence-based practice
IV: Information Management and Application of Patient Care Technology	Informatics
V: Interprofessional Communication and Collaboration for Improving Patient Health Outcomes	Teamwork and collaboration QI

Developed with information from the AACN (2008).

TABLE 2.10 SELECTED ACEN STANDARDS AND QSEN COMPETENCIES

NLNAC STANDARD	QSEN COMPETENCY
4.5. The curriculum includes cultural, ethnic and socially diverse concepts and may also include experiences from regional, national or global perspectives.	Patient-centered care
4.6. The curriculum and instructional processes reflect educational theory, interprofessional collaboration, research, and current standards of practice.	Teamwork and collaboration Evidence-based practice QI
4.10 Students participate in clinical experiences that are evidence-based and reflect contemporary practice and nationally established patient health and safety goals.	Safety QI

Developed with information from the ACEN (2013).

Education to QSEN competencies. Many of the AACN Essentials contain several guidelines for prelicensure curricula, thus the connection to more than one QSEN competency in Table 2.9. ACEN's accreditation standards similarly encourage the integration of QSEN competencies into prelicensure curricula. Table 2.10 connects several of the ACEN standards to QSEN competencies.

QSEN RESOURCES

The QSEN website, http://www.qsen.org, which went live in 2007, has many resources for nurses, nursing students, and nursing faculty. Easily available on the website are the competencies and KSAs for prelicensure nurses and graduate nurses. For each QSEN competency, students will find a continuously updated and very rich annotated bibliography that scans the current literature. These QSEN competency-focused bibliographies are excellent resources for all nurses who are looking for evidence related to a specific QSEN competency. There are more than 50 peer-reviewed learning strategies that can be searched by QSEN competency domain, learner level, learner setting, and strategy type. Learning strategies can be accessed on the QSEN website, http://

www.qsen.org, by clicking on the "Teaching Strategies" link, found under "Faculty Resources." The QSEN website has videos that highlight exemplar cases such as the Lewis Blackman story and the Josie King case. Both of these exemplar cases are potent tools that highlight the vital importance of quality and safety in nursing practice. For nurses who were not educated with a strong foundation in quality and safety, there are faculty learning modules that are available on the website. These faculty learning modules address topics such as appreciating and managing the complexity of nursing work, cognitive stacking, informatics, and other topics relevant for practicing nurses.

The "Related Links" portion of QSEN's website is a virtual goldmine. It quickly links the user to QSEN articles, books, and reports on quality and safety, and additional teaching modules, and scenarios. All of the relevant professional organizations that are making great strides in improving quality and safety in health care, for example, IHI, http://www.ihi.org; Agency for Healthcare Research and Quality Patient Safety Network, http://psnet.ahrq.gov; and the Picker Institute, http://pickerinstitute.org are identified on the QSEN website. QSEN's well-designed website is an invaluable, updated resource for all nurses and nurse educators.

SPECIAL ISSUES OF NURSING JOURNALS THAT HAVE FOCUSED ON QSEN

Two prominent nursing journals, *Nursing Outlook and Journal of Nursing Education*, published QSEN-dedicated issues in late 2009. *Nursing Outlook*'s November/December issue (Volume 57, Number 6) includes articles that focus on the emerging work of QSEN being done by schools of nursing across the county. Nurses who want to learn more about the adoption of QSEN by schools across the county will find this issue of *Nursing Outlook* to be a rich resource. The December 2009 issue of *Journal of Nursing Education* (Volume 48, Number 12) offers articles that address specific QSEN learning strategies, for example, a web-based, near-miss reporting system; and a clinical assessment tool and approaches to target PCC in simulations. This issue also contains articles that address broader aspects of curricula such as the compatibility of QSEN with a competency-based curriculum, methods to assess student learning outcomes, and ideas to incorporate QSEN into fundamentals of nursing. Both nursing journals regularly offer substantive contributions to the emerging body of literature about the importance and logistics of implementing QSEN competencies in nursing curricula.

Critical Thinking 2.3

Go to this link at the IHI website: http://www.ihi.org/knowledge/Pages/HowtoImprove/ScienceofImprovementHowtoImprove.aspx

Read about the Model for Improvement. Consider a unit-based project on an adult patient care unit where a nurse wants to address decreasing the decubitus ulcer rate on her unit. Using the Model for Improvement with its three fundamental questions and its Plan-Do-Study-Act (PDSA) cycle as a model for such a project, answer the following questions:

1. What team members would have important input on this team?
2. Imagine yourself on the QI team. What change are you trying to accomplish?
3. What might be your goal?
4. What data will you collect that will show your changes made a difference?

KEY CONCEPTS

- Historically, a major push for the six competencies of the QSEN initiative came from the IOM report, *Health Professions Education*, where competencies in quality and safety were recommended for all health professions students.
- Dissemination of the competencies in QSEN occurred during the first three phases of the QSEN initiative, between 2005 and 2012. A 2-year QSEN initiative to advance state and regional strategies to create a more highly educated nursing workforce began in 2012.
- All six of the QSEN competencies, that is, PCC, QI, safety, teamwork and collaboration, EBP, and informatics, are integral aspects of nursing clinical practice.
- Each of the six QSEN competencies has KSA elements that help operationalize each competency for practice.
- The QSEN competencies are fundamental components of accreditation standards for nursing programs and can be integrated into the beginning-, intermediate-, and advanced-level nursing courses.
- There are a wide variety of quality and safety resources available for nurses at the QSEN website, www.qsen.org.
- There are several special issues of nursing journals that have focused on QSEN.

KEY TERMS

Rapid response teams
Safety science

DISCUSSION OF OPENING SCENARIO

1. Which members of the interprofessional health care team should be present to review this case?

All members of the interprofessional health care team that care for perioperative patients should be involved in reviewing this case. The oversight of not checking this patient's last dose of Coumadin (warfarin) or her INR blood coagulation level is a significant threat to patient safety. Nurse managers from all of the involved units, that is, the nursing unit where the patient was transferred from preoperatively and the operating room, should be present to review this case. The patient's physicians and surgeons should be present. Anesthesia representation should be present. A representative from the hospital pharmacy, there to examine medication reconciliation, should be present. Bedside nurses from the preop nursing unit where the patient was transferred from, and from the operating room, should be available to review the case.

2. How was patient safety and quality compromised in this case?

Patient safety and quality was severely compromised in this case. There was a lapse in communication about this patient's last dose of Coumadin (warfarin) and her INR lab results. The patient could have bled to death.

3. Which processes of patient care might be reviewed to ensure that this error does not occur again?

Medication reconciliation is the process of verifying patient's medications at points of transfer in the patient care process. Identification of the patient's last medication dose is a standard part of medication reconciliation. This health care team should review this facility's medication reconciliation process for patients going to surgery.

Patient handoffs need to be reviewed in this patient's perioperative care process. When the patient was transferred from the medical–surgical unit to the preop unit, patient handoff report would have been given. Is there a standardized patient handoff format or checklist for this patient transfer that includes an update of medications and lab work? What is nursing and anesthesia's standard process for reviewing diagnostic labs preoperatively? What is the standard process for identifying and monitoring patients who take daily anticoagulants?

CRITICAL THINKING ANSWERS

Critical Thinking 2.1

1. Why is indignity promulgated and tolerated within health care institutions?

Traditionally, patients and families have not been consulted at all stages of care. Not including patients or families in all stages of health care can be perceived as being more efficient and as expediting care. As health care practitioners grow in understanding of the importance of assuring patients their dignity, hopefully tolerance of indignity to patients will decrease. We must all work hard at it.

2. How can families be more authentically included in a patient care experience?

Health care providers can create opportunities for input from patients and families. Have patients and families actively involved in care delivery planning and also in transitions in care. Work to include patients and families in all hospital-based committees.

3. Identify three concrete actions you can take to honor the concept of patient-centeredness.

This answer will vary. Work to include such things as introducing yourself to patients, including the patient in planning for his care, regularly evaluating the care you give to patients, reviewing patient satisfaction surveys, and so on. Always remember...without a patient, a nurse is not needed.

Critical Thinking 2.2

1. What are the factors specific to Lewis's clinical situation that eventually led to Lewis's death?

Here are some of the factors identified:

- Overdose of Toradol (ketorolac)
- No communication among health care team members
- Ignoring the concerns of Lewis's mother
- Ineffective assessment by nurses of Lewis's deteriorating condition

2. What interventions could have been engaged to prevent Lewis's death?
   Interventions that could have been engaged to prevent Lewis's death include:

   - Timely, accurate communication among health care team members
   - Validation of clinical findings among health care team members
   - Validation of Lewis's mother's concerns
   - Accurate, timely assessment of Lewis and subsequent communication to the health care team.

3. How will knowledge of the Lewis Blackman story affect your practice?
   Students' answers will vary on how knowledge of this case affects their practice. Answers may include some of the following:

   - It is important to pay attention to patient's clinical condition and concerns.
   - Do not take a patient situation for granted.
   - Always assess your patients carefully and regularly.
   - Pay attention to family comments and feedback when evaluating your patients.

Critical Thinking 2.3

1. What team members would have important input on this team?
   Team members who would have important input on this team include physicians, hospitalists, physical therapists, nurses, respiratory therapists, occupational therapists, nursing assistants, and so on.

2. Imagine yourself on the QI team. What change are you trying to accomplish?
   You are trying to accomplish decreasing the decubitus ulcer rate on the unit. You must first establish the existing rate of pressure ulcers. Consider what some clinical contributing factors are. What are current unit practices to prevent decubitus ulcers?

3. What might be your goal?
   Your goal would be to decrease occurrence of decubitus ulcers by a certain percentage (e.g., decrease decubitus ulcers rates by 20% each year).

4. What data will you collect to show that your change made a difference?
   You would need to collect data on all patients on the units and measure the change in the decubitus incidence rate over time. It is often helpful to benchmark this rate with other similar units, agencies, and so forth.

CASE STUDY ANSWERS

Case Study 2.1

1. Which QSEN competency would help you in expanding this new graduate nurse's practice?
   This new graduate nurse would benefit from being introduced to the QSEN competency of PCC. QSEN defines PCC as "Recognize the patient or designee as the source of control and full partner in providing compassionate and coordinated care based on respect for patient's preferences, values, and needs."

2. Which resources for this QSEN competency might help you in working with this new graduate nurse?

It would be helpful to look to the QSEN website to find resources on PCC for this new nurse. It might be helpful for this new nurse to read the Picker Institute Report, "Patient-Centered Care: What Does It Take?" Or it might be helpful to search on QSEN's website for a learning activity that focuses on PCC. There are more than 20 learning activities that focus on PCC.

Case Study 2.2

1. How might Gloria build on her existing rapport with the interprofessional health care team to engage them in working to prevent John's decubitus ulcers?

As Gloria cares for John for consecutive shifts, she can build on her rapport with the interprofessional health care team and engage them in working to prevent a decubitus ulcer. It can be useful to share information about national standards and guidelines for decubitus care with the team and come up with a plan specific to John. Gloria can seek input on John's care from the physical therapist to learn about safe activities, from the pharmacist on skin protection products, and from the dietician to identify nutritional strategies for decubitus ulcer prevention. When speaking with the physical therapist and dietician about decubitus ulcer prevention for John, these team members both mention the increase in occurrence of decubitus ulcers on this medical–surgical unit. Gloria decides to work with her manager and the QI department to track the decubitus ulcer rate on her medical–surgical unit for the previous 6 months.

2. How might Gloria use national standards and guidelines to address practice standards on her nursing unit?

Once Gloria has the decubitus ulcer rate on her medical–surgical unit for the previous 6 months, she plans on comparing this decubitus ulcer rate with state and national quality benchmarks for decubitus ulcers. She is also aware that there are many best practices published by the IHI and available on its website, www.ihi.org, for best practices for decubitus ulcer prevention. Once Gloria has the data from her own unit to compare to other national benchmarks, she will work with her nurse manager and the team to identify some additional strategies that can be adopted on her unit. Gloria understands that safety needs to be addressed at the individual clinician level, the unit level, and the total system level.

3. When does an adverse patient outcome move from a quality and safety concern at the individual patient level to a concern of quality and safety at the unit or health care system level?

An adverse patient outcome moves from a concern at the individual patient level to a concern of quality and safety at the unit or health care system level anytime more than one patient is involved, though sometimes the concern is at all levels even when it just involves one individual patient.

Case Study 2.3

1. What patient care processes might you address to attend to this recurring issue?

The patient care processes that you might need to address include:

- Do the nurses on the transferring unit need additional training about the action and timing of preop antibiotics?

- Does the unit use a standardized checklist of preop preparation care that patients should receive on this unit?
- What is the preop patient handoff reporting process?

2. What data might you need to improve care?
    You might start with the following data to improve care:

- Number of patients coming from this unit without preop antibiotics infused
- Volume of surgical patients from this unit/month
- Nurse to patient ratios on this unit

3. Who would you invite to a meeting to address this patient care issue?
    You could invite the following people to a meeting to address this patient care issue:

- Nurse manager from the preop unit where the patients are coming from
- Pharmacist to address availability of preop antibiotics
- Surgeon to address preop orders
- Preop and operative unit nurses to address patient handoff reporting process and the problem of patients not receiving their preop antibiotics.

REVIEW QUESTIONS

Please see Appendix D for answers to Review Questions.

1. The nurse is caring for a newly admitted patient. She introduces herself using her first and last name and asks the patient what his values, needs, and preferences are for this hospital stay. The nurse is practicing which of the QSEN competencies?

    A. EBP
    B. Safety
    C. PCC
    D. Teamwork and collaboration

2. The primary nurse is caring for a patient admitted to the unit from a nursing home with a Stage III decubitus ulcer. In looking at the electronic nurses' notes, she notes a discrepancy in the patient's wound care procedures. The primary nurse calls the wound care nurse to consult and ensure a consistent plan of care. The wound care nurse assesses the patient and provides the necessary information reflecting the standard of care. The primary nurse is practicing which of the QSEN competencies? Select all that apply.

    A. QI
    B. Safety
    C. Teamwork and collaboration
    D. EBP
    E. PCC
    F. Informatics

3. The nurse is transferring his patient from the Postanesthesia Care Unit (PACU) to the surgical unit. He is calling the receiving nurse with patient handoff report. Ensuring patient safety by using the handoff report, he is careful to describe the situation, background, assessment, and recommendation for the patient's continued care. This is an example of assuring patient safety by using which QSEN competency?

   A. Teamwork and collaboration
   B. QI
   C. PCC
   D. Informatics

4. The nurse notices that in her care of the patient a variety of unintentional deviations from her usual care resulted in an adverse patient outcome. She asks for assistance from her manager in analyzing the incidents that occurred in the care of the patient. This is an example of using which QSEN competency?

   A. Safety
   B. QI
   C. PCC
   D. Teamwork and collaboration

5. The nurse is assessing her patient when the medical resident walks into the room and approaches the patient for assessment. The nurse gently reminds the resident to use the hand sanitizer before touching the patient. This reminder is an example of using which QSEN competency?

   A. Safety
   B. QI
   C. PCC
   D. Teamwork and collaboration

6. The nurse is using barcode administration technology to facilitate the administration of medications to her patients. This is an example of how barcode medication administration technology facilitates which QSEN competencies? Select all that apply.

   A. Teamwork and collaboration
   B. Safety
   C. PCC
   D. Informatics
   E. EBP
   F. QI

7. The nurse is participating in a team meeting with her patient, the dietician, physician, and social worker. The nurse recalls the importance of spirituality that the patient had expressed to her and notices that a pastoral care representative is not present. She contacts pastoral care to be included in the meeting. This inclusion is an example of using which QSEN competency?

   A. Teamwork and collaboration
   B. Safety
   C. PCC
   D. Informatics

8. The nurse realizes that her patient's pain management is not effective. She has noticed this with other patients in the past and decides to analyze the unit-based pain control chart posted in the break room. She decides to explore additional pain management options for patients whose pain is not controlled with the usual pain management. Which QSEN competency best describes her approach?

A. Safety
B. QI
C. PCC
D. Teamwork and collaboration

9. In administering medication to her patient, the nurse saw that the medication administration record indicated the dose amount to be 0.5 mg. She immediately double checked the order and confirmed that the dose was supposed to be 0.5 mg. The nurse remembered to always use a zero before a decimal when the dose is less than a whole unit and she updated the medication administration record accordingly. This is an example of using which QSEN competency?

A. Safety
B. QI
C. PCC
D. Teamwork and collaboration

10. The nurse is concerned about his patient's lab values and medication regimen. He uses the electronic health record to obtain trend information about medication doses and resultant lab values and notes that the patient is progressing within normal limits. This use of the electronic health is an example of using which QSEN competency?

A. Teamwork and collaboration
B. Safety
C. PCC
D. Informatics

REVIEW ACTIVITIES

Please see Appendix E for answers to Review Activities.

1. Read your local paper every day for 2 weeks. Identify articles that examine a health care quality or safety issue. Bring these articles to class to discuss with your classmates and instructor. What did you find?
2. Interview three nurses on the unit where you are currently doing a clinical rotation. Ask each nurse, "What is the most pressing patient safety issue on this unit?" Take notes. Compare answers. Discuss the results with your classmates and instructor in postconference. What did you find?

EXPLORING THE WEB

1. The QSEN website offers a wealth of materials for nursing students and faculty alike. Go to www.qsen.org, and on the left side of the homepage, click on "Related Links."
2. Go to the website for the National Patient Safety Foundation (http://www.npsf.org). Use the link at the top of the homepage, click on "For Patients and Consumers." Look at "Key Facts About Patient Safety." Review the facts about wrong-site surgery, medication errors, health-acquired infections, falls, readmissions, and diagnostic errors.

REFERENCES

American Association of Colleges of Nursing (AACN). (2008). *The essentials of baccalaureate education for professional nursing practice.* Retrieved from http://www.aacn.nche.edu/education-resources/BaccEssentials08.pdf

Barton, A. J., Armstrong, G., Preheim, G., Gelmon, S. B., & Andrus, L. C. (2009). A national Delphi to determine developmental progression of quality and safety competencies in nursing education. *Nursing Outlook, 57*(6), 313–322.

Benner, P., Sutphen, M., Leonard, V., & Day, L. (2010). *Educating nurses: A call for radical transformation.* San Francisco, CA: Jossey-Bass.

Cronenwett, L. (2007). *Emory Jowers Lecture on "Quality and Safety Education for Nurses".* Retrieved from http://qsen.org. Slide 10

Cronenwett, L., Sherwood, G., Barnsteiner, J., Disch, J., Johnson, J., Mitchell, P.,...Warren, J. (2007). Quality and safety education for nurses. *Nursing Outlook, 55*(3), 122–131.

Gawande, A. (2007, December 10). The checklist. *The New Yorker.* Retrieved from http://www.newyorker.com/reporting/2007/12/10/071210fa_fact_gawande

Hall, L. W. (2007). *Interprofessional curriculum in patient safety and quality improvement.* Retrieved from http://www.qsen.org/teachingstrategy.php?id=45

Headrick, L. A., Barton, A. J., Ogrinc, G., Strang, C., Aboumatar, H., Aud, M.,...Patterson, J. (2012). Retooling for quality and safety: Integrating quality and safety into the required curriculum at twelve medical and nursing schools. *Health Affairs, 31*(12), 2669–2680. doi:10.1377/hlthaff.2011.012.1

Institute of Medicine (IOM). (1999). *To err is human: Building a safer health system.* Washington, DC: National Academies Press.

Institute of Medicine (IOM). (2001). *Crossing the quality chasm.* Washington, DC: National Academies Press.

Institute of Medicine (IOM). (2003). *Health professions education: A bridge to quality.* Washington, DC: National Academies Press.

Institute of Medicine (IOM). (2011). *The future of nursing: Leading change, advancing health.* Washington, DC: The National Academies Press.

The Institute for Healthcare Improvement (IHI). (2012). *5 million lives campaign.* Retrieved from http://www.ihi.org/offerings/Initiatives/PastStrategicInitiatives/5MillionLives Campaign/Pages/default.aspx

Interprofessional Education Collaborative Expert Panel. (2011). *Core competencies for interprofessional collaborative practice: Report of an expert panel.* Washington, DC: Interprofessional Education Collaborative.

Kovner, C. T., Brewer, C. S., Yingrengreung, S., & Fairchild, S. (2010). New nurses' views of quality improvement education. *Joint Commission Journal on Quality and Patient Safety, 36*(1), 29–35, AP1–AP5.

Leasure, A. R., Stirlen, J., & Thompson, C. (2008). Barriers and facilitators to the use of evidence-based best practices. *Dimensions of Critical Care Nursing, 27*(2), 74–82; quiz 83.

National Quality Forum. (2009). *Safe practices for better healthcare.* Retrieved fromhttp://www.qualityforum.org/Publications/2009/03/Safe_Practices_for_Better_Healthcare%E2%80%932009_Update.aspx

Neily, J., Mills, P. D., Young-Xu, Y., Carney, B. T., West, P., Berger, D. H.,...Bagian, J. P. (2010). Association between implementation of a medical team training program and surgical mortality. *The Journal of the American Medical Association, 304*(15), 1693–1700.

Patterson, K., Grenny, J., McMillan, R., & Switzler, A. (2002). *Crucial conversations: Tools for talkingwhen stakes are high.* New York, NY: McGraw Hill Publishing.

Preheim, G. J., Armstrong, G. E., & Barton, A. J. (2009). The new fundamentals in nursing: Introducing beginning quality and safety education for nurses' competencies. *The Journal of Nursing Education, 48*(12), 694–697.

Scott, K., & McSherry, R. (2009). Evidence-based nursing: Clarifying the concepts for nurses in practice. *Journal of Clinical Nursing, 18*(8), 1085–1095.

Shaller, D. (2007). *Patient-centered care: What does it take?* The Commonwealth Fund. Retrieved from http://www.commonwealthfund.org/Publications/Fund-Reports/2007/Oct/Patient-Centered-Care–What-Does-It-Take.aspx

The 5 Million Lives Campaign. (2006). Retrieved from www.ihi.org

The Joint Commission. (2012). *National patient safety goals 2012.* Retrieved from http://www.jointcommission.org/standards_information/npsgs.aspx

The National League of Nursing Accreditation Commission. (2008). *NLNAC 2008 Standards and-Criteria. Baccalaureate Degree Programs in Nursing.* Retrieved from http://www.nlnac.org/manuals/SC2008_BACCALAUREATE.htm

SUGGESTED READING

Armstrong, G., & Sherwood, G. (2012). Patient safety. In J. Giddens (Ed.), *Concepts based nursing* (1st ed., pp. 434–442). St. Louis, MO: Elsevier.

Armstrong, G., Sherwood, G., & Tagliareni, M. E. (2009). Quality and Safety Education in Nursing (QSEN): Integrating recommendations from IOM into clinical nursing education. In *Clinical nursing education*: Current reflections (pp. 207–227). Washington, DC: National League of Nursing.

Armstrong, G. E., Spencer, T. S., & Lenburg, C. B. (2009). Using quality and safety education fornurses to enhance competency outcome performance assessment: a synergistic approachthat promotes patient safety and quality outcomes. *The Journal of Nursing Education, 48*(12), 686–693.

Avansino, J. R., Peters, L. M., Stockfish, S. L., & Walco, G. A. (2013). A paradigm shift to balance safety and quality in pediatric pain management. *Pediatrics, 131,* e921–e927. doi:10.1542/peds.2012–1378

Cohen, N. L. (2013). Using the ABCs of situational awareness for patient safety. *Nursing, 43,* 64–65. doi:10.1097/01.NURSE.0000428332.23978.82

Dekker, S. (2011). *Patient safety: A human factors approach.* Boca Raton, FL: CRC Press.

Dolansky, M. (2011). Teaching and measuring systems thinking in a quality and safety curriculum. In *Proceedings of the 2011 QSEN National Forum.* Milwaukee, WI (Available on QSEN website under 2011 National Forum Presentation Slides).

Finkelman, A., & Kenner, C. (2012). *Learning IOM. Implications of the Institute of Medicine reports for nursing education.* Silver Spring, MD: American Nurses' Association.

Gawande, A. (2001). *The checklist manifesto: How to get things right.* New York, NY: Henry Holt & Co.

Gawande, A. (2002). *Complications: A surgeon's notes on an imperfect science.* New York, NY: St. Martin's Press.

Gawande, A. (2008). *Better. A surgeon's notes on performance.* New York, NY: Henry Holt & Co.

Henderson, D., Carson-Stevens, A., Bohnen, J., Gutnik, L., Hafiz, S., & Mills, S. (2010). Check a box. save a life: How student leadership is shaking up health care and driving a revolution in patient safety. *Journal of Patient Safety, 6*(1), 43–47.

Hughes, R. G. (2008). *Patient safety and quality: An evidence-based handbook for nurses.* AHRQ Publication No. 08–0043. Rockville, MD: Agency for Healthcare Research and Quality.

Institute of Medicine (IOM). (2004). *Keeping patients safe: Transforming the work environment of nurses.* Washington, DC: National Academies Press.

Kenney, C. (2008). *The best practice: How the new quality movement is transforming medicine.* New York, NY: Public Affairs—A member of the Perseus Books Group.

Ko, H., Turner, T. J., & Finnigan, M. A. (2011). Systematic review of safety checklists for use by medical care teams in acute hospital settings—limited evidence of effectiveness. *BMC Health Services Research, 11,* 211.

Ogrinc, G. S., Headrick, L. A., Moore, S. M., Barton, A. J., Dolansky, M. A., & Madigosky, W. S. (2012). *Fundamentals of health care improvement: A guide to improving your patient's care* (2nd ed.). Oak Terrace, IL: Joint Commission Resources.

St. Onge, J., Hodges, T., McBride, M., & Parnell, R. (2013). An innovative tool for experiential learning of nursing quality and safety competencies. *Nurse Educator, 38,* 71–75. doi:10.1097/NNE.0b013e3182829c7d

The 5 million lives campaign. (2006). Retrieved from www.ihi.org

Wachter, R. M. (2008). *Understanding patient safety.* New York, NY: McGraw-Hill Publishing.

QUALITY AND SAFETY IN HIGH-RELIABILITY ORGANIZATIONS

Pauline Arnold

If a high reliability mindset does not exist among people in an organization, no set of behaviors or rules will ever produce extreme reliability. (Hines, Luna, Lofthus, Marquardt, & Stelmokas, 2008)

Upon completion of this chapter, the reader should be able to

1. Define high-reliability organization (HRO)
2. Understand key concepts in a highly reliable organization
3. Define fair and just culture
4. Recognize organization requirements to be highly reliable
5. Distinguish the underlying factors that impede the health care organization from changing to a culture of high reliability and safety
6. Describe the external driving forces for quality and safety in an HRO
7. Understand internal structures and roles in a health care organization that support a culture of safety and just and fair culture

---

*D*espite intense efforts to eliminate wrong site surgery, it can still occur. When this happens, it is a sentinel event and requires a thorough investigation to determine the underlying cause of the event. The course of action for the investigation includes implementing corrective action plans and collecting data to verify sustained changes. Leadership and the governing board declare that improving the culture of safety in the organization is a priority focus. The culture of safety survey indicates the overall safety *culture appears to be improving in the operating room. Before the year is over, the same organization has another wrong-site surgery involving a different surgeon.*

- *What went wrong and how can this happen after the corrective actions have been implemented to prevent future occurrences?*
- *What organization or unit culture characteristics may contribute to the recurrence of wrong-site surgery?*
- *What can the nurse do to avoid this scenario from repeating?*

An **HRO** (specifically, health care organizations) are those organizations that establish and maintain high quality and safety expectations for patient care delivery and keep rates of quality and safety failures near zero (Weick & Sutcliffe, 2007). A key element of an HRO is the ability to provide consistent care at a high level of excel-

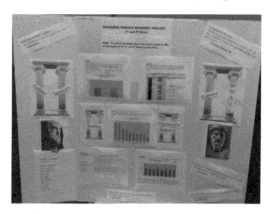

lence over a long period of time. In an HRO, a culture of safety permeates the organization. Each health care worker is mindful of safety in his or her work and patients are not harmed by the care provided. All health care professionals are expected to contribute to the quality and safety of the health care delivery system.

Despite efforts, adverse events and health care errors continue to occur, which may lead to catastrophic outcomes. Progress has been made to close the quality and safety gap of care. Pockets of excellence exist, but they are not widespread and standardized across the health care system. An HRO radically reduces health care system

Quality showcase: Sharing the process improvement story, an interdisciplinary team moving toward high reliability using Lean Six Sigma tools.

failures and effectively responds when a failure does occur. The health care consumer should expect a near-zero rate of failure in key health care processes and outcomes. Nurses play a key role in driving fundamental change to address the challenge of consistently demonstrating high-quality and safe care across care settings and over time. The mentality of delivering high-quality and safe care encourages organizations to become highly reliable and safe systems. The overarching promise of an HRO is to provide safe quality care, to not harm patients, and to deliver on these promises consistently, for every patient, every time.

The purpose of this chapter is to understand characteristics of an HRO. Key concepts, criteria, and essential processes of a highly reliable health care organization are presented. The influence that culture has on being an HRO is examined in terms of impact on quality and safety. Historical context discussion of quality improvement will lead to the evaluation of the external forces driving the mandatory health care changes. An identification of barriers to providing consistent high-quality care is provided. Understanding the internal structures that support a highly reliable organization will assist nurses to become valued contributors to health care reform. Nurses will be able to identify the key structure and roles in an organization that can impact a positive culture.

HROs

A key element to developing and maintaining a high-reliability culture is the premise that every patient will receive the highest quality safe care every single time. To do so requires a fundamental change from fragmented, isolated health care tasks to health care process management and systems thinking. Health care processes are those steps taken when providing care to patients. Managing the health care processes requires minimizing the variation in the tasks and how they are performed. A variation in tasks is how different nurses may take care of the same patient differently when the tasks include assessment, medication administration, and nutrition. For example, one nurse may check a patient's blood sugar reading before breakfast and assessing the patient. Another nurse may assess the patient before giving medications and breakfast. A third nurse may make sure all patients are eating before checking blood sugars then giving medications. The variation is that all three are not following the same health care process. Variations in the sequence of task can impact the patient's outcome. Systems thinking is a way of looking at all health care processes as they relate to each other. Systems thinking considers the interrelatedness of the health care processes and the impact on the outcome.

An HRO has the agility to manage the unexpected and knows that when small things go wrong, it is often a warning signal of a bigger problem. For example, a patient was given a wrong dose of medication causing the patient's blood pressure to drop. In an HRO, this scenario would result in looking at what allowed the nurse to give the wrong dose rather than accepting that the nurse was at fault. The focus is on the medication process and potential problems that may be present allowing a wrong dose to be given. Attentive listening to these early warning signals assists an HRO to manage unexpected failures. At the front line, nurses are typically the first to find the small early warning signs. It is important that nurses are alert and aware of themselves, others, and their environment. An HRO listens to its frontline workers knowing that they hold the key to identifying small problems early.

Five health care process characteristics found in HROs that help to achieve consistent, safe, and high-quality care are described in Table 3.1 (Weick & Sutcliffe, 2007). The characteristics are those elements that, when present, help an organization achieve high reliability.

Preoccupation With Failure

Preoccupation with failure requires the nurse to have knowledge and awareness that the risk of error is always present. An HRO understands that failures can occur and puts processes in place to diminish harm. For example, medication administration is a process that incorporates double checks for high-risk medications such as insulin, anticoagulants (e.g., Lovenox), or narcotics. The presence of double checks, or having another nurse verify medication and dosage, helps support safe medication administration. Another aspect of preoccupation with failure is the ability to feel safe in stopping or reporting any process that the person feels is questionable or unsafe. Reporting of questionable or unsafe practices is key to identifying and fixing problems. Nurses need to have the ability to recognize that an error could occur or that an error has occurred and assume the responsibility to report when an error is recognized.

TABLE 3.1 FIVE HEALTH CARE PROCESS CHARACTERISTICS THAT ARE REQUIRED FOR HROs TO ACHIEVE CONSISTENT, SAFE, AND HIGH-QUALITY CARE

CHARACTERISTICS	ELEMENTS
Preoccupation with failure	• Be alert to near-miss events, recognize weaknesses in health care systems early
Reluctance to simplify	• Recognize the complexity of work. Do not focus on easy-fix causes of failure
Sensitivity to operations	• Recognize the complexity of health care processes • Have situational awareness of the environment, distractions, availability of resources, and supplies • Have an awareness of relationships
Resilience	• Anticipate failure • Determine how to diminish risk of harm to patients • Identify strategies to recover when and adverse event occurs
Deference to expertise	• Use teamwork which recognizes each member's knowledge, skill, and expertise • Invite active participation from health care professionals • Be comfortable in sharing information • Deemphasize hierarchy

Adapted from Weick and Sutcliffe (2007).

The next time you participate in a clinical experience, examine the health care environment based on the characteristics of an HRO described in Table 3.1.

Near-miss events are those process variations that do not affect the outcome or result in an adverse event; however, if there would be a reoccurrence, there is a high probability that it could result in an adverse event (The Joint Commission, 2012). For example, a patient is prescribed morphine sulfate for pain but is allergic to the medication. Although the medication was not given, it was prescribed and is therefore considered a near miss. In an HRO, near misses receive as much attention as a failure to understand what went wrong so that a failure can be avoided in the future. Rewarding the recognition of a near miss by actively addressing the process failures and not punishing a person communicates to the team the value and commitment the organization places on early detection. An HRO commits to improving the health care system before a harmful event occurs.

Reluctance to Simplify

Recognizing the complexity of health care systems and nursing procedures encourages HRO professionals to understand that there are no simple answers to health care process failures. Not accepting easy answers, such as "I forgot" or "I just overlooked it" encourages the organization to search for the underlying causes of failures. Probing below the surface for contributing factors is important to find a real, sustainable solution. For example, if a medication is missed, it is easy to identify that the nurse forgot. When looking deeper into the medication process, the findings might be that the medication was not listed on the medication sheet, was not available from the pharmacy in an electronic medication dispensing system, or the nurse might have set the medication down when attending to another patient. Each of these findings leads the HRO to investigate differently how the medication process broke down to identify areas for improvement.

Sensitivity to Operations

Sensitivity to operations creates an awareness of the situation the nurse is in and the many factors that can influence a nurse's response to actual or potential errors. Factors such as fatigue, distractions, and workload can contribute to a preoccupation that often occurs in the complex workflow of nurses. *Meaningful redundancy* is a term that describes doing the same thing twice. It is meaningful in that the intent is to catch an error before it is committed. Redundancy refers to duplicating a step more than once. Meaningful redundancy is used to describe steps that are taken to reduce the risk of error. For example, withdrawing a dose of insulin and making sure it is the correct dose is the first step. Verifying the dose of insulin with another nurse is considered meaningful redundancy. These steps may be necessary to complement individual safety practices.

Resilience

Because we are human, errors will occur. *Resilience* is a term used to describe the ability to bounce back when something bad happens. For an HRO, the ability to overcome problems, learn from mistakes, and move forward is defined as resilience. The commitment to resilience requires team training and practice. Staff members of an HRO are trained to perform quick situation assessments when an error occurs, work as a team to contain the error, and then take steps to reduce the harm. Simulation learning is one tool to practice responses to errors and prepare health care professionals. Drills for cardiopulmonary resuscitation, environmental disaster, and rapid response teams are health care processes put in place as part of the commitment to resilience. Being able to effectively recover from errors is dependent on having support structures in place before an error occurs so that when an error occurs, health care professionals can work as a team to respond appropriately and efficiently.

Deference to Expertise

In an HRO, healthy teams recognize that each member has the knowledge and skills unique to his or her profession and role. It is important to minimize the authority gradient or hierarchy between caregivers so each one feels valued and secure in his or her role to speak up. Authority gradients refer to positions such as a direct care nurse and the unit manager. Hierarchy refers to levels of power, such as direct care nurses and the physician. In either case, all participants should have equal voice, without fear of punishment resulting from speaking their mind. Deference to expertise in an HRO includes the expectation that team members with the most expertise regarding the issue in that moment have the authority to make any decisions needed regardless of the power hierarchy. For example, one team member may have a piece of information that others do not have, such as a physical therapist's knowledge of an assistive device to help a patient walk. In this case, the other health care workers would acknowledge the physical therapist's expertise when planning care for the patient. It is the knowledge and expertise of the physical therapist that will keep the patient safe. Intimidation or ignoring a team member's expertise can generate anger, indifference, or a failure to respond, which creates opportunities for errors to occur. Open communication with information flowing in all directions among all team members is essential for consistently safe care to be delivered.

CASE STUDY 3.1

A patient requires the insertion of an indwelling urinary catheter to treat urinary retention. The nurse wants to ensure that the patient has a safe experience and that the risk of infection is minimized. Use information from the five HRO health care process concepts to achieve consistent, safe, and high-quality care in Table 3.1 to answer the following questions.

1. *How would the nurse demonstrate her awareness of preoccupation with failure, sensitivity to operations, and deference to expertise?*
2. *How would you engage the patient to assist you in building resilience into your health care process?*
3. *What elements would the nurse document to demonstrate reluctance to simplify?*

FAIR AND JUST CULTURE

A **fair and just culture** is the demonstration of an open, free, and nonpunitive environment, which readily admits its weaknesses and commits to learning from its mistakes (Hughes, 2008). An organization with a fair and just culture recognizes that a potential for error exists. Being fair and just means the organization minimizes blame and punishment. To have a culture of safety, where safe patient care is a priority, the organization must start with building a fair and just culture. This fair and just culture makes reporting of errors safe by holding the individual and the system appropriately accountable. Such accountability does not eliminate individual or organizational responsibility, but rather finds a balance between accountability and creating a learning environment where an organization learns from its mistakes.

According to Reason (1997), a fair and just assessment differentiates between normal human error, at-risk behavior, and reckless behavior. An error that is not intentional and could happen to anyone is a human error. For instance, you have a patient who needs a medication dose. As you walk to the medication room to get the medication, you are interrupted several times and subsequently forget to get the patient's medication. The error was caused by a variety of factors, none of which are intentional acts by the nurse. At-risk behavior is manifested when process shortcuts become a normal variation in the procedure, such as taking shortcuts with the sterile process while inserting a urinary catheter and the patient subsequently acquires an infection. At-risk behavior requires coaching so the individual understands the risks and consequences of the behavior choices. A deliberate choice to not follow a policy is considered reckless behavior. For example, if a nurse knows that a patient requires the assistance of two people to stand and walk but decides to walk the patient alone, it is considered reckless behavior. This is significant when the patient is at a high risk for a fall and the appropriate two-person assistance is not used.

An organization is defined by how blame and punishment occur, which in turn can determine what is reported (Weick & Sutcliffe, 2007). Leaders need to be mindful and not fall into the temptation of blaming individuals. Leaders must look at the organization culture, processes, and the interactions of individuals within the health care systems. Punishing the person does not correct the process problem that allowed the error to occur. Blaming and punishment has a negative consequence that discourages open reporting and communication about errors.

REQUIREMENTS FOR ACHIEVING HIGH RELIABILITY

In Table 3.1, we examined the characteristics of an HRO. Table 3.2 describes the essential requirements needed by an organization to achieve high reliability. This section expands upon the previous section to identify and describe the essential organizational requirements that must be present to achieving high reliability in health care provision.

Committed Leadership

A strong commitment to quality and safety requires the chief executive officer (CEO) of a hospital to provide leadership for a proactive quality safety agenda. The agenda is a plan for the entire organization based on the goal of high-quality safe care for every patient, every time. Executive leaders set the context for the care delivery system and cultivate a supportive environment that considers the environment of the nurse and how nurses interact with the systems within which they work. Leaders encourage nurses and frontline health care workers to engage in problem solving at the point of work. Processes need to be user friendly and efficient.

Safety and quality thrive in an environment of teamwork and respect for all members of the health care team. Frontline health care providers close to the patient and the delivery of care have significant health care process and content knowledge. Not only is it imperative that leaders of an organization value the expertise of frontline health care providers, they need to engage and empower staff to function as leaders for the quality and safety efforts.

TABLE 3.2 THREE ORGANIZATIONAL REQUIREMENTS FOR ACHIEVING HIGH RELIABILITY

1. Leadership commitment to zero major quality failures
2. Safety culture embedded into the organization
3. Robust process improvement to fix flawed processes

From Dr. Chassin's Keynote at the fourth International High Reliability Organizing Conference. © The Joint Commission, 2011. Reprinted with permission.

REAL-WORLD INTERVIEW

Several key practices move an organization toward high reliability. First, a patient-centered mission provides the foundation for a culture of safety and guides both decisions and interventions, which increase reliability. Second, strong administrative support of culture of safety efforts, with a low-or-no tolerance stance for safety indiscretions is essential for maintaining high reliability. Third, all direct caregivers, as well as all other staff, must accept personal responsibility for sustaining and continually improving the organization's reliability. Lastly, involving the patient and family in culture of safety efforts enhances staff and organizational efforts, while encouraging patient self-empowerment and self-responsibility for protecting their own safety.

Rose Flinchum, MSEd, MS, CNS, RN, BC-ADM, CDE
Clinical Diabetic Educator, Indiana University (IU)
Health La Porte Hospital, La Porte, Indiana

Culture of Safety

A **culture of safety** is described as a culture that combines individual and group values, attitudes, and ways of behaving that identify the commitment to an organization's endeavors toward safety and safe practice (Hughes, 2008). The organizational culture of safety is defined by the shared values and practices of the organization. A mission-focused adaptable organization with clear values, high integrity, and a strong trust relationship is positioned to have a culture of safety. The culture of safety, as well as quality, drives the high-reliability mindset for leaders. A culture of safety includes having strong teams to work on improving safe health care delivery and demonstrates a learning organization mentality. A learning organization mentality describes an organization that learns from previous mistakes to improve health care delivery. In addition, an organization with a strong culture of safety establishes ways of reporting errors by health care providers that is blame free and without punishment.

Nurses at the Sharp End

The majority of errors that occur in health care are related to organizational factors, known as the "blunt end." Clinicians, such as nurses, are considered the "sharp end," where errors materialize. For instance, if a wrong medication were given to the patient the focus of blame would be on the nurse. Upon further analysis of the error, it was identified that there was an error in transcription and an error resulting from two patients on the unit having the same name. All of these smaller errors resulted in the nurse giving the wrong medication. Historically, nurses were treated differently if they were involved in an error or an adverse event. Being at the sharp end means that the nurse is usually the last line of defense against health care errors (Hughes, 2008). To eliminate nurses at the sharp end of blame, it is essential that a culture of safety be established that values nonpunitive reporting. Focusing on the cause of errors such as systems and process factors that allow an error to occur helps develop a culture of safety.

Learning Organization

The learning organization views each failure as an opportunity to learn from mistakes. Organizational learning and culture change are always connected. The frequency of adverse event reporting provides information about the organization culture and the willingness to learn from events and near misses. For example, Hospital A has 30 reported near misses and five errors. Hospital B has no reports of near misses and only two errors. You may think that Hospital B is doing well. Consider this, Hospital A has an anonymous reporting system that allows the person to report a near miss or error, allowing an investigation of the problem. Hospital B, on the other hand, does not have anonymous reporting and health care providers fear punishment if they report a near miss or error. This example demonstrates how reporting errors and near misses can assist in understanding a problem rather than hiding that a problem exists. An HRO avoids placing individual blame to build an attitude of system failures and finding long-lasting solutions. In the past, organizations dealt with adverse events by eliminating the person from employment, staff education, and focusing attention on the problem or problems that resulted from the adverse event. These approaches failed to sustain any improvement over time.

Critical Thinking 3.1

According to Dr. Chassin, president of The Joint Commission Center for Transforming Health Care, the safety culture must be embedded into a health care organization. Consider the culture of an organization you have experience with or perform a web search on an organization to find its values statement.

1. What are the written values of the organization and what are the values demonstrated by the employees' behavior?
2. Is there alignment between the written values and the demonstrated values?
3. How does the alignment of the values support the organization's readiness for a culture of high reliability?

Human Factors Engineering

Understanding human characteristics is important to sustain improvements. **Human factors engineering** is the discipline concerned with understanding human characteristics and applying that knowledge to the design of systems that are reliable, safe, efficient, and comfortable to use (Gosbee & Gosbee, 2010). A simple example concerns the computerized charting system found in the clinical setting. Initially, computers were located in the nurse's station requiring nurses to write their assessment on a piece of paper then transfer the information into the computer charting system. To make charting more efficient for the nurse, some hospitals mounted laptops on carts with wheels. By doing so, nurses were able to take their charting to the patient's bedside. This simple step encouraged nurses to spend more time at the bedside and eliminated inefficiencies with charting. Understanding human characteristics assists with achieving simplicity, safety, and efficiency. Incorporating human factors engineering science in health care work processes can decrease frustration, inefficiencies in providing care, and help to minimize the risk of errors. Human factors engineering takes into consideration the nurse's interaction with supplies and equipment in his or her environment. For example, nurses frequently search for supplies, human factors would suggest that because humans make color association, color-coding certain types of supplies would make them easier to locate.

Improving processes using human factors engineering science takes into consideration the nurses' physical ability and how they interact within their environment. It also takes into account policies and procedures, which provide standardized directions on how to perform work duties. A review of the process requires the determination of whether or not the policy or procedure is capable of being followed with the current workflow and availability of supplies and equipment. When the effort needed to complete the task is high, it is less likely to occur or to occur without a work-around.

Work-Around

A **work-around** bypasses an essential step or problem when the planned steps in the process are not working (Gosbee & Gosbee, 2010). For example, the policy for medication withdrawal on the unit states that medications will be removed for one patient and immediately administered to that patient. If a nurse is running behind schedule and is having trouble keeping up with patient care tasks, the nurse may withdraw more than one patient's medications, placing the other patient's medications in a pocket. This action may seem efficient and saved the nurse time by withdrawing two patients' medications simultaneously, but it also increased the risk for a medication error. Now the nurse has two patient's medications with the potential for mistakenly giving a patient the wrong medication. Using human factors engineering concepts, the process of medication withdrawal would be examined. Results might include changing the medication process by having the patient's medications available in a locked medication storage area in the patient's room. The organization that examines the current medication process, looks at innovative ways to address problems, and considers the effect on the nurse's work is exhibiting characteristics of a learning organization. Simplifying the required steps to perform a task can increase adherence to safe practices. In addition, reducing distractions that take the attention away from performing the task and minimizing interruptions that interfere with task performance will support the learning efforts of the individual and the organization (Gosbee & Gosbee, 2010).

An effective culture of safety is based on mutual trust among physicians, nurses, other health care professionals, and administration. A culture of safety requires that a fundamental change from the past bureaucratic structure of leaders telling people what to do has to occur. This involves listening to what caregivers say about providing safe, high-quality care, and then finding ways to meet their needs. In a culture of safety, the patient is the central focus. Interprofessionals concentrate on doing the right thing for every patient. Frontline caregivers frequently have the knowledge and wisdom to find solutions for safe quality care. The frontline staff (e.g., nurses, certified nursing assistants) are the gatekeepers of quality safe care. A culture of safety requires that frontline staff are engaged and actively working toward promoting safety. An organizational value of teamwork drives how work is structured, divided, and rewarded. Leadership sets the expectation and creates the environment where teamwork can flourish, creating the framework for a culture of safety.

Process Improvements

An HRO has a strong commitment to health care process improvement. Becoming an HRO requires a systematic look at the complexity of the health care process, identification of the root causes of failures in the health care process, implementation of solutions, measuring and monitoring outcomes from the implemented solutions, and then building ways to sustain the improvement. It is important to recognize when a health care process needs improvement versus when an entirely new process is required. A critical element is the engagement of patients and their families to assist in health care process improvements to merge quality and service efforts. The use of systematic process improvement methodologies and tools such as Six Sigma and Lean discussed in Chapter 7, and Baldrige discussed later in this chapter, assist in driving the high-reliability changes

In an HRO, health information technologies help support and sustain the quality and safety efforts. Hospital leaders often apply information technology (IT) to faulty health care processes and hope to prevent error with technology. An example is the use of electronic medication systems and bar coding. Each of these encourages compliance with medication policies while supporting safe medication practices. For instance, we are taught as nursing students that the patient's armband must be checked every time we administer medications. Bar-coding technology requires the nurse to scan the patient's armband and then scan each medication. The patient's medication list and name are located on a database that the technology accesses. Bar coding reduces the number of wrong medication, wrong dose, wrong time, and wrong patient medication errors before they reach the patient. Technology can only help and assist health care process improvements when applied appropriately. A focus on a safe and efficient health care process design using technology to support and sustain any improvement is critical.

REAL-WORLD INTERVIEW

An electronic health record (EHR) provides an improved foundation of clinical information upon which an organization can build more reliable clinical workflows for the delivery of high-quality, safe patient care. Paper records by their nature are fragmented often requiring sifting through many volumes to extract the needed data to appropriately treat the patient. An EHR allows for real-time abstraction of data and the generation of alerts so that the clinician can more reliably provide the correct care for each particular patient. One of the key practices necessary for an organization to move toward high reliability is the careful integration of human and electronic workflows.

Jeffrey E. Anderson, MD, MS
Chief Medical Information and Quality Officer
IU Health La Porte Hospital, La Porte, Indiana

Reporting of Events

In a fair and just culture, reporting of safety events is a professional responsibility for all health care providers. The scope of reported events includes near misses, adverse, and sentinel events. A near-miss safety event allows an opportunity to improve health care processes before harm occurs. An **adverse event** is an undesired or intended consequence of the care provided, such as a significant decrease in blood pressure after the wrong dose of medication is given. **Sentinel events** are unexpected outcomes or risk of an outcome involving death or serious physical or psychological injury (The Joint Commission, 2012).

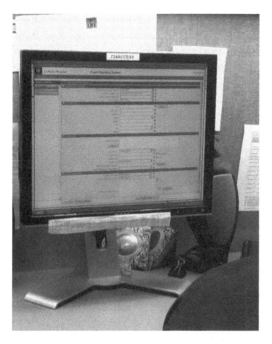

Nursing reports a safety event with an online reporting system, which allows anonymous reporting.

HROs depend on voluntary reporting of events as an indicator of safe delivery of care. Reporting has its limitations, as it is dependent both on the recognition of the safety event and the safety event report being completed. It is estimated that by using only voluntary reporting and error tracking, only around 10% to 20% of all errors are reported in health care delivery organizations (Classen, Lloyd, Provost, Griffin, & Resar, 2008). In an HRO, a multifaceted reporting approach is needed that is comprehensive and provides accurate measurements of errors and near misses. The Institute for Healthcare Improvement (IHI) Global Trigger Tool helps health care organizations get a clearer understanding of the safety of care by measuring risk and harm at the hospital level.

The Global Trigger Tool uses specified care triggers as indicators that an adverse event may have occurred. If the indicators are present, then the chance of harm increases (Griffin & Resar, 2009). For example, "transfer to a higher level of care" is one of the triggers. A patient is transferred to the ICU from a medical–surgical unit due to a rapid drop in blood pressure and decreased level of consciousness. This would cause activation of the trigger and a review of the chart to see what happened to the patient. The review would examine what happened, when it happened, and could it have been avoided. There are more than 50 triggers that are consolidated into categories, which include provision of care, surgical, ICU, perinatal, medication, and emergency department. The categories and triggers can be viewed at www.ihi.org, click on the knowledge tab, select tools, and the Global Trigger Tool is located as a link on the page (you will need to register to use the free tool). Triggers may include care interventions such as the movement of a patient to the critical care unit, or the use of a medication reversal agent. In an HRO, voluntary reporting investigation results and the global trigger results are shared with health care providers and process improvement changes are put into protocols, policies, and procedures to reduce the chance of future events occurring.

Critical Thinking 3.2

Visit the website www.ihi.org to access the Global Trigger Tool.

1. What patient signs and symptoms would you look for that could potentially indicate an adverse event has occurred?
2. What new physician orders may suggest an adverse event has occurred?
3. What actions would you as a nurse take to mitigate the harm of an adverse event?

BARRIERS TO HIGH RELIABILITY AND SAFETY

Achieving high reliability in an organization can pose challenges. The culture and traditions of a health care organization can pose a barrier to becoming an HRO. Workplace intimidation and disruptive behaviors can oppose the creation of an HRO. Blending of professional health care subcultures, that is, unit, department, and team, into a common professional culture may create challenges for high-reliability minded leaders. Managing the enculturation of quality and safety principles into an organization requires an understanding of the values, beliefs, and past successes as well as hierarchies of the organization. In addition, the ability to measure outcomes related to high reliability and lack of robust health IT systems can undermine the ability to achieve high reliability and safety.

Culture and Traditions

The overall culture of an organization is a reflection of past learning experiences. Revising the cultural patterns of basic assumptions and beliefs is difficult, time consuming, and anxiety provoking. If a past experience with reporting an error resulted in punishment, it may deter future reporting of errors. The fear of punishment can be a significant barrier to error reporting. Changing culture requires a significant leadership commitment to focus on processes and systems that lead to the error rather than on individual blame. Changing a long-standing tradition of blame and punishment takes considerable time.

Workplace Intimidation and Disruptive Behavior

Workplace intimidation, making others feel fear, timid, and inferior, destroys the trust environment that is essential for a culture of high reliability. Intimidation is created by what The Joint Commission has identified as disruptive behaviors or behaviors that do not support a culture that makes safety a priority (The Joint Commission, 2012). A culture of safety is a necessary element of an HRO. Intimidation behaviors such as refusing to answer a question, not answering a page, using nonverbal gestures of pointing, and raising your voice need to be eliminated in an HRO to build the critical component of trust.

Critical Thinking 3.3

The Joint Commission (2008) has defined disruptive behavior as any behavior that does not support a culture of safety. Go to The Joint Commission website, http://www.jointcommission.org, type in "sentinel alert" in the search box at the top right corner. Select "Sentinel Alert #40: Behaviors that undermine a culture of safety."

1. Identify nursing behaviors that may be defined as disruptive, including nurse to nurse, nurse to patient, nurse to physician, physician to nurse, nurse to other health care team members.
2. Identify recommended strategies to address disruptive behaviors.
3. What is nursing's role in creating an intimidation-free work environment?

Accepting disrespectful or disruptive behavior of any health care provider, nurse, or staff member is a potential threat to a high level of quality and safety for an organization. Human behavior will naturally want to return to the comfort of how things were traditionally done. It is essential that committed leaders recognize and manage unwanted behavior to change a culture.

Interprofessional Complexity

The complexity of the health care environment creates challenges for the HRO. The safety of patient care relies on effective coordination and communication among the diverse interprofessional health care teams. Members of the same interprofessional team may use different terminology and come from very diverse educational preparation. These barriers create a challenge in making decisions required for high-quality safe care. The complex dependency of one health care process on another health care process requires coordination of efforts across the continuum. For example, the coordination of interprofessional health care processes is essential for a safe transition when preparing a patient to be discharged from the acute care setting to the home environment. Extensive coordination and clear communication among the entire health care team facilitates post-hospital services the patient may require, the prescriptions to obtain, follow-up appointments to make, patient and family understanding of care instructions, and to ensure that the appropriate transportation is in place.

History and Traditions

The history and traditions of the organization set the stage for becoming an HRO. Some health care organizations may have assumptions and beliefs that high reliability is not achievable in health care organizations. The complexity of the work and past history of the organization may overwhelm the organization. The past history of how improvements were made in the health care organization can limit future improvements for an organization seeking to be an HRO. For instance, a nurse is preparing an insulin injection at the medication station. When reaching for an insulin syringe, the nurse discovers that insulin and tuberculin syringes are mixed together in the same container. Using the wrong syringe would result in a medication error. The last time a medication error was made on the unit, the nurse was suspended for 3 days. Due to the punishment associated with the medication error, the nurse decides to separate the insulin and tuberculin syringes into two containers rather than reporting the near miss. In this example, the organization does not have the opportunity to examine why the two syringes were mixed together in the same container since the nurse fixed the problem. Without knowledge of the near miss, no actions can be taken to prevent the problem from occurring again.

Hierarchies

The traditional hierarchical roles of physicians, nurses, and organizational leadership along with the use of a medical model of care create a challenge to implement the HRO principles. The traditional hierarchical role of the physician was based on a medical model of care, which is physician-driven health care delivery. Traditionally, the physician was the leader in the provision of health care. Patient care protocols and algorithms were physician driven. This did not always allow for open questioning and communication regarding the integrated care of the patient. In contrast, the HRO values the perspective of all health care team members. In doing so, the HRO works toward eliminating power hierarchies, allowing for open communication among the interprofessional health care providers.

Measuring a Culture of Safety

Measuring a culture of safety is often challenging. To date, there are no clear culture of safety measures that demonstrate validity and reliability. Many organizations use a culture of safety survey tool to capture the perspectives of the health care provider. Effective use of the tool is still in the infancy stage. The Agency for Healthcare Research and Quality (AHRQ) has made a survey tool available to measure the culture of safety on their website, http://psnet.ahrq.gov/primer.aspx?primerID=5. Although the survey is called Patient Safety Culture, it measures the culture of safety. Results are used to

- Raise staff awareness about patient safety
- Diagnose and assess the current status of patient safety culture
- Identify strengths and areas of opportunity for patient safety culture improvement
- Examine trends in patient safety culture change over time
- Evaluate the cultural impact of patient safety initiatives and interventions
- Conduct internal and external evaluations

IT

A barrier can exist regarding IT. The use of health IT for the documentation of care and the gathering of quality and safety information is essential. Additionally, health care technology systems provide a means for reporting errors and near misses. The lack of health IT can impede progress to an HRO. Devoting scarce resources in a health care organization to implement technology systems that require significant capital expense and ongoing maintenance cost is a challenge.

EXTERNAL INFLUENCES FOR CHANGE

Greater transparency by health care organizations in reporting quality measures is mandated by government and requested by the health care consumer and payers. The Institute of Medicine (IOM) defines transparency as "making available to the public, in a reliable and understandable manner, information on the health care system's quality, efficiency and consumer experience with care, which includes price and quality data, so as to influence the behavior of patients, providers, payers and others to achieve better outcomes (quality and cost of care)" (American College of Physicians, 2010). Transparency is the sharing of the costs and outcomes of health care with consumers to help the consumer make informed choices about selecting health care providers (http://archive.hhs.gov/valuedriven). The premise behind transparency is holding health care providers and organizations accountable for quality care. In other purchase transactions, consumers can easily obtain information about cost and value to make informed purchases. The health care business is required to follow the same practice of transparency. Public awareness of medical errors, poor quality outcomes, and perceived low value are driving changes in health care.

Leapfrog, a business consortium, is a public reporting mechanism on health care organization's performance on quality and safety measures. Payers (insurance companies) and the public use the information from Leapfrog to make informed health care decisions. Leapfrog is a voluntary reporting agency that collects and publishes quality information. The Leapfrog consortium works on behalf of the public and employers to inform Americans about the performance of hospitals on quality measures. The Leapfrog group promotes full disclosure of hospital performance information and helps provide employers with information to provide the best health care benefits to employees (www.leapfroggroup.org).

Health care costs have escalated in response to poor quality of care patient outcomes, health care medical errors, and waste. Historically, organizations were rewarded for the volume of health care services delivered instead of for their achievement of high-quality and safety outcomes. For example, a hospital was reimbursed for the number of appendectomies performed regardless of the outcome. Now, certain quality outcomes must be achieved to receive reimbursement. The Department of Health and Human Services (HHS) and the Centers for Medicare and Medicaid Services (CMS) are currently charged with the task of assuring quality health care through accountability and transparency. The Affordable Care Act of 2010 requires CMS to hold organizations accountable for quality measures as viewed in Table 3.3 (CMS, 2011).

As of January 2013, CMS had over 375 quality measures in place that span across various settings and types. Settings include hospital inpatient, hospital outpatient, nursing homes, home health, and dialysis centers. Types include physician quality reporting systems (PQRS), dialysis or end-stage renal disease, Part D prescription drug benefits administered by private health plans, and Medicare Advantage (insurance plans provided by private insurers approved by Medicare; CMS, 2011). Additional measures are added regularly and expanded to include other settings such as ambulatory surgery centers. These quality measures are creating the foundation for health care reimbursement through pay-for-performance (P4P) or value-based purchasing (VBP) programs.

In P4P and VBP programs, payers (insurers) calculate reimbursement for services provided by measuring the completion of specific interventions and paying for the outcomes achieved. For example, patients with acute myocardial infarction are prescribed to take an aspirin every day. This is an example of a specific intervention. The outcome is the absence of subsequent heart damage from a blocked coronary artery. Through VBP, the CMS calculates reimbursement for hospitals for the quality of care provided to Medicare patients. To read more about VBP, go to the CMS website at www.cms.gov and type value-based purchasing in the search box at the upper-right-hand corner.

P4P and VBP have already substantially changed the quality of health care delivery. Future efforts by CMS will encourage better coordination and integration of care across multiple settings. Accountable Care Organization models focus on the delivery of care across an episode of illness with special emphasis on chronic disease management and end-of-life care. Care delivery across the health care continuum will emphasize vulnerable points of patient care transitions. Accountable

TABLE 3.3 CENTERS FOR MEDICARE AND MEDICAID SERVICES QUALITY MEASURES

MEASURE	DEFINITION	EXAMPLE
Efficiency of care	The correlation between resources needed to provide quality care and the quality outcomes from the delivery of health care services	• Cost of care per Medicare beneficiary
Structure of care	Monitors the presence of a mechanism or system is in place that supports the delivery of quality health care	• Presence of electronic health records (EHRs) or electronic prescribing systems • Participation in quality measures databases such as the National Database for Nursing Quality Indicators (NDNQI)
Process of care	Evaluates whether the patient received certain elements of care as defined by evidence-based health care related to the patient's diagnosis	• Documentation that aspirin was given for all patients admitted with myocardial infarction (heart attack)
Intermediate outcome	Examines the results of health care processes during the hospital stay that support patient outcomes	• Measurement of Hgb AIC results for patients with diabetes
Outcome	Monitors the morbidity and mortality rates resulting from a disease	• Mortality rates for specific patient populations such as patients with heart failure • Agency for Healthcare Research and Quality and research patient safety indicators which include mortality for specified procedures
Patient-centered care	Tracks the patient's experience with the health care organization and health care providers	• Survey of patient's perception of the care received

care focuses on the health care provided across multiple care settings. Outcome measurements include successful transitions of care for the patient to a different care setting (e.g., a patient is discharged home with home health care) and resources used. Health care professionals at each care setting must be engaged to deliver high-quality safe care to every patient, every time, and across all settings and locations.

The Joint Commission is currently focused on ensuring that quality measures are effective in promoting improved outcomes for the patient. Every health care organization that seeks The Joint Commission accreditation must meet specific criteria in their measures of quality. The Joint Commission has adopted the Donabedian conceptual framework of assessing the health care structure, work processes, and outcomes of care as the foundation of how to structure quality of care measurement (Chassin, 2011). During 2011, The Joint Commission extensively reviewed its quality measure criteria and identified four key measurement criteria to drive improvement. These key criteria for measurement address what needs to be present in health care organizations to achieve accreditation.

1. Measures had to have a strong foundation of research that links the measure to an improved outcome. The recommended care intervention has to have evidence in research with a correlation between the intervention and the desired outcome.
2. Measurement had to accurately determine whether the evidence-based care was provided. Care can be provided and documented as a bundle; therefore, each individual step would not be measurable. Bundles are groupings of interventions that when done together, increase the likelihood of achieving the desired outcome.
3. Measures had to address a process that was in close proximity to the outcome. For example, the smoking cessation measure did not adequately reflect whether the patient discontinued smoking, just that the education was provided.
4. Measures had to have minimal or no unintended consequences (Chassin, Loeb, Schmaltz, & Wachter, 2010). For example, for patients with a lab confirmation diagnosis of pneumonia, the evidence supports the administration of antibiotics within 4 hours of diagnosis. The measurement is "antibiotics administered within 4 hours of diagnosis." This measurement had the unintended consequence of providers focusing more on meeting the 4-hour time limitation than on waiting for test results. Many times the lab results indicated that an antibiotic might not have been needed.

Along with the public reported quality and safety measures, many states are now requiring some form of mandatory reporting of specified adverse events. The National Quality Forum has identified a list of 28 adverse events, also called never events, which should never occur in health care. They are grouped into six categories; surgical, product or device related, patient protection, care management, environmental, and criminal. The list is evolving as more events are added. To view the complete list of adverse events, go to http://psnet.ahrq.gov, click on the tab Patient Safety Primers, and scroll down to Never Events. Many states use this list as a guide for the required reporting of data.

Public Recognition of Quality Achievements

In the race to achieve and maintain high levels of quality, organizations are seeking marks of distinction that set them apart from other health care organizations. The Baldrige award recognizes organizations that have improved and sustained organizational results. The purpose of this award in health care is to challenge organizations to improve their effectiveness of care and health care outcomes to pursue excellence, which moves organizations toward becoming an HRO. Go to http://www.nist.gov/baldrige/enter/health_care.cfm to learn more about the Baldrige Health Care Criteria for Performance Excellence.

The designation by the American Nurse's Credentialing Center (ANCC) as a Magnet™ organization denotes nursing excellence and may factor into payer negotiations for reimbursement. An organization that has nursing firmly grounded in the Magnet components found in Chapter 1 will be positioned to achieve high-quality outcomes and transition to a highly reliable health care system (ANCC, 2008).

CASE STUDY 3.2

A nurse works for an organization that has achieved Magnet designation. The nurse is a member of the Quality and Safety Unit Practice Council. As a member of the Council, the nurse is assigned the task of educating nursing and other peers on how the Magnet designation supports and helps the organization become an HRO. Complete a web literature search on the Magnet components and correlate the key Magnet principles to the HRO concepts.

1. *How do the Magnet components support the organizational requirements for high reliability?*
2. *How do the Magnet components align with the HRO process concepts?*
3. *How do the Magnet components support a culture of safety?*

In a Magnet-designated hospital, the chief nursing officer (CNO) is an active leader in creating an HRO by establishing strategic goals in conjunction with the hospital's executive team for quality and safety. These goals support the organization's commitment to zero major quality failures. Transformational leadership and structural empowerment require the active engagement of nurses. For example, nurses serve on committees at the unit, department, and organizational levels. Nurses also participate on quality improvement teams to find innovative solutions to move health care into the future. Exemplary professional nursing practice with evidence-based new knowledge, innovation, and improvements provide the framework to sustain improvements. Sustained empirical outcomes will move an organization on the journey to becoming an HRO.

REAL-WORLD INTERVIEW

For an organization to achieve Magnet designation, it must exhibit many characteristics of an HRO. Nursing is embedded within an organizational culture and cannot achieve this important status without a strong organizational framework and leadership support. The Magnet Designation Program translates into a workplace that values nursing, promotes excellence, and focuses on the patient receiving the highest quality of care. For a hospital or system to achieve Magnet status, it must be sensitive to opportunities in both systems and work processes that influence, impact, and improve patient care. Magnet status identifies a learning organization that has a mindset of continuous evaluation and improvement. Magnet status demonstrates an organization that is committed to nursing and improving patient care.

Jo Ann Brooks, PhD, RN, FAAN, FCCP
Vice President of System Quality, IU Health, Indianapolis, Indiana

INTERNAL STRUCTURES AND ROLES TO SUPPORT AN HRO

To become an HRO, an internal organization infrastructure needs to support the goals and strategies of the organization. The governing body, typically the board of directors, must set the priority for quality and safety. Implementing quality and safety initiatives requires an executive team that is committed to lead the organization on the journey to high reliability and excellence. Physicians must be engaged at all levels of the quality and safety infrastructure. A human factors engineer (HFE) may be engaged in an HRO as a support professional. HFE is an interprofessional approach that looks at the safety and efficiency of work systems. The HFE will examine how people, policies, technology, and work structures interact to improve quality, safety, efficiency, and reliability of health care provision. The HFE can also function as educators and project consultants for clinical effectiveness and quality improvement teams.

In an HRO, the ideal situation is to have the quality and safety committee led (or chaired) by the CEO. This structure provides a liaison between the executive level and direct-care level of a health care organization. The chair of the quality and safety committee must provide leadership for all quality and safety initiatives. An interprofessional membership often includes physicians, nurses, pharmacists, a patient safety officer, risk management, customer service, infection control, and a community member. Multiple committees, defined in Table 3.4, can exist to support the overall work of the quality and safety committee.

In addition to the committees described in Table 3.4, certain departments also support an HRO infrastructure. The quality and patient safety departments often encompass multiple functions such as quality and safety reporting for public reporting, as well as database submissions for benchmarking, process improvements, clinical documentation, infection prevention, and control. The quality and safety departments also support peer review, regulatory and accreditation compliance, risk management, and customer service. The case management and social services department facilitates a safe discharge plan for the patient. Utilization review activities are often combined into the case management department. An example of a quality and safety infrastructure to support an HRO can be viewed in Figure 3.1.

The infrastructure is also supported by key positions in the organization. Not all health care organizations will have every position described but most will have a majority of the positions. A patient safety officer is the quality and safety leader at the executive level. The patient safety officer provides leadership for error prevention, error identification and reporting, and reduction of the severity of harm. The role of the patient safety officer closely aligns to risk management. The risk manager has the responsibility to protect the assets of the organization by undertaking activities to identify, evaluate, and reduce the likelihood of patient injury, and the risk of loss to the organization. In the journey to high reliability, several roles have emerged or expanded in health care organizations. A quality analyst functions as an expert in the process improvement methodologies and tools. A clinical documentation expert assesses and supports documentation processes to ensure that they accurately reflect the patient's condition and the level of service required to meet the patient's care need. A customer service expert provides leadership to ensure that the patient receives respectful and coordinated care and to facilitate a process to address complaints that may arise when failure to meet patient's health care expectations occur.

With health care quality and safety changing to HROs and the focus on coordinated health care across multiple providers and settings, many organizations are developing transitional care departments. The role of this department is to focus on

TABLE 3.4 COMMITTEES THAT SUPPORT QUALITY AND SAFETY

Medical Staff Executive Committee	Supports medical staff processes and clinical quality improvement.
Credentials Committee	Ensures that qualified competent providers practice in the organization.
Infection Control Committee	Provides leadership for the infection prevention and control program.
Utilization Review Committee	Provides leadership for the appropriate resource management of patient care. Review of the medical necessity for patient care and the appropriate levels of care are key responsibilities. The Committee ensures the management of the appropriate admission status of the patient, i.e, inpatient, outpatient, or observation based on the severity of the patient's illness.
Medical Staff Peer Review Committee	Conducts retrospective reviews of patient care to identify opportunities for improvement and to share what was learned with other providers.
Nursing Peer Review Committee	Conducts retrospective reviews of nursing patient care to identify opportunities for improvement and to share what was learned with other providers.
Pharmacy and Therapeutics Committee	Provides the leadership for safe medication processes.
Environment of Care Committee	Provides leadership for the facility's safety management program.
Ethics Committee	Provides support for ethical dilemmas that may present themselves in health care and in research activities. May be combined with the Institutional Review Board Committee.
Institutional Review Board Committee	Responsible for ensuring that all research practices are safe and follow standard guidelines for the conduct of research. May be combined with the Ethics Committee.

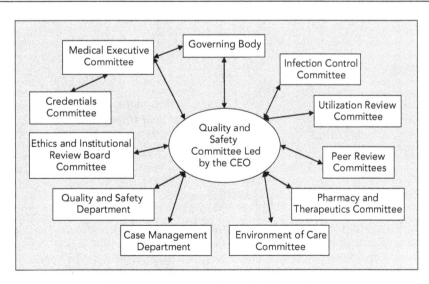

FIGURE 3.1 Example of an organization quality and safety infrastructure to support an HRO.

CEO, chief executive officer.

safe transitions within the health care system. An initial primary focus is on the transition from hospital to home for patients with chronic disease and end-of-life issues to ensure that health care is provided seamlessly. Transitional care nurses help coordinate care between transitions to different care settings such as hospital to home health care and assist patients to navigate the complex health care system. A well-defined organization infrastructure that promotes teamwork and communication supports the transition to an HRO.

KEY CONCEPTS

1. An HRO targets near-zero rates of failure.
2. Process concepts required to become an HRO include preoccupation with failure, sensitivity to operations, deference to expertise, resilience, and reluctance to simplify.
3. To achieve high reliability, an organization must have strong leadership commitment, an established culture of safety, and a well-developed quality improvement program.
4. A fair and just culture differentiates between human error, at-risk behavior, and reckless behavior.
5. A fair and just culture requires no-blame reporting and a commitment to be a learning organization.
6. The organizational culture, traditions, hierarchy, disruptive behaviors, complexity of health care, and the lack of health IT systems are barriers to achieving consistent, high-quality and safe health care outcomes.
7. The VBP and P4P links quality and safety outcomes to payment and The Joint Commission accountability measure program is linked to accreditation.
8. The organization's infrastructure must provide support to achieve high reliability.

KEY TERMS

Adverse event	Human factors engineering
Culture of safety	Near-miss event
Fair and just culture	Sentinel event
HRO	Work-around

DISCUSSION OF OPENING SCENARIO

1. What went wrong and how can this happen after the corrective actions have been implemented to prevent future occurrences?

   To avoid sentinel events requires a mindfulness by every team member. There has to be a mindfulness of the complexity of the process and anticipation that things can and do go wrong. Improving the culture of safety is not enough, there has to be consistency, every single time, with all safety standards. Lessons learned from near misses and past events need to be shared. It requires a team effort where every member is safe to speak up when something is wrong. All team members including physicians need to embrace the mindset of safety. Collection of data is not enough; action needs to be taken based on the data. The health care team should be held accountable for following the established policies and procedures.

2. What organization or unit culture characteristics may contribute to the recurrence of wrong-site surgery?

A committed leadership sets expectations and holds all team members accountable. A culture of lack of accountability, fear, mistrust, without teamwork could all contribute to an error-prone culture.

3. What can the nurse do to avoid this scenario from repeating?

Nursing can provide the leadership to ensure that policy and procedure are followed. Nursing can enforce the established safety standards such as implementation of the World Health Organization Surgical Check List. Nursing needs to report noncompliance by any team member. Nursing can stop the time out if not all team members are actively engaged in the timeout procedure. Nursing needs to be the advocate for the patient, engage the patient in the preparation process to assist the patient to have a safe surgical experience.

CRITICAL THINKING ANSWERS

Critical Thinking 3.1

1. What are the written values of the organization and what are the values demonstrated by the employees' behavior?

The written values are of little use if they are not driving the behaviors of the employees.

2. Is there alignment between the written values and the demonstrated values?

The alignment of the values is essential to create the environment and the consistency in behaviors required for high reliability.

3. How does the alignment of the values support the organization's readiness for a culture of high reliability?

It requires that employees "walk the talk."

Critical Thinking 3.2

1. What patient signs and symptoms would you look for that could potentially indicate an adverse event has occurred?

Signs and symptoms that may indicate an adverse event has occurred may be changes in vital signs, changes in patient status such as skin color, nausea, diarrhea, bleeding, signs and symptoms of a stroke, changes in mental status, the development of a pressure ulcer, and/or there may be a change in behavior requiring restraint use. The patient may experience sudden weakness and it could trigger a fall.

2. What new physician orders may suggest an adverse event has occurred?

A physician's order to transfer to a higher level of care, or a medication order to counteract another medication, the sudden discontinuance of a medication, additional unanticipated lab work, or an order to transfuse blood products may indicate an adverse event.

3. What actions would you as a nurse take to mitigate the harm of an adverse event?

Nurses can mitigate the harm from an adverse event by early recognition of potential triggers. Recognition, assessment, and communication with the physician is essential. Knowledge regarding medication actions and interactions can prevent an adverse event. Safety measures should be implemented to prevent additional harm. Patient and family education and listening to the patient's concerns can prevent error. Complete and accurate documentation to communicate the patient's event is essential.

Critical Thinking 3.3

1. Identify nursing behaviors that may be defined as disruptive, including nurse to nurse, nurse to patient, nurse to physician, physician to nurse, nurse to other health care team members.

Any behavior that does not promote teamwork can be considered disruptive. Intimidating behavior toward another nurse, a patient or any team member, such as pharmacist, respiratory therapist, or any support staff is considered disruptive. Passive aggressive behavior, such as not answering a question, condescending answers to questions; and nonverbal communication, such as eye-rolling, finger pointing, and so on can be considered disruptive. Verbal outbursts or aggressive behavior are disruptive. Knowingly withholding pertinent information from the patient or another member of the health care team can be considered disruptive and can cause medical error. Patients should be invited and encouraged to speak up regarding their care and if they have any care concerns.

2. Identify recommended strategies to address disruptive behaviors.

Recommended strategies to address disruptive behavior are to ensure policy exists that defines behavior expectations and holds all team members accountable to follow policy. All team members need to be educated on behavior expectations and the behaviors that will not be tolerated. There must be enforcement of zero tolerance for intimidating and disruptive behaviors. Organizations must have a reporting method along with a safety net for reporting. Leaders and patient advocates round and observe team behaviors. There must be conducting of nonthreatening interventions that creates individual awareness of the behavior that has occurred.

3. What is nursing's role in creating an intimidation-free work environment?

Nursing has a specific role in creating a functional high-reliability environment. Nurses have to treat other nurses with respect and encourage open dialogue of behavior expectations. Nurses need to be free to speak up and report when they witness disruptive and intimidating behavior among nurses as well as among other team members.

CASE STUDY ANSWERS

Case Study 3.1

1. How would the nurse demonstrate her mindfulness in the preoccupation with failure, sensitivity to operations, and deference to expertise?

   The nurse would demonstrate her mindfulness by gathering all the required supplies to have them readily available. She would double check the order and make sure she identified the criteria of why a catheter was needed. She would use the two-patient identifiers to ensure that the right patient is identified.

   She would set up her field to work and keep her catheter uncontaminated. She would assess the situation and determine if assistance was required to safely complete the intervention. The environment check would indicate if she has adequate lighting to complete the insertion. The nursing assistant may be needed to assist and should feel free to speak up if an issue is identified.

2. How would you engage the patient to assist you in building resilience into your health care process?

   Engaging the patient is essential to have cooperation in completing the task. Patient education regarding the order and the why of the catheter can provide the opportunity to request the patient's cooperation. Patient education should include catheter care and maintenance and the monitoring of intake and output. If the patient is able, he or she can remind other health care workers of the safety measures.

3. What elements would the nurse document to demonstrate the reluctance to simplify?

   The nurse would document the time, date, size of the catheter inserted, how the patient tolerated the procedure, patient education, the color, and consistency of the urine. This is important to create the baseline and communicate it to caregivers so they are able to recognize when a change may occur, indicating a potential adverse event. To avoid a catheter-associated urinary tract infection the catheter should be used only for approved criteria and removed as soon as possible. The nurse needs to document the ongoing need for the catheter daily.

Case Study 3.2

1. How do the Magnet components support the organizational requirements for high reliability?

   The five Magnet components, transformational leadership; structural empowerment; exemplary professional practice; new knowledge, innovations and improvements; and empirical outcomes align with the three organizational requirements for high reliability. Committed leadership aligns with transformational leadership. Leadership is crucial for strategic planning and the prioritization of quality and safety goals. To be an HRO the leaders have a strong commitment to quality and safety. Structural empowerment, exemplary professional practice and new knowledge, innovations and improvements align with the safety culture of the organization. The professional nurse is engaged and vested in improving clinical practice through incorporating evidence-based practice for patient care. The nurse bases his or her patient care interventions on new knowledge, innovations, and research to improve clinical practice. Process improvements to fix broken processes lead to exemplary empirical outcomes. The quality and safety culture of the organization is recognized in the Magnet designation.

2. How do the Magnet components align with the HRO process concepts?

HRO CONCEPTS	MAGNET COMPONENTS
Preoccupation with failure	Exemplary professional practice, new knowledge, innovations
Reluctance to simplify	Exemplary professional practice, new knowledge, innovations
Sensitivity to operations	Exemplary professional practice
Resilience	Structural empowerment
Deference to expertise	Transformational leadership and structural empowerment

The nurse's active engagement in her professional practice, recognizing the complexity of care processes, and the ability to fail, using the evidence-based protocols, creating a culture of open communication and teamwork will set the baseline for an HRO. Teamwork with pharmacists, therapists, and other support staff assists in creating an environment where broken processes can safely be identified.

3. How do the Magnet components support a culture of safety?

The components support a culture of safety by demonstrating the committed leader in a transformational leadership role. Open communication regarding safety events, using evidence-based protocols, and implementation of the fair and just culture principles are part of the safety culture. Transformational leadership, structural empowerment, and exemplary professional practice provide a framework for the culture of safety to thrive.

REVIEW QUESTIONS

Please see Appendix D for answers to Review Questions.

1. Which of the following is not a key theme found in an HRO?

A. Culture of belief that all patients should receive the best possible care every time

B. Leadership commitment to quality and safety throughout an organization

C. A strategic goal to bring errors to as close to zero as possible

D. Belief that nurses are key to changing a culture of an organization

2. Which statement about an HRO is false?

A. HROs seek to standardize health care practices.

B. HROs use systems thinking to look at health care practices.

C. HROs understand that tasks are independent and often need to be isolated.

D. HROs know that when small things go wrong it is often a sign of a larger problem.

3. A nurse is asked how the culture of an organization affects quality, safety, and performance improvement. Which response best demonstrates an understanding?

A. "We have a committee on our unit that looks at patient outcomes, practice issues, and most recently, the number of falls on our unit. Our unit director lets us figure out the best way to fix the problem and suggest changes."

B. "A couple of nurses got together last night to look at the number of falls on our unit. We are concerned about the problem and think there is a better way to do it."

C. "I saw an article about falls on a unit like ours. I took the article to work to show my unit director but she said the solution isn't feasible on our unit."

D. "Our fall rates are so high that the physical therapist formed a committee to address the issue then came back to the nursing staff with some recommendations for changes in our care delivery."

4. Which of the following is an example of human factors engineering on a nursing unit? Select all that apply.

A. Color-coded scrubs based on the person's role and profession (i.e., nurses wear blue, laboratory personnel wear tan, dietary representatives wear red)

B. Placing laptop computers on movable stands with the ability to connect to the wireless network for charting

C. Placing notices about patient satisfaction surveys in the break room

D. Having a box of insulin syringes next to the medication withdrawal area

E. Enclosing the nurse's station with one entryway to eliminate walkthrough traffic

F. Highlighting lab values that are out of normal ranges in the computer system

5. An external driving force for change to a high-quality, safe, and reliable organization includes patient-centered care. An example of a patient-centered care force is:

A. Number of hospital-acquired pressure ulcers on a medical–surgical unit

B. Monitoring trends in brain natriuretic peptide (BNP) for heart failure patients

C. Relating monthly staffing levels on a given unit to the number of falls on the same unit

D. Number of respondents stating they were "very satisfied" with their care on their patient satisfaction survey

6. Which of the following points are essential to developing a culture of high reliability and safety?

A. Empower interdisciplinary committees with the autonomy to make changes to patient care practices

B. Organize a team to look at complex care processes to simplify them

C. Create a team to suggest electronic evidence databases accessible at the point of care

D. Establish a peer review process that examines disruptive behaviors by physicians

7. Which of the following is a function of the quality and patient safety department?

A. Submitting data to regulatory agencies

B. Ensuring the ethical delivery of safe patient care

C. Overseeing the Institutional Review Board

D. Ensuring the proper distribution of resources

8. Establishing a fair and just culture requires that the organization commits to a nonpunitive reporting of errors. Which of the following best represents this philosophy?

   A. Medication errors are reported through a "hot line" that asks what happened and who was involved. A report is sent to the unit director.
   B. All medication errors are reported through a computer system. A quality department representative gets a report about the event without names.
   C. Reporting medication errors includes notifying the unit director of the incident and the persons involved.
   D. When a medication error occurs, a form is completed and cosigned by the charge nurse then forwarded to the risk management department.

9. What are the four key measurement criteria to drive quality improvement as outlined by The Joint Commission? Select all that apply.

   A. Measurements must be tested for applicability to the health care process.
   B. Research evidence must support the intervention and improved patient outcomes.
   C. Measurements must accurately demonstrate that interventions were provided.
   D. Research evidence must be evaluated against a standard.
   E. Measurements must address a process that is in close proximity to the outcome.
   F. Measures must not have an unintended consequence.

10. Which of the following hospital scenarios best demonstrates principles of an HRO?

    A. All employees feel comfortable reporting errors and near misses to their unit director.
    B. Nurses are counseled when a near-miss or adverse event occurs by their department manager.
    C. Employees are required to complete a form when a near-miss or adverse event occurs. Follow-up is done by the patient safety officer and reported to the director of the area.
    D. Process improvements are interprofessional and meetings are well attended.

REVIEW ACTIVITIES

Please see Appendix E for answers to Review Activities.

1. During one of your clinical experience, ask the nurses if they have ever reported an error. Ask them to describe the processes in place for reporting errors. Based on what you have learned, is the reporting method blame free? What happens when an error is reported? Compare your responses with those of a classmate.
2. Use Table 3.1, which describes the five process concepts of an HRO to deliver high-quality, safe care, to complete the following activity. Evaluate a hospital's ability to meet each of the five process concepts by interviewing a variety of employees such as nurses, pharmacist or pharmacy tech, physical therapists, laboratory technician, certified nursing assistant or other direct care provider, or support personnel. What examples are given to demonstrate that the five concepts are present or absent in the hospital? Compare your responses with those of your classmates.

3. Review Table 3.1. How does being preoccupied with failure reduce the risk of harm? What steps can be taken to maximize patient safety? Why is it important for all health care providers to feel safe in their work environment? Why is important for all health care providers to contribute to decision making?

4. Review the external forces that currently influence the need for change in quality and safety. How does transparency influence quality and safety? How does coordination across multiple care settings influence improved patient care? What key criteria did The Joint Commission identify in establishing accountability measures?

EXPLORING THE WEB

1. Go to the website www.ahrq.gov. Click on the Quality and Patient Safety link on the left side of the page. Select Patient Safety and Medication Errors from the list of links. Select Surveys on Patient Safety Culture to view the Culture of Safety Survey tools.

2. See the National Quality Forum website, www.qualityforum.org (June 18, 2013), to view the current list of approved measurement standards and the list of 28 adverse events that should never happen in a health care setting.

3. See The Joint Commission website, www.jointcommission.org (June 18, 2013), for further reading on quality and safety measurement in highly reliable organizations.

REFERENCES

American College of Physicians. (2010). *Health care transparency—Focus on price and clinical performance information.* American College of Physicians Policy Paper. Retrieved from http://www.acponline.org/advocacy/where_we_stand/policy/transparency.pdf

American Hospital Association. (2009). *Hospitals in pursuit of excellence: A guide to superior performance improvement.* Retrieved from www.ahaqualitycenter.org

American Nurses's Credentialing Center (ANCC). (2008). *Magnet recognition program manual; recognizing nursing excellence.* Silver Springs, MD: American Nurses Association.

Centers for Medicare and Medicaid Services (CMS). (2011). *Roadmap for quality measurement in thetraditional medicare fee-for-service program.* Retrieved from https://www.cms.gov/qualityinitiativesgeninfo/downloads/QualityMeasurementRoadmap_OEA1–16_508.pdf

Chassin, M. R. (2011). *Dr. Chassin's keynote at the 4th international high reliability organizing conference.* Video presentation May 11, 2011. Retrieved from www.jointcommission.org

Chassin, M. R., Loeb, J. M., Schmaltz, S. P., & Wachter, R. M. (2010). Accountability measures: Usingmeasurement to promote quality improvement. *New England Journal of Medicine, 363,* 683–688.

Classen, D. C., Lloyd, R. C., Provost, L., Griffin, F. A., & Resar, R. (2008). Development and evaluationof the Institute for Healthcare Improvement Global Trigger Tool. *Journal of Patient Safety, 4*(3), 169–177.

Gosbee, J. W., & Gosbee, L. L. (2010). *Using human factors engineering to improve patient safety: Problem solving on the front line* (2nd ed.). Oakbrook Terrace, IL: Joint Commission Resources.

Griffin, F. A., & Resar, R. K. (2009). *IHI Global Trigger Tool for measuring adverse events* (2nd ed., IHI Innovation Series white paper). Retrieved from www.IHI.org

Hines, S., Luna, K., Lofthus, J., Marquardt, M., & Stelmokas, D. (2008). *Becoming a high reliability organization: Operational advice for hospital leaders.* (Prepared by the Lewin Group under Contract No. 290–04–0011.) AHRQ Publication No. 08–0022. Rockville, MD: Agency for Healthcare Research and Quality.

Hughes, R. G. (2008). Nurses at the "sharp end" of patient care. In R. Hughes (ed.), *Patient safety and quality: An evidence-based handbook for nurses* (pp. 7–36). AHRQ Publication No. 08–0043. Rockville, MD: Agency for Healthcare Research and Quality. Retrieved June 18, 2013 from http://www.ahrq.gov/qual/nurseshdbk

Reason, J. (1997). *Managing the risks of organizational accidents*. London, England: Ashgate.

The Joint Commission. (2008). *Sentinel event alert: Behaviors that undermine a culture of safety*. Retrieved from http://www.jointcommission.org/assets/1/18/SEA_40.PDF

The Joint Commission. (2012). *Joint Commission hospital accreditation standards*. Oak Brook, IL: Joint Commission Resources.

Weick, K. E., & Sutcliffe, K. M. (2007). *Managing the unexpected: Resilient performance in an age of uncertainty* (2nd ed.). San Francisco, CA: Jossey-Bass.

SUGGESTED READING

Conner, M., Duncombe, D., Barclay, E., Bartel, S., Borden, C., Gross, E.,...Ponte, P. R. (2007). Creating a fair and just culture: One institution's path toward organizational change. *The Joint Commission Journal on Quality and Patient Safety, 33*(10), 617–624.

Dekker, S. (2011). *Patient safety: A human factors approach*. Boca Raton, FL: CRC Press Taylor and Francis Group.

Graban, M. (2008). *Lean hospitals: Improving quality, patient safety and employee satisfaction*. Boca Raton, FL: CRC Press Taylor and Francis Group.

Henriksen, K., Dayton E., Keyes, M. A., Carayon, P., & Hughes, R. G. (2008). Understanding adverse events: A human factors framework. In R. Hughes (Ed.), *Patient safety and quality: An evidence-based handbook for nurses* (pp. 67–85). AHRQ Publication No. 08–0043. Rockville, MD: Agency for Healthcare Research and Quality. Retrieved from http://www.ahrq.gov/qual/nurseshdbk

Marx, D. (2009). *Whack a mole; the price we pay for expecting perfection*. Plano, TX: By Your Side Studios.

Pepe, J., & Cataldo P. J. (2011). *Manage risk: Build a just culture*. Retrieved from http://www.just-culture.org/downloads/manage-risk.pdf

Spath, P. L. (2011). *Error reduction in healthcare: A systems approach to improving patient safety* (2nd ed.). San Francisco, CA: Jossey-Bass.

Stolzer, A. J., Halford, C. D., & Goglia, J. J. (2011). *Implementing safety management systems in aviation*. Burlington, VT: Ashgate Publishing.

Wakefield, M. K. (2008). The quality chasm series: Implications for nursing. In R. Hughes (Ed.), *Patient. safety and quality: An evidence-based handbook for nurses*. Chapter 4. AHRQ Publication No. 08–0043. Rockville, MD: Agency for Healthcare Research and Quality. Retrieved June 18, 2013 from http://www.ahrq.gov/qual/nurseshdbk

4

PATIENT SAFETY

Christine Rovinski-Wagner and Peter D. Mills

Understanding safety requires the ability to understand that every patient care event has the ability to go wrong and result in harm to patients and staff. The greatest opportunity for nurses to prevent inadvertent harm lies in their ability to effectively uncover and report potentially unsafe patient care situations. A strong sense of professional integrity will provide you with the conviction to remain vigilant and the courage to report unsafe situations before harm occurs. (M. C. Labson, personal communication, January 8, 2012)

Upon completion of this chapter, the reader should be able to

1. Define safety
2. Discuss quality structures, processes, and the monitoring of outcomes related to a safe health care environment
3. Describe the components necessary to create a culture of safety in a health care environment, that is, leadership, measurement, risk identification and reduction, and teamwork
4. Describe how utilization management (UM) supports a culture of safety
5. Discuss the overuse, underuse, and misuse of health care services
6. Describe the difference between a personal approach and a system approach to patient care safety
7. Discuss strategies that reduce variation in health care delivery and standardize the provision of safe patient care
8. Identify characteristics of organizations that sustain and spread health care safety
9. Discuss safety initiatives in health care, that is, workforce bullying, health care rankings, safe staffing, medication safety, hand hygiene, safe patient handling and mobility (SPHM), suicide prevention, environmental safety, safe patient handoffs, and rapid response teams (RRT)
10. Discuss safety for health care staff

*M*r. Williams is an 82-year-old man with resolving pneumonia. He lives alone and has a residual right-sided weakness from an old cerebral vascular accident. During the 2 days that Mr. Williams has been under your care, you have observed him borrowing salt from his roommate's tray, forgetting to use his walker, and insisting on reusing other patient's cloth handkerchiefs because he states that it is better for the environment. The physical therapy and social work consults have not been completed.

- What actions could you take as an individual person to support Mr. Williams's safety?
- What actions could you take within your health care system to support Mr. Williams's safety?

*S*afety is the process of minimizing risk of harm to patients and providers through both system effectiveness and individual performance (QSEN Institute, 2012). Safety does not occur naturally or without effort. When a nurse accepts a patient care assignment, the nurse will use a health care system's structures and processes to ensure safe, high-quality patient outcomes (Table 4.1). Safe health care environments use all of their system's resources as well as personal individual resources to create, nurture, and sustain safety. A safe health care system allows quality problems to be identified and fixed before patient and/or staff is harmed.

"Maintaining safety reflects a level of compassion and vigilance for patient welfare that is as important as any other aspect of competent health care" (Stone, Hughes, & Dailey, 2008). Safety has major financial consequences for patients, providers, insurers, family, and/or caregivers. Using Agency for Healthcare Research and Quality (AHRQ) patient safety indicators, researchers estimated the excess length of stay for postoperative sepsis to be approximately 11 days at a cost of almost $60,000 per patient (Zhan & Miller, 2003). The length of hospital stay is also associated with an increase in risk of harm to patients (Wilson et al., 2012). Postoperative sepsis and other hospital-acquired infections such as postoperative sepsis are a major contributor to patient morbidity and mortality (Yaneva-Deliverska, 2011). The way to improve safety is to learn about causes of error and use this knowledge to design safe systems of care to "make errors less common and less harmful when they do occur" (Institute of Medicine [IOM], 2001).

In this chapter, we define and discuss safety and describe four components necessary to create a culture of safety in a health care environment, that is, leadership, measurement, risk identification and reduction, and teamwork. The role of UM in patient safety and the overuse, underuse, and misuse of health care services are discussed. The difference between a person approach and a system approach to the process of eliminating harm to patients will be reviewed. We introduce strategies that reduce variation in health care delivery and standardize the provision of safe patient care. Organizations that sustain and spread health care safety will be identified. We discuss safety initiatives in health care, that is, workforce bullying, health care rankings, safe staffing, medication safety, hand hygiene, SPHM, suicide prevention, environmental safety, safe patient handoffs, and RRT. Finally, we discuss safety for health care staff.

COMPONENTS NEEDED FOR SAFETY

Safety flourishes best when it is part of an organization's culture of safety. The term *culture* broadly relates to the norms, values, beliefs, and assumptions shared by members

TABLE 4.1 NURSING IN A SAFE, HIGH-QUALITY HEALTH CARE ENVIRONMENT

ELEMENT	ELEMENT EXAMPLES	USE OF ELEMENTS
Structure—The setting where health care occurs. Includes physical facility structures, ventilation, equipment, human resources, staffing, etc.	• Patient care environment (clean air, safe environment) • Staffing guidelines • Access to supervisor support • High-reliability quality environment • Just culture • Assignment sheets	• The nurse assesses the patient environment, staffing, and access to interprofessional team and supervisor to assure patient safety and quality care before beginning patient care. • The nurse and interprofessional team structure the health care environment and develop standards to deliver quality patient care with a high degree of reliability. • When errors in patient care occur, the interprofessional team reports them and reviews them in a just, fair-minded spirit that realizes that errors are often system problems, not just individual problems. Errors often call for review of the entire system that led to the error not just review of the individual involved. • The nurse utilizes assignment sheets to communicate elements of patient care to the interprofessional team.
Process—All actions in health care delivery. Includes the process of diagnosis, treatment, the technical way care is delivered and the interpersonal way care is delivered.	• Delegation policies and procedures • Evidence-based patient care standards, guidelines, bundles, etc. • Priority setting	• Delegation policies reflect The Five Rights of Delegation of the National Council of State Boards of Nursing (National Council of State Boards of Nursing, Inc., 1997). The Five Rights of Delegation specify leadership and supervisor involvement, chain of command, and the actions to take when delegating care. They also specify follow-up and remediation when indicated. • The nurse and interprofessional team follow policy and procedure and evidence-based patient care standards, guidelines, bundles, and so on, when giving patient care. • The nurse and interprofessional team set priorities when delivering patient care processes to ensure patient safety.
Outcomes—The effects of health care on patients. Includes changes in knowledge, behavior, health status, and patient satisfaction.	• Patient-centered care • Patient satisfaction • Patient safety • Quality of patient care • Staff safety	• The nurse and interprofessional team monitor the following outcomes on an ongoing basis: patient clinical outcomes, patient satisfaction, patient safety, staff safety, staff satisfaction, staff adherence to policy and procedure and evidence-based standards, and key health care structures and processes.

Created with information from the Agency for Healthcare Research and Quality Patient Safety Network (2013) and Kelly (2013).

of an organization or a distinctive subculture within an organization (Martin, 2002; Schein, 1985).

The term **culture of safety** refers to the extent to which individuals and groups will

- Commit to personal responsibility for safety
- Act to preserve, enhance, and communicate safety concerns
- Strive to actively learn, adapt, and modify both individual and organizational behavior based on lessons learned from mistakes
- Strive to be honored in association with these values (von Thaden & Gibbons, 2008).

For example, a nurse comes on duty and is assigned four empty patient rooms to monitor. The nurse checks supplies, suction equipment, and patient monitors. The nurse clarifies responsibilities with the physician, other nurses, and nursing assistive personnel. The nurse verifies that the emergency cart has been stocked according to the emergency cart checklist. Then the nurse is ready for patient arrival, having ensured that the structures and processes are in place to ensure the outcomes of patient safety and quality patient care.

In a culture of safety, a personal responsibility for safety means that individuals, groups, and organizations are attentive to situations that may cause harm to a patient or other person. Safety concerns are preserved, enhanced, and communicated. Potentially harmful situations are followed up with thoughtful action and good communication. Individual persons and organizations strive to actively learn, adapt, and modify their behavior within the organization's work structure to address issues that threaten patient and staff safety and learn new behaviors based on lessons learned from mistakes. Participation in educational offerings and committee activities about safety and the tools and strategies that reduce the risk of harm to patients and staff is part of the individual's responsibility in a culture of safety. So, too, is role-model behaviors that support safety values and recognizing and honoring when others do the same. A culture of safety in a health care organization allows for the greatest reduction in accidental harm to patients. A culture of safety allows for health care delivery that is replicable and reliable regardless of the day of the week, area of patient care, patient transfers, or patient background. A culture of safety has at least four components: leadership, measurement, risk identification and reduction, and teamwork.

Leadership

Leadership creates a culture of safety in which employees are empowered to report safety hazards. In a culture of safety, employees feel confident that there will be no negative consequences to communicating perceived safety problems up and down the power hierarchy. Leaders are personally involved in seeking and understanding the gaps in patient safety, making safety a priority, and providing the resources needed to close any performance gaps in providing safe, high-quality care. In a culture of safety, successful hospital boards and leaders use specific measures of safe performance to drive quality improvement (QI), they hold managers accountable for high levels of quality and safety, they learn from best practices in the health care field, and they implement new knowledge within their organizations.

Measurement

The second component of a culture of safety is measurement. Measurement provides information and feedback to leadership and clinicians about a culture of safety and its clinical outcomes. Clinical outcomes associated with patient safety such as patient falls and risk-adjusted mortality and morbidity are tracked, measured, and analyzed. In-hospital mortality in healthy patients who were not expected to die based on the condition of the patient upon admission is reviewed. Measurement and analysis of how and what clinicians feel about their work environment is also reviewed and can predict whether nurse and patient safety outcomes will be positive or negative. A more positive culture of safety has been associated with fewer adverse events (Mardon, Khanna, Sorra, Dyer, & Famolaro, 2010).

Risk Identification and Reduction

Risk identification and reduction, the third component of a culture of safety, studies human error and reduces factors that contribute to human error. Risks are identified both prospectively (looking forward) and retrospectively (looking backward). The study of any human error associated with these risks analyzes the different factors contributing to the ways that humans make mistakes. Human factors engineering uses what we know about the way humans think, how humans' minds and bodies work, and how humans interact with the environment to make products and processes that are safer to use. Unconscious human safety errors, for example, forgetting to give a medication to a patient or picking up the wrong medication syringe, derive from a breakdown in an automatic human behavior or a temporary lapse in memory. These unconscious human errors can be influenced by both environmental external factors such as distractions, noise, time pressure; and internal factors such as fatigue, expectations about the future, and anxiety. Conscious human safety errors involve a breakdown in a human's decision-making process, for example, a work-around. **Work-arounds** occur when one does not follow the rules and/or works around the rules or correct actions of a patient care process or a work process in order to save time (Table 4.2).

Human beings are prone to making safety errors because we have a limited capacity in our short-term memory. Safety improves when we use strategies to reduce reliance on memory. For example, a patient with congestive heart failure (CHF) will be at risk if intake and output amounts are not documented at the time they are measured. It is unlikely that the intake and output amounts can be accurately remembered at the end of a busy shift because human beings have a limited capacity to recall facts. In addition, humans are susceptible to a bias in thinking, which can distort our perceptions. For example, if you have been using a specific type of infusion pump on one unit and then you float to another unit, you may assume that the new unit has the same infusion pump. You can use your bias in thinking and make a programming error on the new infusion pump and give the wrong dose of medication if you don't check directions for the new infusion pump. It is probably impossible to eliminate all human errors in health care. However, it is possible and very important to work to design a

TABLE 4.2 WORK-AROUND EXAMPLES

CORRECT ACTION	WORK-AROUND
Follow-up on an alert from an electronic medication administration system about a potentially dangerous drug interaction.	Override an alert from an electronic medication administration record about a potentially dangerous drug interaction.
Read the label of a medication pulled from the drawer in an electronic medication administration system to ensure the "right medication."	Assume that the medication in the drawer is correct and not check the label of a medication pulled from the medication drawer.
Return shared blood pressure cuffs to a central access area when staff has to share the equipment.	Hide the blood pressure cuff so that it is only handy for one clinician.
Bar-code patient medications into an electronic medication administration record at the time the patient takes the medication.	Have another copy of patient wristbands in the nursing station and bar-code them all at once, then pass the medications.
Check a patient every 15 minutes as prescribed.	Record all 15-minute patient checks at the beginning of the shift.

culture of safety that can catch as many errors as possible before any potential harm caused by errors reach the patient. For example, white boards used to communicate that are placed on the unit and in patient rooms can reduce the risk of errors that occur through misinterpreted or unclear communication between nurses and physicians (Timmel et al., 2010).

Teamwork

Teamwork, the fourth component of a culture of safety, must be valued and be evident in health care. For safe care to be delivered in today's highly complex health care systems, it is critical for clinicians to collaborate in interprofessional teams of nurses, physicians, pharmacists, dieticians, and so on. It is often impossible to safely deliver care, monitor patients, document treatments, and manage changes in the health status of multiple patients while working alone. Interprofessional teams can back each other up, identify potential safety hazards, and provide patient care effectively. For good working teams to exist, there must be mutual respect, understanding of respective roles, and trust. For example, when an attending physician asks a student nurse to accompany the medical resident team on morning rounds and provide the nursing assessment about the patient, the physician is showing respect and trust for the student as part of the health care team.

Crew resource management (CRM) is a program that has taught airline pilots precise methods to speak up in a manner that is specific, direct and concise, and designed to resolve operational conflicts in real time. These same methods have been imported to health care practice. One method is called "3Ws©," that is,

- What I see
- What I'm concerned about
- What I want

For example, "What I see" is that the patient's blood pressure is 90/50. "What I'm concerned about" is that the patient is bleeding internally. "What I want" is for you to come and evaluate the patient immediately. Nurses can use the "3Ws" to avoid sub-optimal forms of team communication, and gain timely resolution to clinical concerns and conflicts (Sculli, Fore, Neily, Mills, & Sine, 2011; Sculli et al., 2013). The "3Ws" tool is an entry point for issuing an assertive and professional safety challenge.

REAL-WORLD INTERVIEW

One ineffective form of communication is called "hinting and hoping." Here, a nurse would make a subtle and oblique statement about a safety concern, for example, "I sure don't like that blood pressure." Then the nurse would hope the team decision maker understands the meaning of the hint and acts on it promptly. This communication method is rarely effective. Using the "3Ws", nurses can relay feedback that is specific, direct, and concise in real time. When the "3Ws" are used, there is little doubt on the part of the physician what the nurse's concerns are and what the nurse wants to occur to keep the patient safe.

Gary L. Sculli MSN, ATP
Director of Clinical Training Programs, Patient Safety Program Manager
VHA National Center for Patient Safety, Ann Arbor, Michigan

Critical Thinking 4.1

While doing their monthly review of outcome measurements, the nurse executive at a hospital identifies that falls and associated patient and staff injuries on a medical unit have steadily increased over the past 3 months. The nurse executive meets with the unit staff to discuss the issue. Several of the nurses suggest the implementation of a comprehensive unit-based safety program (CUSP; Agency for Healthcare and Research and Quality, 2013). The nurse executive agrees, asks what resources are needed to accomplish this, and facilitates getting the resources. The unit staff implement the interprofessional CUSP program, monitor the unit's fall rate and associated patient and staff injuries, and provide reports to the nurse executive and other hospital leadership on a regularly scheduled basis. The fall rate on the unit demonstrates a sustained decrease as well as no associated patient or staff injuries. Hospital leadership implements the CUSP program facility wide and invites the CUSP unit staff to share their knowledge and experience with the rest of the hospital.

1. What actions by the nurses demonstrated individual responsibility for supporting a culture of safety?
2. What actions by leadership empowered the staff on the medical unit?
3. What actions of the unit staff demonstrated teamwork?

EVIDENCE FROM THE LITERATURE

Citation

Neily, J., Mills, P. D., Young-Xu, Y., Carney, B. T., West, P., Berger, D. H.,…Bagian, J. P. (2010). Association between implementation of a medical team training program and surgical mortality. *Journal of the American Medical Association, 304*(15), 1693–1700.

Discussion

A training program was implemented to improve patient safety related to surgical care. Using CRM theory from the field of aviation, the surgical staff of physicians, nurses, and technicians were trained to work together as a team; challenge each other when they identified safety risks; conduct preoperative briefings and postoperative debriefings; and implement other communication strategies. At the end of 1 year, a Safety Attitudes Questionnaire, completed by the participants, showed improvement in working conditions, perceptions of management, job satisfaction, safety, and teamwork. Undesirable patient care events were avoided. Patient outcomes including morbidity and mortality were improved.

Implications for Practice

An interprofessional health care team training program that teaches staff how to effectively use the principles of teamwork and collaboration improves the culture of patient safety.

THE ROLE OF UM IN SUPPORTING A CULTURE OF SAFETY

UM, is a process of patient case management using criteria such as the McKesson InterQual® criteria to evaluate a patient's level of care from hospital admission to discharge. UM supports patient safety. Prolonged hospital stays are associated with a higher frequency of complications and increased risk of hospital acquired conditions including infections and skin breakdown. UM provides the information needed to know if, given his or her current status, the patient could receive health care services in a different level of care, such as at home (Table 4.3). UM also facilitates cooperative teamwork and communication among the patient's health care providers. The utilization manager reviews objective patient and clinical data, imaging studies, and laboratory findings. This information, along with the service intensity, or the amount and type of health care services provided to the patient, is compared to evidence-based standards for patient care.

The UM comparison helps evaluate whether the amount and type of hospital resources used are appropriate for a particular patient and don't vary from the standards. Evidence-based recommendations are made by UM to the patient's health

TABLE 4.3 UTILIZATION MANAGEMENT

DIAGNOSIS	PATIENT INFORMATION FROM MEDICAL RECORD	INTERPROFESSIONAL TEAM DISCUSSION	UTILIZATION REVIEW
Pneumonia	Day 5 of hospitalization. Chest x-ray shows left lower lobe infiltrate resolving; temperature 98.8 F. Oxygen saturation between 96% and 99%. Patient remains on oral antibiotics.	Physician: There are no medical contra-indications to discharge. Nurse: Patient no longer using prn oxygen. There have been no instances of labored respirations observed by staff or reported by patient. Physical therapist: Patient is ambulating in corridors at least 4 times/day and is using a cane appropriately. Social worker/Case manager: Home health care referral completed. Patient's wife will drive him home.	Patient no longer meets acute care InterQual Day 5 continuing stay criteria for pneumonia as temperature is below 99.4 F, oxygen saturation is above 91%, and there are no complications or active comorbidities.

Created with material from McKesson InterQual Evidence-Based Clinical Content (n.d.).

care team and the patient may be transferred to a different level of care as a result. For example, a patient with an exacerbation of chronic obstructive lung disease may be transferred from an intensive care unit (ICU) to a medical patient care unit as his breathing improves and his need for hourly respiratory therapy interventions and one-to-one nursing care decreases. A culture of patient safety, as evidenced through measurements of shorter patient lengths of stay and reduced patient readmissions to the hospital, is supported through the application of evidence-based decisions to patient care delivery. The patient receives the health care services and supplies that are no more or less than the patient needs at that particular point in time. Criteria such as the McKesson InterQual criteria are not used in isolation to measure the appropriateness of the patient's level of care. Clear and effective communication among the interprofessional health care team is also essential. For example, an interprofessional team caring for a group of surgical patients meets daily to discuss each patient's readiness for discharge or transfer. The team reviews and, as necessary, revises the care plans to support each patient's progress toward a timely and appropriate discharge. The nurse caring for the patient contributes information about the patient's pain and symptom management and learning needs.

The findings from UM reviews are tracked and measured to help leadership determine if patients are consistently admitted to the most appropriate level of care, transitioned to the most appropriate level of care, and discharged in a timely manner to help prevent patient readmission to the hospital. For example, hospital leadership at an acute care hospital approves creation of a substance abuse residential rehabilitation unit after analyzing utilization review data showing that a large number of patients admitted to the medical unit for detoxification are readmitted for another detoxification within 30 days of discharge. Further examination of the utilization review data revealed a lack of available residential substance abuse rehabilitation facilities. The utilization review data enabled leadership to improve the continuum of health care services provided to people with substance abuse problems.

REAL-WORLD INTERVIEW

UM assesses 100% of all patients admitted to Veterans Affairs (VA) Medical Centers in Illinois, Wisconsin, and Upper Michigan using McKesson's standardized, evidence-based InterQual criteria. This assures that patients are admitted to the correct level of care. Our goal is to assure that each veteran receives the right care, at the right time, and in the right setting. InterQual criteria are used in approximately 4,000 hospitals across the United States as well as in health care facilities internationally. There are different criteria for various levels of care; for example, patients cared for in an intensive care setting are evaluated against criteria specifically defined for this level of care. InterQual criteria are applied to review patients in acute as well as nonacute levels of care.

An example of using the InterQual criteria with an acutely ill, hospitalized patient with CHF here at the VA is as follows: Each patient is reviewed by UM staff on admission and every day of their hospitalization to assure that the criteria are met for the designated level of care. A patient with CHF must meet one of the admission criteria such as elevated heart rate or low oxygen saturation, along with evidence of CHF treatments and interventions. Then, to stay in the hospital, the patient must meet criteria that include clinical findings related to CHF such as continued low oxygen saturation or an exacerbation of patient comorbidities (e.g., elevated blood sugar), along with the interventions to address the clinical findings. Finally, before we discharge the patient, the patient must meet the discharge criteria; for example, oxygen saturation and vital signs stability are within normal limits for the patient.

Most hospitals and insurance companies in the United States use InterQual criteria or similar criteria to assure that patients are admitted to the appropriate level of care, that they transition to the most appropriate level of care, and that they are discharged in a timely manner following the InterQual Transition Plan Guidelines to help prevent a readmission to the hospital.

A primary function of the UM review process is to identify and address system barriers to achieving the right care, at the right time, and in the right setting. All barriers are documented and analyzed to improve the efficiency and effectiveness of the care provided to veterans. We use the VA Team-Aim-Map-Measure-Change-Sustain (VA-TAMMCS) model to achieve this. A Team of individuals who are

(continued)

involved in the improvement opportunity is formed. The team develops a specific, measurable *Aim* that focuses on decreasing or eliminating the barrier. The team develops a flow *Map* of the current process as well as a *Map* of the ideal state. The team then measures the process both before and after improvements are made to assure that *Changes* made result in improvement. Improvements are made to the process and finally, actions are taken to assure that improvements are hardwired into the work flow process to *Sustain* the gains that have been achieved.

Anna Marie Lieske, MS, RN
Veterans Integrated Service Network 12, Utilization Management Manager
Milwaukee VA Medical Center, Milwaukee, Wisconsin

OVERUSE, UNDERUSE, AND MISUSE OF HEALTH CARE SERVICES

Overuse, underuse, and misuse of health care services were identified by the Congressional Budget Office as items that undermine efficiency and patient safety (Orszag, 2008). **Overuse of health care services** occurs when a health care service is provided even though it is not justified by the patient's health care needs, for example, a surgical procedure is performed on a patient even though the procedure was not clinically appropriate. Underuse of health care services occurs when a health care service is not provided even though it would have benefited the patient, for example, a patient who has a heart attack is not prescribed a beta-blocking drug at discharge from the hospital. **Misuse of health care services** occurs when incorrect diagnoses, medical errors, and avoidable health care complications occur, for example, a patient acquires an infection during a hospitalization. Overuse, underuse, and misuse of health care services all have the potential to cause harm or an adverse event to a patient (Orszag, 2008).

CASE STUDY 4.1

A 68-year-old male patient was admitted to the hospital 7 days ago with a non-hemorrhagic cerebral vascular accident. The patient's ability to walk, transfer, and move about were minimally affected. The patient's course of treatment and care was uneventful until the patient experienced an exacerbation of his gout. Although medically stable for discharge to a skilled nursing facility for rehabilitation, the patient is refusing to get out of bed or go to physical therapy due to severe foot pain from the gout exacerbation. You are the patient's primary nurse. Your father had gout and he had given you a good idea of the pain a patient with gout feels. The UM nurse says that the patient no longer meets continued stay criteria on an acute care hospital unit and should be discharged.

1. *Which members of the interprofessional clinical team should you conference with to discuss the situation?*
2. *What actions can you take to facilitate this patient's discharge, both personally and as part of the system?*

PERSON APPROACH VERSUS A SYSTEM APPROACH TO PATIENT CARE SAFETY

When an adverse patient care event occurs, it is possible to analyze what happened in one or two ways, that is, with a person approach to safety and/or with a system approach to safety. Too often in health care, we have taken only a **person approach to safety** in which we only blame the person at the end of the long chain of errors for making an error that caused an adverse event from overuse, underuse, or misuse of health care services. A **system approach to safety** takes a broader look at an adverse event, looks at the total context in which the adverse event took place, and considers how to prevent future occurrences through improvement in the total health care system. For example, in a person approach to safety, a nurse who gave the wrong dose of a medication might be fired. In a system approach to safety, the total system of medication administration would be reviewed, for example, the materials, patient characteristics, process/methods, and people involved in medication administration would be reviewed using root cause analysis and a fishbone diagram (Figure 4.1). A system approach to safety does not just review an individual nurse's practice. It considers what elements of the total system should be modified to prevent medication administration problems is the future.

In a culture of safety, leadership fosters both a person approach and a system approach to safety. Sometimes leadership will examine trends from a large group of similar adverse events, such as falls. Data from fall events for a 3- to 6-month period are combined and reviewed. The fall events are separated into subsets of injury levels such as falls causing serious injury and falls causing less serious injury. This separation into injury subsets allows differentiation of the critical fall factors, for example, time, location, medications, environmental conditions, and so on, during the aggregate review of the falls. An aggregate review is a multistep review process in which critical factors from a group of similar adverse events, for example, falls occurring

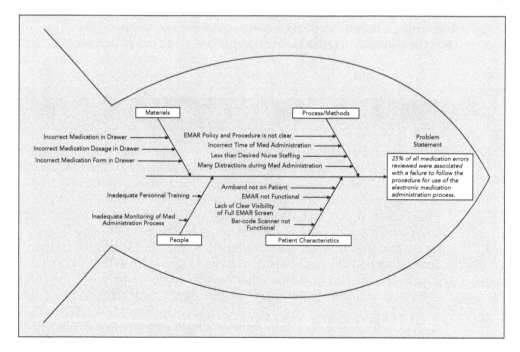

FIGURE 4.1 Use of a fishbone diagram to review materials, process/methods, people, and patient characteristics to improve quality in a health care system.

EMAR, electronic medication administration record.

Constructed by author.

in a specific time period are analyzed together. Based on this aggregate review, common root causes of the falls are identified and actions are developed to reduce their occurrence. The advantage of this aggregate review of falls is that the actions taken to improve care are based on data from multiple adverse events and so are more likely to address problems common to many of them

TERCAP (Taxonomy of Error, Root Cause Analysis, and Practice Responsibility)

TERCAP is an initiative of the National Council of State Boards of Nursing (NCSBN, 2013). TERCAP is a national nursing adverse event database designed to collect the practice breakdown data from state boards of nursing to identify the root causes of nursing practice breakdown from individual person and system causes. In using TERCAP categories to identify and analyze the root cause of a problem, a nurse could construct a fishbone diagram (Figure 4.2) that includes nurse characteristics, patient characteristics, system factors, practice breakdown, or other optional questions (NCSBN, 2013).

Practice breakdown categories may include safe medication administration, documentation, attentiveness/surveillance, clinical reasoning, prevention, intervention, interpretation of authorized provider's orders, and professional responsibility/patient advocacy. System factors may include communication, leadership/management, backup and support, environment, other health team members, staffing issues, and the health care team.

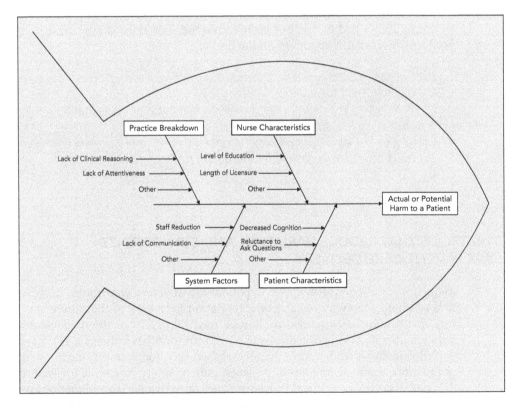

FIGURE 4.2 Fishbone diagram using TERCAP.

TERCAP, taxonomy of error, root cause analysis, and practice responsibility.
Categories developed with information from NCSBN (2013).

REAL-WORLD INTERVIEW

I wish I knew in my early years as a physician the role of systems failure in patient safety. I think it would have been helpful to know that most serious harm is caused by systems failures, not incompetent people.

Bradley V. Watts, MD, MPH
Director, VA Interprofessional Fellowship in Patient Safety
White River Junction, Vermont
Associate Residency Training Director for Psychiatry
Dartmouth Medical School, Hanover, New Hampshire

CASE STUDY 4.2

An 81-year-old male was admitted to the hospital for an acute exacerbation of his chronic obstructive pulmonary disease. He also has high blood pressure and is on several medications to control it. He uses a walker to ambulate and becomes confused at night, especially in unfamiliar environments. On his first night of admission, he got up to use the bathroom in his room, began urinating on the way to the bathroom, slipped on his urine, fell, and fractured his right hip. He had a call light and bed alarm, but by the time the staff arrived after hearing the bed alarm, he was already down on the floor.

1. *What could the staff have done differently that may have prevented this harm to the patient?*
2. *What role could communication have played in this scenario?*
3. *Are there any individual and/or system actions that would guarantee a safe patient outcome?*
4. *Use Table 4.1 and identify a few structures, processes, and outcomes that should be set up and periodically reviewed for this type of patient.*

STRATEGIES THAT REDUCE VARIATION AND STANDARDIZE SAFE PATIENT CARE DELIVERY

Reducing variation or differences in patient care delivery contributes to creating a culture of safety. One way to categorize variation is to look at the differences in health care that cannot be explained by illness, medical needs, or the dictates of evidence-based medicine. This is called unwarranted variation (Wennberg, 2011). Unwarranted variation includes underuse of evidence-based care, for example, inconsistent offering of pneumococcal vaccination to patients; patient safety concerns, for example, when different aspects of a surgical procedure vary and correlate to a higher or lower occurrence of death; preference-sensitive treatments, for example, using shared decision making with patients versus using just the physician's personal preference for selection of a treatment; and supply and utilization concerns, for example, providing a specialty health care service just because it is easily available (McCue, 2003).

When patterns of patient care delivery vary widely, safety is compromised and patient clinical outcomes suffer. UM, discussed earlier, is one process in a culture of safety that reduces variation in health care delivery. Two other effective ways to reduce variation in patient care delivery are simplification of work processes and standardization of simplified work processes. **Simplification of work processes** is the act of reducing a work process to its basic components and, in so doing, making it easier to complete the work and to understand it. Simplification of work processes requires that only the essential elements of a work process are retained. For example, when you take a patient's vital signs, you take their temperature and monitor their pulse and respirations. You then check the patient's blood pressure reading and ask him to identify his level of pain on a scale of 1 to 10. Collecting this vital sign data in this format simplifies the work process, decreases the likelihood for variation in the data set of "vital signs," and improves the understanding of vital signs among health team members.

Standardization of simplified work processes in an organization facilitates safety, QI, and accurate communication by using a single set of terms, definitions, and/or practices, for example, bundles, routines, checklists, pathways, protocols, and guidelines to reduce variation in patient care delivery (Table 4.4). Standardization of simplified work processes is associated with improved quality and reduced hospital complications (Stermer, 2011).

ORGANIZATIONS THAT SUSTAIN AND SPREAD HEALTH CARE SAFETY

There are many organizations that sustain and spread health care safety outcomes by reducing variation in health care practices (Table 4.5). They collect, analyze, disseminate, and share evidence-based best practices. These organizations welcome organizational membership and participation by nurses involved in the development and use of standardized clinical practice tools and strategies.

SAFETY INITIATIVES IN HEALTH CARE

Safety initiatives are programs that use standardized clinical practice tools and strategies and focus on reducing health care errors and improving patient safety in selected areas of health care (Table 4.6).

Safety initiatives are often initiated by hospital leadership in a culture of safety. Employees are encouraged to communicate perceived safety issues up and down the power hierarchy of the hospital. Effective communication among health care professionals in the work setting is essential to patient safety.

Avoidance of Workforce Bullying

One of the most lethal deterrents to effective communication is workforce bullying. **Workforce bullying** refers to ongoing negative behaviors and negative verbal and nonverbal communications that nurses and other interprofessional team members may inflict on each other such as rolling their eyes, sighing deeply or turning away every time a team member speaks, not returning phone calls, being reluctant to answer questions, and using a condescending tone of voice. A new nurse or team member is particularly susceptible to workplace bullying. A new team member may avoid staff interactions necessary for patient care as a means of avoiding workforce bullying.

TABLE 4.4 STANDARDIZED AND SIMPLIFIED WORK PROCESSES USED IN PATIENT CARE

CLINICAL TOOL	DESCRIPTION	EXAMPLE
Bundle	A small set of uncomplicated evidence-based practices, which are interventions that have enough scientific support to be considered standards of care.	Use of a central line bundle daily to review the necessity of patients' central lines with prompt removal of unnecessary lines, for example, Implement the IHI Central Line Bundle. Available at http://www.ihi.org/knowledge/Pages/Changes
Routine	A series of actions that ordinarily is followed in a given situation.	Use of a patient identification routine to identify patients who have the same last name by using both their first and last names and ensuring that this information is shared and highlighted shift-to-shift, for example, Relay Safety Reports at Shift Change. Available at http://www.ihi.org/knowledge/Pages/Changes
Checklist	A list of reminders that help reduce health care variation by compensating for errors in human memory.	Use of a surgical safety checklist by the nurse and anesthetist to confirm the patient's name, procedure, and where the incision will be made before the skin is cut for surgery, for example, a surgical safety checklist to reduce morbidity and mortality in a global population. Available at http://www.nejm.org/doi/full/10.1056/NEJMsa0810119
Pathway	An evidence-based algorithm or map that provides recommendations for clinical management and decision-making based on the patient's status and needs.	Use of a community-acquired pneumonia pathway to give specified antibiotics for patients admitted to the hospital with community-acquired pneumonia, for example, community-acquired pneumonia pathway and order set, Society of Hospital Medicine. Available at http://www.hospitalmedicine.org/AM/Template.cfm?Section=Quality_Improvement_Tools&Template=/CM/HTMLDisplay.cfm&ContentID=4233
Protocol	Predetermined steps of care management for a single clinical condition. It can be individualized to a patient's needs.	Use of a pressure ulcer treatment and prevention protocol to identify a pressure ulcer prevention plan that includes interventions that minimize or eliminate friction and shear, minimize pressure with off-loading, manage moisture, and maintain adequate nutrition and hydration, for example, Pressure Ulcer Treatment and Prevention Protocol, Agency for Healthcare Quality Research. Available at http://www.guideline.gov/content.aspx?id=36059
Guideline	A range of interprofessional evidence-based guidelines for the diagnosis, management, or prevention of specific diseases or conditions that meet the needs of most patients in most circumstances. A guideline is individualized to the patient.	Use of a Management of Diabetes Mellitus in Primary Care guideline to individualize the frequency of self-monitored blood glucose levels based on the frequency of insulin injections, hypoglycemic reactions, level of glycemic control, and patient/provider use of the data to adjust therapy, for example, Management of Diabetes Mellitus in Primary Care, Department of Veteran Affairs. Available at http://www.healthquality.va.gov/diabetes_mellitus.asp

TABLE 4.5 ORGANIZATIONS THAT SUSTAIN AND SPREAD HEALTH CARE SAFETY

ORGANIZATION	UNIQUE FEATURE
The National Guidelines Clearinghouse, http://guideline.gov	Helps providers and patients locate, compare, and learn about current best practice guidelines.
The Registered Nurses Association of Ontario, http://www.rnao.org	Provides personal digital assistant (PDA) downloads of a wide range of nursing best practice guidelines.
Guidelines International Network (G-I-N), http://www.g-i-n.net	Provides the world's largest international guidelines library website.
The Cochrane Collaboration, http://www.cochrane.org	Uses a systematic methodology to assess health care research.
U.S. National Library of Medicine National Information Center on Health Services Research and Health Care Technology (NICHSR), http://www.nlm.nih.gov/hsrinfo/quality.html	Collects, stores, analyzes, retrieves, and shares information on health services research, clinical practice guidelines, and on health care technology, including the assessment of such technology.
Joanna Briggs Institute, http://joannabriggs.org	Applies a cyclical process to the assessment, analysis, and sharing of evidence-based nursing and health care information. Develops evidence in various formats for nursing, allied health, and health care professionals as well as support information for consumers.

Sometimes a new team member will adopt the behaviors of workforce bullying, seeing it as the "norm" or as a way to survive in the workplace. Some team members quit rather than work in an environment tolerant of workforce bullying. Patient safety is in jeopardy when workforce bullying occurs. In addition, team members regularly leave an organization when workforce bullying occurs. Staffing patterns may be impacted. Recruitment of new staff may be difficult for an organization when team members share their stories about workforce bullying experiences with the health care community. Confronting workforce bullying in an organization is difficult but necessary. The American Association of Critical-Care Nurses Healthy Work Environment Initiative, http://www.aacn.org, and the American Psychiatric Nurses Association Task Force on Workplace Violence, http://www.apna.org, provide strategies for helping nurses productively deal with workforce bullying and create a healthy and safe work environment.

Critical Thinking 4.2

Think about the past several years of your nursing education. Focus on your classroom discussions and clinical debriefing sessions.

1. Were there times when you grew tired of hearing from a particular peer?
2. How did you respond?
3. Were any of your behaviors consistent with workforce bullying?

TABLE 4.6 A SAMPLING OF HEALTH CARE SAFETY INITIATIVES

INITIATIVE	EXAMPLE	SPONSORING ORGANIZATION
Medication safety	Avoid abbreviations that are associated with frequent misinterpretation and medication errors, for example, qd, MS, PCA, and so on.	Institute for Safe Medication Practice (ISMP) Error-Prone Abbreviation List. Available at http://www.ismp.org/tools
Core measures	Provide all patients with heart failure with discharge instructions that include guidelines for medications (dose and schedule), activity, weight management, diet, symptom management, and plan for follow-up.	The Joint Commission, Heart Failure, core measures. Available at http://www.jointcommission.org
Surgical care improvement project	Use a safer method (electric clippers or hair removal cream—not a razor) to remove hair from surgical patients needing hair removal from the surgical area before surgery.	Centers for Medicare and Medicaid Services Timely and Effective Care/Surgical Care. Available at http://www.hospitalcompare.hhs.gov
Safe patient handling	Prevent falls during patient ambulation by using gait belts with handles.	Association of Safe Patient Handling Professionals Ten Strategies for Reducing Patient Handling Injuries. Available at www.asphp.org
Comprehensive unit-based safety program	Partner a senior hospital executive with a medical–surgical unit to improve communication and educate leadership.	Agency for Healthcare and Research and Quality Comprehensive Unit-Based Safety Program (CUSP). Available at http://www.ahrq.gov/professionals/quality-patient-safety/cusp/index.html
Hand-off communication project	Emphasize key information when handing off or transferring a patient to another clinician.	The Joint Commission Center for Transforming Healthcare. Available at www.centerfortransforminghealthcare.org
Alarm fatigue	Consider new alarm signal technologies, for example, wireless notification devices/pagers, split-screen monitors.	The Johns Hopkins Hospital. Available at http://www.hopkinsmedicine.org/news/using_data_to_drive_alarm_improvements.html

Comparison of Health Care Rankings

Comparison of health care rankings provides leadership with a broad picture of a hospital's culture of safety. Health care rankings are issued by diverse groups of organizations. These rankings are listed in Chapter 1. The rankings use patient outcome data to measure and compare the safety of different health care facilities and organizations, nationally and worldwide. Health care rankings provide leadership with national and international benchmark data. Leadership can use the data to focus their efforts and resources to improve safety by reducing risks to patients. For example, Hospital A shows a higher occurrence of hospital-acquired infections than other similar hospitals. Leadership conducts an in-depth analysis of their hospital-acquired infections, identifies a large turnover in staff, and implements an immediate and aggressive hospital-wide education program about how to reduce transmission of communicable diseases between patients and health care workers. Some of the health care rankings include rankings of preventable hospitalizations; rankings of the occurrence of adverse events, such as patient deaths or hospital-acquired infections; rankings of health care systems' comparison of total health expenditure to health performance; and rankings of the health care provided to patients who pose technical or high-risk challenges, for instance, due to age and physical infirmity.

Comparisons of health care outcomes take on different meanings when reviewed with regional, ethnic, and racial variations. It is important to recognize the context of the comparison information and how it applies to your particular practice setting and patient population. Learn the details that describe your patient population and your health care work setting. You will be better equipped to evaluate health care safety in a way that is meaningful to you, your nursing practice, and your patients.

Critical Thinking 4.3

Go to the Centers for Medicare and Medicaid Services (CMS) website, Hospital Compare, at http://www.hospitalcompare.hhs.gov. Enter your zip code in the designated section, select "general," and click on "find hospital." Click on the "quality of care" tab. Select two hospitals that have checkmarks in the patient safety column, and click on the "compare" button. Review the patient safety findings for each hospital. When you are done, click on the "about the data" tab and review the information there.

1. Is there a difference between the hospitals?
2. How does this information influence your perspective about either of the hospitals?

Safe Nurse Staffing

Safe nurse staffing is associated with better patient care and safety outcomes, especially outcomes related to patient mortality; failure to rescue a patient from his or her deterioration, death, or permanent disability from a complication of health care or an underlying illness; and other patient outcomes sensitive to nursing care.

TABLE 4.7 PATIENT ACUITY AND NURSE STAFFING RATIOS

UNIT TYPE	TYPE OF PATIENTS	NURSE-TO-PATIENT STAFFING RATIO
Medical–surgical care unit	Patients who require less care than that which is available in intensive care units, step-down units, or telemetry units and receive 24-hour inpatient general medical services, postsurgical services, or both general medical and postsurgical services.	1:5 or fewer
Telemetry unit	Patients who require more care than patients in medical–surgical units and have, or are suspected of having, a cardiac condition or a disease requiring the electronic monitoring, recording, retrieval, and display of cardiac electrical signals.	1:4 or fewer
ICU	Patients who require intensive care and need medical technology to aid, support, or replace a vital function of the body that has been seriously damaged and specialized equipment and/or personnel providing for invasive monitoring, telemetry, or mechanical ventilation, for the immediate amelioration or remediation of severe pathology.	1:2 or fewer

Compiled from California Code of Regulations (22CCR, 70053.2 and 70217) (2014).

Nurse staffing plans are guidelines that identify the number of nurses needed to provide safe and adequate care in a given health care setting. Nurse staffing plans are associated with patient acuity measurements. **Patient acuity** refers to the degree of health care service complexity needed by a patient related to their physical or mental status (Table 4.7). For example, patient acuity is higher for a patient who has a central line infusion than for a patient who is receiving oral medications, as the higher acuity patient with a central line infusion will need more nursing resources to provide safe care. Likewise, patients in an ICU have higher acuity and need more clinical attention due to the instability of their conditions than patients on a telemetry unit. Thus a patient care unit with high patient acuity such as an ICU will require more nursing staff to provide safe care. The lower acuity telemetry patient care unit requires less staffing.

The nursing hours per patient day (NHPPD) calculation, used worldwide and one of the National Database of Nursing Quality Indicators (NDNQI), computes nurse staffing, that is, registered nurse (RN) and/or licensed practical nurse (LPN) staffing. The NHPPD calculation provides a measurement to compare to the desired patient acuity guidelines in the nurse staffing plan. To calculate the NHPPD, add the total nursing hours worked by all nurses on a day and divide the total nursing hours by patients on the same day, based on the midnight census. The result is the nursing hours needed to care for each patient each day on the unit.

For example, 14 nurses worked on Friday on a same-day procedure unit. All nurses worked an 8-hour shift to staff the 35-bed unit that is open 12 hours daily. The unit cared for 40 patients on Friday. The number of NHPPD is 2.8 hours. To calculate the NHPPD, multiply the hours worked by each nurse by the number of nurses (8 multiplied by 14 equals 112 total nursing hours). Divide the total nursing hours by the number of patients cared for (112 divided by 40 equals 2.8 NHPPD). Neither the number of beds on the unit nor the 12 hours the same-day unit is open are used in the calculation.

NHPPD staffing calculation can provide retrospective information for an aggregate analysis of adverse events, for example, to determine if a relationship exists between the number of patient falls during a shift and the NHPPD. If the number of patient falls increases when nursing staffing is low, this is an unsafe situation and nurses need to take action to provide safe care for patients.

Critical Thinking 4.4

You work in a long-term care facility in a 30-bed unit. Most of the patients are elderly and ambulatory with chronic medical conditions and mild to moderate cognitive impairment. You arrive for your evening shift and learn that the other nurse scheduled has called in sick. The evening supervisor says that she is unable to find another nurse to work with you but she will send you two extra licensed nursing assistants. This gives you a total of four licensed nursing assistants and yourself for the unit's staffing. The evening supervisor adds that you should call her if you have any problems. She says she is sure you will do fine and she will see you during her regular rounds.

1. What criteria will you use to assess this situation from a safety perspective?
2. Is there enough staff to provide safe patient care?
3. If you feel this is an unsafe situation, what actions will you take as an individual nurse and/or as a nurse in a health care system?
4. Is this an environment for safety?
5. What types of structures or processes should you build into this patient care unit?
6. What outcomes should be monitored?

Having more nurses does not guarantee better outcomes (Shuldham, Parkin, Firouzi, Roughton, & Lau-Walker, 2009). More nurses with higher level of basic nursing education such as a bachelor's degree and the use of standardized evidence-based clinical pathways might lead to better patient outcomes. Researchers from the University of Pennsylvania found that surgical patients in Magnet™ hospitals had 14% lower odds of inpatient death within 30 days and 12% lower odds of failure-to-rescue compared with patients cared for in non-Magnet hospitals. The study authors conclude that these better outcomes were attributed in large part to investments in highly qualified and educated nurses, including a higher proportion of baccalaureate prepared nurses (McHugh et al., 2013). Leadership commitment to safe nurse staffing levels and effective nurse retention strategies such as zero tolerance for workforce bullying may also influence the achievement of better and safer patient outcomes due to the stability of clinical staff (Aiken, Clarke, Sloane, Lake, & Cheney, 2008).

REAL-WORLD INTERVIEW

I would like to see more nurses being aware of "accidents waiting to happen." For example, if there is an uneven surface in the floor, nurses can report that problem, so a patient doesn't trip and fall. The nurse should speak up. The nurse's perspective is important. Reporting unsafe situations can help change a system and prevent future adverse events.

Julia Neily, RN, MS, MPH
Associate Director, VA National Center for Patient Safety, Field Office
White River Junction, Vermont

Medication Safety

Improved medication safety outcomes are seen in health care facilities that implement prospective and retrospective risk identification and reduction activities, such as working with the Institute for Safe Medication Practice (ISMP), to prevent harm to patient or staff. The ISMP, www.ismp.org, is an independent patient safety organization devoted entirely to medication error prevention and safe medication use. The ISMP sponsors a confidential, voluntary medication error reporting program and data bank on the same website, which allows expert analysis of system causes of medication errors. This facilitates identification and sharing of the best evidence-based practices (EBPs) to improve medication safety. For example, an accidental programming by a pediatric nurse of an infusion pump for 10 times the dose ordered was reported to the ISMP data bank. The ISMP issued evidence-based recommendations on their website for improving patient safety during pediatric administration of IV acetaminophen, including using "smart" IV infusion pump technology when giving maximum dosages of medications and requiring pharmacy preparation of medication doses that are different from the usual strength available commercially.

Hand Hygiene

Another risk reduction strategy in a culture of safety is a focus on hand hygiene. Hand hygiene is the single most effective way to prevent the spread of health care associated infections. Hand hygiene is well-suited for prospective and retrospective risk identification and risk reduction through direct observation. The Centers for Disease Control (CDC) and the World Health Organization (WHO) have issued guidelines for hand hygiene that include having the patient remind providers to wash their hands. Research reveals the compliance of health care workers with hand hygiene protocols is low (McGuckin, Govednik, & Waterman, 2010). Nurses may sometimes think that certain types of physical contact with patients are less likely to require hand washing, such as checking blood pressure or straightening bed linens. Staff are often reluctant to correct or remind coworkers to wash their hands. When done with tact and a professional demeanor, communication from one health care clinician to another about hand hygiene is not only appropriate but can also be effective in improving hand hygiene compliance (Pittet, Allegranzi, & Boyce, 2009). One commercial system, the HyGreen Hand Hygiene Recording and Reminding System, available at http://www.hygreeninc.com, electronically records all hand hygiene events in a hospital and reminds all health care workers to wash their hands between patients. HyGreen gives hospitals a tool to effectively monitor adherence to hand hygiene protocols. For example, a hand hygiene report can be generated showing daily compliance percentages by staff —with specific identification of staff. This facilitates individualized education of health care workers about hand hygiene and how it contributes to a culture of safety. The hand wash system should not be used to penalize persons. Instead, the system should be used to help staff understand that their actions will either support or diminish a safe health care environment.

SPHM

The American Nurses Association (ANA) Safe Patient Handling and Mobility (SPHM) Working Group has added the words "and mobility" to the more common term of "safe patient handling," to include the emerging evidence-based concept of progressive mobility for the patient as an end goal, rather than simply the "handling" of patients (ANA, 2013). SPHM initiatives include evidence-based recommendations (ANA, 2013) for improving patient and staff safety associated with physical movement. Appropriate safe patient handling equipment, ergonomic training and patient assessment protocols, encouragement of staff participation, and leadership support to obtain necessary resources such as ceiling mounted patient lifts, have been identified as being effective in reducing harm to patients and staff (Veterans Health Administration, 2011).

Suicide Prevention

Suicide prevention involves prospective and retrospective risk identification and risk reduction for individual patients and high-risk populations such as patients on inpatient mental health units. It is likely that nurses in all areas of the hospital will encounter suicidal patients and need to understand how to care for them and how to avoid an inpatient suicide (The Joint Commission, 2010). Of the reported suicides reported to The Joint Commission between 1995 and 2010, 14% occurred in the nonbehavioral health units of general hospitals such as medical or surgical units, the ICU, and oncology and 8% occurred in the emergency department (ED) of general hospitals (The Joint Commission, 2010).

The primary patient risk factors for suicide include previous suicide attempts and suicidal thoughts; a mental health diagnosis; physical health problems, especially problems with a poor prognosis; and social stressors, such as relationship, financial, or legal problems. In addition, patients who are agitated, overwhelmed, and desperate or hopeless about the future are at higher risk for suicide (Tischler & Reiss, 2009).

When working with a patient whom you think is suicidal, ask if the patient is thinking about hurting himself or herself or committing suicide. If the patient's answer is yes, notify the patient's provider or the psychiatry department per your facility's protocol so that a more thorough patient evaluation can be done. In the meantime, ensure that the patient does not have access to sharps, ropes, medications, or other means of self-harm and that the patient is under continuous observation until he or she can be moved to a safer environment. Suicide prevention includes removing clothes hooks and unnecessary doors from a psychiatric unit since these could be used for a suicide by hanging. Most often, suicidal patients are only feeling suicidal for a short period of time. It may be a moment of desperation when they are feeling hopeless about the future or devastated by recent losses or overwhelming social stressors. The job for clinicians is to get these patients through this time without allowing the patients to hurt or kill themselves.

CASE STUDY 4.3

A 25-year-old female patient was admitted to the hospital after cutting her wrists with a steak knife in her home. The lacerations were severe and required sutures. She also sustained a mild head injury after passing out and falling due to blood loss. Because of her health care problems, she was admitted to the medical floor for observation directly from the ED. The first night of her admission, she was found in the bathroom with several additional superficial lacerations. Her injuries were treated and she was placed on one-to-one observation for the rest of the night. She was transferred to the psychiatric unit in the morning.

1. *Was there any way to avoid this inpatient suicide attempt?*
2. *How could the environment have been changed by the individual nurse and by the health care system to increase this patient's safety?*

Environmental Safety

A safe health care environment minimizes potential errors and maximizes safe health care practice. Nursing care units must be accommodating to patient needs. Door alarms alert staff on a health care unit that has cognitively impaired inpatients when a patient goes through a door. Pressure-sensitive bed and chair alarms alert staff to patient movement and facilitate interventions to prevent falls when a patient doesn't call for transfer assistance. A safe health care environment controls noise and keeps distractions to a minimum so that staff can focus on patient care.

Safe Patient Handoffs

A health care process that requires teamwork and is vulnerable to human errors and adverse events is the patient handoff. A **patient handoff** is the transfer of responsibility for a patient from one clinician to another and involves sharing current information that is pertinent to the patient's care with time allowed for discussion, questions, and clarification. A patient handoff happens any time a clinician or team taking care of a patient transfers the patient to another clinician or team to continue their care or provide a different type of care. For example, a patient comes into the ED and is seen by the triage nurse. The nurse takes information and does a patient handoff of information to the ED doctor who sees the patient. If the ED doctor decides to admit the patient, another patient handoff takes place between the ED doctor and the clinicians on the patient care unit. If the patient needs surgery, there is another patient handoff to the surgery team and then a patient handoff from the surgery team back to the patient care unit. At shift change, there is a patient handoff as one nurse transfers the patient's care to another nurse. Each time the patient's care is transferred to another clinician, another opportunity for critical information to be lost or misunderstood occurs. Research in the area of patient handoffs has identified numerous barriers to effective patient handoffs, for example, breakdowns in communication, no standardized format for the handoff, limitations of equipment used, such as voice recorders, interruptions and distractions, not enough time or staff, complex patients, limits to human memory, and fatigue (Riesenbery, Leitzsch, & Cunningham, 2010).

TABLE 4.8 SBARR

What is the situation?	Mr. Jones has normal saline running at 75 mL/hour. I am going to an hour-long safety in-service program.
What is the background?	I hung the normal saline infusion bag an hour ago. Mr. Jones said that his arm was "bothering" him. I put his arm on a pillow.
What is the assessment?	The normal saline infusion is running without a problem; the insertion site in his left arm is not red, swollen, or tender. He has his call bell, is able to use it, and knows that you will be covering for me.
What is the recommendation?	Please assess Mr. Jones and the normal saline infusion site several times during the next hour.
What is the response?	I will make rounds on Mr. Jones in about 10 minutes.

Created with information from SBARR (Kaiser Permanente, 2011).

While there are not yet any high-quality research studies to support specific best practices in the area of patient handoffs, standardized checklists are effective tools to help the nurse remember what information is important to share with a another nurse (Cohen & Hilligoss, 2010; Riesenbery et al., 2010). For example, a nurse leaving the unit uses a simplified and standardized work process, such as a checklist, to share information about a patient who has parenteral fluids infusing, thus supporting safe patient care. The **Situation, Background, Assessment, Recommendation, and Response (SBARR) patient reporting tool** is an example of a simplified and standardized work process used by a clinician to ensure patient safety when handing a patient over to another clinician for continued care (Table 4.8).

RRT

RRT in a hospital are typically composed of an interprofessional team of critical care nurses, physicians, and respiratory therapists, and are called at an early stage of a patient's clinical deterioration in the hopes of preventing a cardiac arrest or an unexpected death. A RRT allows staff to obtain additional assistance when the patient's condition appears to be worsening (Chan, Jain, Nallmothu, Berg, & Sasson, 2010). Teamwork is the cornerstone to successful use of RRT, a safety mechanism to reduce harm to patients. RRTs differ from a cardiac arrest or code blue team, which is called in response to a cardiac or respiratory arrest that has already occurred. While RRTs have been widely implemented and appear to be helpful, there is controversy regarding their measurable effectiveness in reducing hospital mortality. It is hoped that RRTs prevent failure to rescue. **Failure to rescue** occurs when clinicians fail to notice patient symptoms or they fail to respond adequately or quickly enough to clinical signs that may indicate that a patient is dying of preventable complications in a hospital. Timely identification of deteriorating cardiac, neurologic, or respiratory status with prompt and appropriate subsequent action can avoid serious adverse events in patients.

SAFETY FOR HEALTH CARE STAFF

Safety is an important concern for health care staff as well as patients. Health care staffs face a number of serious safety hazards, including blood-borne pathogens and biological hazards, potential chemical and drug exposures, waste anesthetic gas exposures, respiratory hazards, ergonomic hazards from lifting and repetitive tasks, laser hazards, and workplace violence, hazards associated with laboratories, and radioactive material and x-ray hazards. Safe health care environments control the scope and variety of chemicals in the facility, including those chemicals used for cleaning and those chemicals used in treating patients with cancer. Distribution of chemicals in a safe environment is limited to areas that have a facility-approved need to use the particular hazardous chemical. For example, in a safe health care environment, only housekeeping would have access to cleansing solutions used to clean rooms where patients with *Clostridium difficile* have stayed. In a culture of safety, all employees know which chemicals are in their work areas, how to use the chemicals appropriately, and how to access the related material safety data sheets (MSDS) at their facility. MSDS can also be accessed at websites such as http://www.ehso.com/msds.php. MSDS contains information on the chemical makeup, use, storage, handling, emergency procedures, and potential health effects related to a hazardous material. This is the information that identifies how to reduce the risk of harm caused by chemicals.

In 2010, the health care and social assistance industry reported more work-related injury and illness cases than any other private industry sector—653,900 cases. That is 152,000 more cases than the next industry sector, manufacturing. In 2010, the incidence rate for work-related nonfatal injuries and illnesses in health care and social assistance was 139.9. The incidence rate for nonfatal injury and illnesses in all private industry was 107.7 (OSHA, 2013).

Nursing aides, orderlies, and attendants had the highest rates of musculoskeletal disorders of all occupations in 2010. The incidence rate of work-related musculoskeletal disorders for these occupations was 249 per 10,000 workers. This compares to the average rate for all workers in 2010 of 34 (U.S. Department of Labor, 2012). The consequences of work-related musculoskeletal injuries among nurses are substantial and primarily due to patient handling (OSHA, 2013). A safe health care environment reduces the risk of harm to patients and staff by using assistive patient handling equipment that helps lift, transfer, and reposition patients to reduce the potential for musculoskeletal injuries, doing specific patient assessments, and using algorithms to determine the safest way to lift, and move each individual patient (OSHA, 2009). Developing a culture of safety for staff as well as for patients is an important consideration in health care organizations today (Table 4.9).

TABLE 4.9 SAFETY RISK AND REDUCTION FOR HEALTH CARE STAFF

RISK CATEGORY	RISK EXAMPLE	RISK REDUCTION EXAMPLE
Biological	Infections caused by needle sticks	Assure presence of impervious containers for needles and other sharp objects
Chemical	Drugs used in the treatment of cancer	Assure availability of a Class II Type A or B biological safety cabinet for mixing chemotherapeutic drugs
Physical	Ionizing radiation	Monitor maintenance and radiation logs
Ergonomic	Patient handling	Use an electric-powered, sit-to-stand device
Psychological	Shift work	Develop permanent shift assignments

Compiled from https://osha.europa.eu/en/sector/healthcare. Developed with material from the European Agency for Safety and Health at Work (n.d.).

KEY CONCEPTS

- Quality structures, processes, and the monitoring of outcomes leads to a safe health care environment.
- A culture of safety encourages the implementation of safety initiatives by individuals and health care systems to reduce and prevent harm to patients and staff.
- A culture of safety has four necessary components: leadership, measurement, risk identification and reduction, and teamwork. A culture of safety reduces variation and standardizes the provision of safe patient care.
- UM facilitates patient safety and teamwork.
- Overuse, underuse, and misuse of health care services increases the incidence of patient harm.
- A culture of safety is strengthened by a system approach to analysis of adverse events and work processes.
- Several organizations sustain and spread health care safety.
- Multiple safety initiatives are used to improve patient care, that is, workforce bullying, health care rankings, safe staffing, medication safety, hand hygiene, safe patient handling, suicide prevention, environmental safety, safe patient handoffs, and RRT.
- Developing a culture of safety for staff as well as for patients is an important consideration in health care organizations today.

KEY TERMS

Culture of safety
Failure to rescue
Misuse of health care services
Overuse of health care services
Patient acuity
Patient handoff
Person approach to safety
Patient reporting tool
Rapid reponse team

SBARR
Safety initiatives
Simplification of work processes
Standardization of simplified work processes
System approach to safety
Underuse of health care services
Utilization management
Work-arounds
Workforce bullying

DISCUSSION OF OPENING SCENARIO

1. What actions could you take as an individual person to support Mr. Williams's safety?

Mr. Williams's readiness for discharge home is questionable. It is probably not safe for him to live alone. A completed consult by physical therapy will give the team more information about the degree of Mr. Williams's debilitation and its effect on his residual weakness. An occupational therapy consult could provide further information about the patient's ability to safely manage his activities of daily living. The therapists could recommend a more appropriate disposition for Mr. Williams, that is, a rehabilitation or nursing home facility. A completed consult by social work would also identify Mr. Williams's wishes regarding his care after discharge. The social worker's information would be tailored to the disposition plan and would support a safe discharge. If Mr. Williams is going to a rehabilitation or nursing home facility, the social worker would ensure that the appropriate information is shared with the receiving facility.

2. What actions could you take within your health care system to support Mr. Williams's safety?

You could confer with the patient's physician, the utilization review nurse and the nursing case manager about your observations. Confer with physical therapy and social work to share your observations and concerns and make a request for priority completion of their consultations. You can also review your facility's discharge planning policy and procedure and talk to your nurse manager about the discharge planning to assure safety for this patient.

CRITICAL THINKING ANSWERS

Critical Thinking 4.1

1. What actions by the nurses demonstrated individual responsibility for supporting a culture of safety?

The nurses demonstrated individual responsibility for supporting a culture of safety by suggesting a CUSP focused on falls and by monitoring the unit's fall rate and associated patient and staff injuries.

2. What actions by leadership empowered the staff on the medical unit?

The staff on the medical unit were empowered when leadership agreed with their suggestion, asked what resources the staff needed, facilitated getting those resources, and asked the staff to share their experience and knowledge with the rest of the hospital.

3. What actions of the unit staff demonstrated teamwork?

The unit staff demonstrated teamwork by implementing the interprofessional CUSP and providing regular follow-up reports to hospital leadership.

Critical Thinking 4.2

1. Were there times when you grew tired of hearing from a particular peer?

Many of us have a tendency to not look at our own behavior when responding to someone we are tired of hearing from. To be an effective member of a nursing or interprofessional team, we must be willing to examine our own behavior and see ourselves as others see us.

2. How did you respond?

When we respond, we must avoid being quick to label a peer as tiresome. Look for ways to work together. Note that this is a team responsibility.

3. Were any of your behaviors consistent with workforce bullying?

Our verbal and nonverbal behaviors will define our professional selves more than anything else we do. Accepting responsibility for a culture of safety and avoidance of workforce bullying starts within.

Critical Thinking 4.3

1. Is there a difference between the hospitals?

Hospital patient care outcomes are indicators of health care quality and safety. Outcome measures can be used to decide if you want to receive care or work at a particular health care facility.

2. How does this information influence your perspective about either of the hospitals?

There are frequently significant differences between hospitals and this information can influence yours and your patients' perspectives about the hospitals. However, this information is not something the general public generally uses in selection of a health care system. As a nurse, you have the opportunity to educate others about the health care quality resources available to them and the importance of their using these resources in making health care decisions.

Critical Thinking 4.4

1. What criteria will you use to assess this situation from a safety perspective?

When assessing this situation from a safety perspective, you might want to review criteria such as what tasks/interventions are usually done by the nurses during the evening shift, how long do those tasks/interventions take to complete, what are the priority elements of patient care needed now, what is the impact that the time required to complete tasks/interventions will have as the evening progresses, what will you do in an emergency, and so on.

2. Is there enough staff to provide safe patient care?

The regular staffing pattern of two nurses to provide safe patient care is likely based on required staffing criteria and a standardized staffing calculation based on patient acuity.

3. If you feel this is an unsafe situation, what actions will you take as an individual nurse and/or as a nurse in a health care system?

If you feel that you are in an unsafe situation, alert your supervisor. Identify priority patient needs. Provide justification for your safety concerns based on your objective assessment. Be specific in your request for help. As a follow-up action, approach your supervisor about having a team organized to create a backup safety plan in case of similar unsafe situations in the future. For example, the plan for safety should address elements of structure, process, and outcome to build an environment for safety.

4. Is this an environment for safety?

Be sure to always alert your supervisor and the chain of command when dealing with patient safety concerns. If this situation occurs more than once, hospital leadership must review and improve their environment for safety.

5. What types of structures or processes should you build into this patient care unit?

    The environment for safety could include a list of nurses who are willing and able to be called in to work on short notice (structure), a standard operating procedure for deciding the safest nurse-to-patient ratio for the unit (process), and measurement of medication errors, patient falls, and staff injuries by shift (outcome).

6. What outcomes should be monitored?

    Other outcomes to be monitored include outcomes related to patient satisfaction, clinical outcomes, patient access, and so on.

CASE STUDY ANSWERS

Case Study 4.1

1. Which members of the interprofessional clinical team should you conference with to discuss the situation?

    An interprofessional clinical team conference would ideally include the utilization review nurse, the nurse case manager, the social worker, the attending physician or other medical team members, involved family members, and the patient.

2. What actions can you take to facilitate this patient's discharge, both personally and as part of the system?

    To facilitate this patient's discharge, both personally and as part of the system, talk to the patient to elicit any concerns he might have about his pending discharge. Be sure his pain management concerns are being dealt with. Ask the physical therapist to meet with you and the patient to identify what the patient can do with your assistance and/or supervision to ensure that he doesn't regress in his physical ability. Provide positive recognition of any increased activity by the patient.

    While the attending physician will order the patient's continued stay or discharge, you have the responsibility of helping to evaluate the patient's needs and his ability to achieve a safe discharge.

Case Study 4.2

1. What could the staff have done differently that may have prevented this harm to the patient?

    The staff could have given the patient a low bed and good access to the call signal. They could have conducted regular toileting rounds to take the patient to the bathroom on a regular schedule. They could have anticipated that the patient would try to get to the bathroom on his own since he was known to be confused. It may have been that his blood pressure medication was causing orthostatic hypotension and that also contributed to his fall. This could have been assessed more carefully to ensure patient safety.

2. What role could communication have played in this scenario?

    The staff could have communicated with the patient and with each staff member to identify the patient's needs and discuss what the staff planned to do to keep the patient safe. This would have been respectful of the patient's abilities and might have encouraged the patient's engagement in safety efforts.

3. Are there any individual and/or system actions that would guarantee a safe patient outcome?

There are limited individual and/or system actions that completely guarantee patient safety especially in relation to falls. Staff evaluation and alertness along with a culture of safety can, however, minimize the chance of falling and associated injuries.

4. Use Table 4.1 and identify a few structures, processes, and outcomes that should be set up and periodically reviewed for this type of patient.

A few structures that could be set up and periodically reviewed for this type of patient include safe staffing and bed alarms. A few processes would include regular patient care rounds, assurance of side rails, toileting assistance, and so on. A few outcomes to review would be anything related to the morbidity and mortality of patients at risk for falls.

Case Study 4.3

1. Was there any way to avoid this inpatient suicide attempt?

The staff should have done a thorough nursing evaluation and also had a psychiatric evaluation of the patient completed. They should have kept the patient on one-to-one suicide observation while in the medical unit.

2. How could the environment have been changed by the individual nurse and by the health care system to increase this patient's safety?

All sharp instruments and equipment should have been removed from the patient's room and bathroom. A check for potential injury items and contraband should have been performed. A risk-reduction patient suicide safety protocol should have been initiated to increase this patient's safety.

REVIEW QUESTIONS

Please see Appendix D for answers to Review Questions.

1. You have been asked to participate on a hospital safety committee that will be conducting a review of falls. At the first meeting, a review of the data shows the majority of falls all occurred on one medical unit. In a culture of safety, the next committee action would be which of the following?

A. Reeducate all the nurses in the hospital about fall risk reduction.
B. Report the nurse whose patients had the most falls to the nursing office.
C. Review the process of care delivery on the medical unit with all the falls.
D. Interview all of the nurses whose patients fell.

2. A patient is treated in the ED after a car accident. The patient says to the nurse, "I don't think I would do it but sometimes, like now, I think about ways to kill myself." Of the following, which should be the nurse's priority safety action?

A. Contact the hospital's psychiatry service.
B. Remove the patient's access to means of self-harm.
C. Keep the patient under continuous observation.
D. Alert other staff members about the patient's statement.

3. The nurse administered the wrong dose of heparin to a patient. This is classified as which of the following?

   A. Deliberate error
   B. Close call
   C. Adverse event
   D. Biased action

4. You are assisting another nurse in providing complex wound care to an alert and attentive patient. The nurse does not wash her hands between the first change of gloves and is in the middle of giving the wound care. Which of the following would be your most appropriate safety action?

   A. Do nothing. The nurse has many years of experience and knows more than you.
   B. Inobtrusively remind the nurse that her hands need to be washed between glove changes.
   C. Do nothing. Report the event to your supervisor immediately after care completion.
   D. Offer the nurse a hand sanitizer at the next glove change in the procedure.

5. The nurse is covering for another nurse who has to attend a committee meeting. During the medication administration process, the nurse notices an alert about a potentially dangerous drug interaction for a patient who has been hospitalized and taking the medication for a week. What is the nurse's safest action?

   A. Override the alert on the electronic medication administration record.
   B. Check with the pharmacy about the alert before giving the medication.
   C. Call the physician and ask for a clarification of the medication order.
   D. Administer the medication since the patient has probably been receiving it for a week.

6. A patient with a known cardiac history tells the nurse that he feels very tired, he can feel his heart beating, and he doesn't seem to be able to concentrate. The nurse assesses his vital signs and notes that the patient's blood pressure is much higher than usual and he is beginning to complain of chest pain. Which action should the nurse take to ensure the patient's safety?

   A. Call the RRT.
   B. Ask another nurse to assess the patient.
   C. Notify the patient's physician.
   D. Continue to assess the patient.

7. The nurse is caring for a patient with orthostatic hypotension and mild dementia with some forgetfulness. Which of the following would create a safe environment for this patient? Select all that apply.

   A. Skid-resistant floor mat
   B. Dim lighting in the patient's room
   C. Ceiling-mounted transfer equipment
   D. Bed alarm
   E. Chair alarm

8. Whenever Nurse Jones speaks, some members of the team roll their eyes, cross their arms, and sigh heavily. This is an example of which of the following?

    A. Boredom
    B. Workplace bullying
    C. Fatigue
    D. Rudeness

9. The nurse is writing a care plan for a patient who has a sacral pressure ulcer and is at risk for developing several more pressure ulcers due to limited mobility. Which of the following includes standardized clinical patient care and might be most useful? Select all that apply.

    A. Routine
    B. Bundle
    C. Core measure
    D. Protocol
    E. Checklist

10. There are eight RNs working on a medical–surgical unit. All nurses work 8-hour shifts to cover the 24-hour unit. Today's patient census at midnight was 32. What is the correct calculation for the number of NHPPD?

    A. 1.6
    B. 3.8
    C. 6.0
    D. 2.0

REVIEW ACTIVITIES

Please see Appendix E for answers to Review Activities.

1. Calculate and compare the NHPPD for 1 day in 2 different weeks at your assigned clinical unit. What did you find?
2. Identify one clinical tool used at your clinical agency that reduces variation in patient care. Ask staff what might occur if the tool was not used or was not used appropriately.
3. Use the SBARR format to give a handoff report on your patients to another nurse at lunch time. Are there differences in the process between your use of the SBARR format compared to other handoffs you have done without the SBARR format?

EXPLORING THE WEB

1. Go to the site for The Joint Commission, http://www.jointcommission.org. Find the current year's patient safety goals that are applicable to your assigned health care setting. Identify differences based on setting of care.
2. Go to the National Quality Forum website, http://www.qualityforum.org. Select the measuring performance tab. Find and review the list of safe practices contributing to better health care.
3. Read about Pennsylvania's Color of Safety Task Force and risk reduction associated with the use of color-coded patient wristbands on http://www.patientsafetyauthority.org. Find the safety web links to your state.

4. Search the Cochrane Collaboration site for patient care guidelines in an area of nursing that interests you on http://www.cochrane.org.

REFERENCES

Agency for Healthcare Research and Quality (AHRQ). (2013). *How to use the CUSP toolkit.* Rockville, MD: AHRQ. Retrieved from http://www.ahrq.gov/professionals/education/curriculum-tools/cusptoolkit/toolkit/index.html

Agency for Healthcare Research and Quality Patient Safety Network. (2013). *Making Healthcare Safer II: An updated critical analysis of the evidence for patient safety practices.* Retrieved from https://www.ahrq/research/findings/evidence-based-reports/patientsafetysum/html

Aiken, L., Clarke, S. P., Sloane, D. M., Lake, E. T., & Cheney, T. (2008). Effects of hospital care environment on patient mortality and nurse outcomes. *Journal of Nursing Administration, 38*(5),223–229.

American Nurses Association (ANA). (2013). *Safe patient handling.* Retrieved from http://www.nursingworld.org/handlewithcare

California Code of Regulations. (2014). *Nurse-to-patient staffing ratio regulations.* Retrieved from http://www.cdph.ca.gov/services/DPOPP/regs/Pages/N2PRegulations.aspx

Chan, P. S., Jain, R., Nallmothu, B. K., Berg, R. A., & Sasson, C. (2010). Rapid response teams: A systematic review and meta-analysis. *Archives of Internal Medicine, 170*(1), 18–26.

Cohen, M. D., & Hilligoss, P. B. (2010). The published literature on handoffs in hospitals: deficiencies indentified in an extensive review. *Quality and Safety in Health Care, 19*(6), 493–497.

European Agency for Safety and Health at Work. (n.d.). *Health and safety of healthcare staff.* Retrieved from https://osha.europa.eu/en/sector/healthcare/index_htmlmanagedhealthcareexecutive.modernmedicine.com/managed-healthcare-executive/news/ clamping-down-variation

Institute of Medicine (IOM). (2001). *Crossing the quality chasm: A new health system for the 21st century.* Washington, DC: National Academy Press.

Kaiser Permanente. (2011). *SBAR technique for communication: A situation briefing model.* Retrieved from http://www.ihi.org/knowledge/Pages/Tools/SBARTechniqueforCommunicationASituationalBriefingModel.aspx

Kelly, P. (2013). Unpublished manuscript.

Mardon, R. E., Khanna, K., Sorra, J., Dyer, N., & Famolaro, T. (2010). Exploring relationships between hospital patient safety culture and adverse events. *Journal of Patient Safety, 6*(4), 226–232.

Martin, J. (2002). *Organizational culture: Mapping the terrain.* Thousand Oaks, CA: Sage.

McCue, M. T. (February, 2003). *Clamping down on variation.* Managed Healthcare Executive. Retrieved from http://managedhealthcareexecutive.modernmedicine.com/managed-healthcare-executive/news/ clamping-down-variation

McGuckin, M., Govednik, J., & Waterman, R. (2010). *Six years of monitoring hand hygiene events and sanitizer usage in United States: a multicenter study using product volume measurement.* Atlanta, GA: International Conference on Healthcare Associated Infections.

McHugh, M. D., Kelly, L. A., Smith, H. L., Wu, E. S., Vanak, J. M., & Aiken, L. H. (2013). Lower mortality in magnet hospitals. *Medical Care, 51*(5), 382–388. doi:10.1097/MLR.0b013e3182726cc5

McKesson InterQual Evidence-based Clinical Content. (n.d.). *Improve quality and efficiency with clinical decision support.* Retrieved from http://www.mckesson.com/payers/decision-management/interqual-evidence-based-clinical-content/interqual-evidence-based-clinical-content

National Council of State Boards of Nursing. (1997). *The five rights of delegation.* Retrieved from https://www.ncsbn.org/fiverights.pdf

National Council of State Boards of Nursing. (2013). *Nursing Regulation in the US: TERCAP.* Retrieved from https://www.ncsbn.org/441.htm

Neily, J., Mills, P. D., Young-Xu, Y., Carney, B. T., West, P., Berger, D. H.,…Bagian, J. E. (2010). Association between implementation of a medical team training program and surgical mortality. *Journal of the American Medical Association, 304*(15), 1693–1700.

Occupational Safety and Health Administration. (2009). *Guidelines for nursing homes: Ergonomics for the prevention of musculoskeletal disorders*. OSHA 3182–3R 2009. Retrieved from https://www.osha.gov/ergonomics/guidelines/nursinghome/final_nh_guidelines.pdf.

Orszag, P. (2008). *The overuse, underuse, and misuse of health care*. Washington, DC: Congresssional Budget Office. Retrieved from http://www.cbo.gov

Pittet, D., Allegranzi, B., & Boyce, J. (2009). The World Health Organization guidelines on hand hygiene in health care and their consensus recommendations. *Infection Control and Hospital Epidemiology, 30*(7), 611–622.

QSEN Institute. (2012). *Pre-licensure KSAs: Safety*. Retrieved from http://qsen.org/competencies/pre-licensure-ksas/#safety

Riesenbery, L. A., Leitzsch, J., & Cunningham, J. M. (2010). Nursing handoffs: A systematic review of the literature. *American Journal of Nursing, 110*(4), 24–36.

Schein, E. (1985). Organizational culture and leadership. San Francisco, CA: Jossey-Bass.

Sculli, G. L., Fore, A. M., Neily, J., Mills, P. D., & Sine, D. M. (2011). The case for training veterans administration frontline nurses in crew resource management. *Journal of Nursing Administration, 41*(12), 524–530.

Sculli, G. L., Fore, A. M., West, P., Neily, J., Mills, P. D., & Paull, D. E. (2013). Nursing Crew Resource Management: A follow up report from the Veterans Health Administration. *Journal of Nursing Administration, 43*(3), 122–126.

Shuldham, C., Parkin, C., Firouzi, A., Roughton, M., & Lau-Walker, M. (2009). The relationship between nurse staffing and patient outcomes: A case study. *Journal of Nursing Studies, 46*(7), 986–992.

Stermer, B. (2011). *Early goal-directed therapy reduces sepsis complications and mortality*. Retrieved from http://www.ihi.org/knowledge/Pages/ImprovementStories/EarlyGoalDirectedTherapy ReducesSepsisComplicationsandMortality.aspx

Stone, P. W., Hughes, R. G., & Dailey, M. (2008). Creating a safe and high-quality health care environment. In R. G. Hughes (Ed.), *Patient safety and quality: An evidence-based handbook for nurses* (pp. 594–603). Rockville, MD: Agency for Healthcare Research and Quality.

The Joint Commission. (2010). *Sentinel event alert 46: A follow-up report on the prevention of suicide*. Retrieved from http://www.jointcommission.org/assets/1/18/SEA_46.pdf

Timmel, J., Kent, P. S., Holzmueller, C. G., Paine, L., Schulick, R. D., & Pronovost, P. J. (2010). Impact of the Comprehensive Unit-based Safety Program (CUSP) on safety culture in a surgical inpatient unit. *The Joint Commission Journal on Quality and Patient Safety, 36*(6), 252–260.

Tischler, C. L., & Reiss, N. S. (2009). Inpatient suicide: Preventing a common sentinel event. *General Hospital Psychiatry, 31*(2), 103–109.

U.S. Department of Labor, Occupational Safety & Health Administration. (2012). *What is healthcare?* Retrieved from http://www.osha.gov/SLTC/healthcarefacilities/index.html

Veterans Health Administration. (2011). *VHA national patient safety improvement handbook 1050.01*. Retrieved from http://www.va.gov/vhapublications/ViewPublication.asp?pub_ID=2389

von Thaden, T. L., & Gibbons, A. M. (2008). *The safety culture indicator scale measurement system (SCISMS)*. Technical Report HFD-08–03/FAA-08–02. Savoy, IL: University of Illinois, Human Factors Division.

Wennberg, J. E. (2011). Time to tackle unwarranted variations in practice. *British Medical Journal, 342*, d1513. http://dx.doi.org/10.1136/bmj.d1513(Published 17 March 2011)

Wilson, R. M., Michel, P., Olsen, S., Gibberd, R. W., Vincent, C., El-Assady, R., ... Larizgoitia, I. (2012). Patient safety in developing countries: Retrospective estimation of scale and nature of harm to patients in hospital. *British Medical Journal, 344*, e832. Retrieved from http://dx.doi. org/10.1136/bmj.e832 /bmj.e832

Yaneva-Deliverska, M. (2011). Patient safety and healthcare associated infections. *Journal of IMAB—Annual Proceeding (Scientific Papers), 17*, book 1.

Zhan, C., & Miller, M. R. (2003). Excess length of stay, charges, and mortality attributable to medical injuries during hospitalization. *Journal of the American Medical Association, 8*(290), 1868–1874.

SUGGESTED READING

Agency for Healthcare Research and Quality (AHRQ). (2013, March). *Making health care safer II: An updated critical analysis of the evidence for patient safety practices*. Pub. No. 13-E001–1-EF. Rockville, MD: Author.

AHRQ. (2013). *How to use the CUSP toolkit*. Agency for Healthcare Research and Quality, Rockville, MD. http://www.ahrq.gov/professionals/education/curriculum-tools/cusp-toolkit/toolkit/index.html

American Nurses Association (ANA). (2011). *Health and safety survey*. Retrieved from http://www.nursingworld.org/2011HealthSurveyResults.aspx

American Nurses Association (ANA). (2013). *Safe patient handling and mobility: Interprofessional national standards*. Silver Spring, MD: American Nurses Association.

Benner, P. E., Malloch, K., & Sheets, V. (2010). *Nursing pathways for patient safety*. National Council of State Board of Nursing. St. Louis, MO: Mosby Elsevier.

Blouin, A. S., & McDonagh, K. J. (2010). Framework for patient safety. *Part 1. Journal of Nursing Administration, 10*(1), 397–400.

Blouin, A. S., & McDonagh, K. J. (2011). A framework for patient safety. *Part 2. Journal of Nursing Administration, 41*(11), 450–452.

Institute of Medicine (IOM). (2013). *Keeping patients safe: Transforming the work environment of nurses*. Washington, DC: The National Academies Press.

Robert Wood Johnson Foundation. (2011). *Nurses are key to improving patient safety*. Retrieved from www.RWJF.org

Sculli, G. L., & Sine, D. M. (2011). *Soaring to success: Taking crew resource management from the cockpit to the nursing unit*. Danvers, MA: HCPro.

Tierney, S. J. (2010). Nursing unit staffing: An innovative model incorporating patient acuity and patient turnover. University of Massachusetts Medical School. Graduate School of Nursing Dissertations. Paper 18. Retrieved from http://escholarship.umassmed.edu/gsn_diss/18

INTERPROFESSIONAL TEAMWORK AND COLLABORATION

Gerry Altmiller

It's less of a thing to do…and more of a way to be. (Unknown Participant, Quality and Safety Education for Nurses Collaboration, Chicago, June 2007)

Upon completion of this chapter, the reader should be able to

1. Define interprofessional team
2. Describe how a rapid response team (RRT) contributes to patient safety
3. Identify the benefit of collaborative interprofessional teams on patient outcomes
4. Discuss strategies and techniques to maximize effective interprofessional communication
5. Describe resources interprofessional teams can employ to improve quality and safety for patients
6. Describe how reflection contributes to positive patient outcomes
7. Identify the characteristics of effective interprofessional teams
8. List the three steps of the Team*STEPPS*™ Delivery System
9. Describe how informatics has benefited interprofessional team's ability to more efficiently and effectively solve problems
10. Discuss strategies the nurse can implement to include the patient as a partner on the interprofessional team

*A*patient's family approaches the nurse's station and verbalizes concerns regarding their family member's care. Their greatest concern is the patient's lack of energy following surgery to correct a bowel obstruction. They are concerned because the patient is elderly and *hasn't been out of bed for 2 days. He is not eating even though he has diabetes. They ask to speak to the people in charge of the patient's care.*

- *What do you know about the members of the interprofessional team caring for the patient?*
- *How will you bring the patient's immediate problems to the appropriate interprofessional team member's attention?*
- *How will you know you are approaching the correct interprofessional team member?*
- *How can the interprofessional team work together to address this patient's needs?*

With the increasing complexity of patient care, it is clear that no one person can address a single patient's needs. It takes an interprofessional team of people working together, each contributing their individual expertise for the well-being of the patient. Care for the patient extends beyond the hands-on care provided by direct caregivers. To be effective, patient care requires the coordinated services of many people, some not even directly involved with the patient, yet all focused on one thing, a positive experience, and outcome for the patient.

This chapter describes what an interprofessional team is and discusses the characteristics that make a team most effective. It describes how at the very center of the interprofessional team is the patient and the patient's family and how their individual

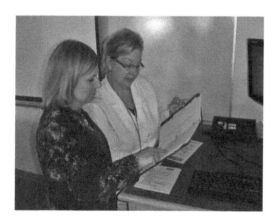

Interprofessional collaboration on the hospital floor.

preferences influence the decisions that the team makes as they assist the patient in achieving optimal patient outcomes. Within this goal of putting the patient front and center of the interprofessional health care team, strategies for how best to include the patient as a partner are presented. This chapter highlights resources that can be utilized as well as strategies that individuals and institutions can implement to create an environment where effective interprofessional communication facilitates patient safety and improves the overall quality of the care provided to patients, including the use of RRTs. With the increasing emphasis on quality and safety, techniques to improve communication between interprofessional health care team members have gained new importance. Tools, techniques, and strategies for communication aimed at facilitating patient safety and quality of care are stressed on, including the use of reflection by the nurse and other members of the interprofessional health care team as a means of improving patient outcomes. Likewise, Team*STEPPS* is presented as an effective way to ensure interprofessional health care teams are able to communicate with each other to promote situational awareness and patient safety. Strategies to create and develop effective team functioning is identified in this chapter. In addition, this chapter discusses how the World Wide Web has increased the availability of resources to support improved interprofessional communication and the dissemination of information. Informatics has contributed to effective teamwork by making information available at a moment's notice so that team members can exchange ideas to solve problems.

Nursing holds a vital position on the health care team, contributing to the plan of care, delivering nursing services, and providing that vital link between the patient, the patient's family, and the other members of the health care team. Skilled communication by the nurse and other members of the interprofessional health care team promote the exchange of clear and concise information, which allows the team to react quickly and appropriately to meet patients' needs.

WHAT IS AN INTERPROFESSIONAL TEAM?

A team is a group of individuals who work together for a common goal. In health care, the interprofessional team consists of people who have a stake or interest in and contribute to the well-being of the patient. An interprofessional team not only includes those directly involved in the patient's physical care such as the physicians, nurses, and family members, but it also includes those who provide support services such as pharmacists, social workers, dieticians, and those from departments such as housekeeping, radiology, the laboratory, transport services, and physical and occupational therapy. It is important to recognize the value of all these interprofessional team members' contribution to the patient's care.

RRTs

Interprofessional teams in the hospital setting may be brought together to focus on identified problems and find solutions. This can happen on a patient care unit or in other areas of the hospital. One common example of an effective team in the hospital is a **rapid response team** (RRT). An RRT is a team made up of specific health care professionals with specialized skills, who can mobilize and deliver immediate patient assessment and intervention if needed at the patient's bedside any time of day or night, 7 days a week at the beginning signs of a deterioration of a patient's health status. The RRT is separate from a "code" or resuscitation team that is also made up of specialized interprofessional team members who would respond to cardiac and/or respiratory arrest. The RRT was recommended to improve patient safety and quality by the Institute for Healthcare Improvement (IHI) with the intention of preventing deaths outside of the ICU (IHI, 2012). RRTs may be structured differently within different institutions, but most RRTs consist of a physician, critical care nurse, and respiratory therapist, along with other designated interprofessional members, as needed. RRTs support an institution's nurses by providing immediate support and assistance for all patients with deteriorating conditions. RRTs may be summoned to a patient's bedside by anyone, including family members. Providing RRT support allows for early intervention at the first sign of deterioration in patients, before they become critically ill or experience a cardiac arrest.

BENEFITS OF COLLABORATIVE INTERPROFESSIONAL TEAMS

At the center of the interprofessional health care team are the patient and the patient's family. Patient-centered care ensures that the patient is an integral part of the team and is central in all interactions and decisions. With patient-centered care, the interprofessional team acknowledges patient preferences regarding care and acknowledges their individual health values and priorities. Without the patient, there would be no need for the team.

Nurses have not always been considered members of the interprofessional health care team; traditionally they have taken direction from hospital administrators and physicians rather than directly contributing to a collaborative plan of care. Nurses were charged with direct patient care and focused mostly on providing patient hygiene under the direction of the physician. Differences in educational requirements prevented even routine tasks such as obtaining a patient's blood pressure from being delegated to the nurse. Nurses did not have a role in advocating for the patient and physicians did not confer with nurses regarding any aspect of the patient's care. The interprofessional relationship was strictly one of orders being dictated by the physician team member and orders being carried out by the nursing team member.

Gender issues have also contributed to the lack of interprofessional **collaboration** or the ability to effectively work together. In the past, males traditionally assumed the physician role while nurses have primarily been female. Much has changed in recent decades with both males and females assuming roles as physicians and nurses, independent of gender. Females still dominate the nursing profession, however, with the U.S. Department of Labor reporting in 2008 that males made up only 6.6% of the nursing workforce (U.S. Department of Health and Human Services, 2010a). In comparison, females now make up almost 25% of the current physician workforce (U.S. Department of Health and Human Services, 2010b).

Economic issues have also contributed to the lack of interprofessional collaboration. Nurses represent the largest segment of the hospital-based employee workforce and have been paid as hourly workers by the hospital. Physicians have been community based and have managed their practice as a business, directly billing their patients and the insurance companies. Some of this is changing as the expanding roles of nurses have created opportunities for hospital-based nurses and for advanced practice nurses in all areas of health care. Both these groups of registered nurses (RNs) have increased their education and have contributed to bridging the gap between nurses and physicians. Greater requirements in prelicensure education of nurses have also resulted in a bedside nurse that is able to assess, plan, implement, and evaluate care provided to patients, making the nurse a more valuable team member.

Nursing knowledge is based on science combined with the art of caring for the individual needs of patients. Nursing brings a holistic perspective to patient care. The connection of the nurse to the patient and family through close and continued interaction allows nurses to understand and advocate for patient concerns and needs regardless of their practice level. Nurses can build rapport between patients and the team and facilitate collaboration between the interprofessional health care disciplines involved in the patient's care. Nurses' knowledge of the patient experience allows them to identify subtle changes in the patient's condition and act quickly to prevent complications of illness. The ability of the nurse to function proactively helps to reduce unnecessary costs to hospitals as well as improve patient satisfaction and outcomes.

Nurses need to recognize the value of this perspective and acknowledge the positive impact they have on patient outcomes. It is important that nurses articulate the value of this positive effect on patient satisfaction as well as the financial benefit that nurses bring to the institutions they serve to enhance their role as contributing team members and to advance the profession of nursing.

Recognizing the value of nursing, the Institute of Medicine (IOM) in collaboration with the Robert Wood Johnson Foundation (RWJF), published its report, *The Future of Nursing: Leading Change, Advancing Health* (IOM, 2010). This report identified the barriers that prevent nurses from being able to respond to the rapidly changing health care system. It also validated the important role that nurses play in the delivery of seamless, high-quality, affordable health care to all. The four key recommendations from the report were focused on the role that nursing should play in providing care (Table 5.1).

TABLE 5.1 *THE FUTURE OF NURSING: LEADING CHANGE, ADVANCING HEALTH*

FOUR KEY RECOMMENDATIONS

1. Nurses should practice to the full extent of their education.
2. Nurses should achieve higher levels of education through an improved education system that promotes seamless academic progression.
3. Nurses should be full partners with physicians and other health care professionals in the redesign of health care.
4. Better data collection and information infrastructure is necessary for effective workforce planning and policy making.

Advancing Health Care Through Improved Education

Although educational differences exist among interprofessional team members, it is important to recognize that each team member brings a perspective to the team that represents specialized knowledge from his or her discipline. For physicians, the educational requirements include a baccalaureate degree with an additional 4 years of medical school, followed by a year of internship in clinical practice, and 2 years of residency. Medical specialization adds additional years of training and fellowship. For nurses, there are varied levels of educational requirements for entry into practice. These include a 3-year diploma school education, a 2-year associate degree education, and a 4-year baccalaureate degree education as well as master's completion programs. Other health care disciplines have varied educational degree requirements as well. No matter the educational degree requirements, each health care discipline needs to collaborate with the other disciplines to provide the highest quality care for the patient. While concepts of interprofessional collaboration are included in the educational process of each health care discipline, Petri (2010) notes a more deliberate approach to interprofessional learning would foster a enhanced group dynamic as well as a shared commitment to collaboration that recognizes the value of other disciplines.

To support the appreciation of each health care discipline's perspective, expertise, and values, many programs now include an integration of interprofessional education as part of their curriculum. **Interprofessional education** is the opportunity for multiple health care disciplines to learn together in the same learning environment simultaneously, gaining a greater understanding for each discipline's role and contributions. A common example of this is medical and nursing students taking an ethics class together or participating in a communication exercise as part of an orientation program.

REAL-WORLD INTERVIEW

Health care providers have limited educational preparation for complex care coordination across disciplines that are necessary in today's increasingly complex delivery system. Challenging patient health conditions mean no one discipline can be responsible for the entire spectrum of care, yet, health professions' education remains primarily a professional individual silo experience where each

(continued)

REAL-WORLD INTERVIEW (continued)

discipline is educated together and learns separately from the other health care disciplines. To effectively care for and coordinate care delivery, interprofessional health care professionals require repeated blended educational experiences to achieve the four interprofessional educational competencies:

- Understand the scope of responsibilities of each team member
- Maintain ethical conduct and quality of care within the team to develop respect and trust
- Communicate effectively with patients, families, and health care team members
- Utilize teamwork behaviors in executing patient care requirements

Complex health care work environments are driven by little understood human factors including intricacies of communication and behavior. These are important for sharing critical information and coordination among the team. Knowing what each health care discipline can contribute during the stress of a health care intervention is a critical factor in delivering safe care. A well-developed self-awareness allows team members to function alternately as leader or follower, as appropriate to the situation and individual competence. Health care is a team sport involving multiple individuals in the delivery of safe care.

Gwen Sherwood, PhD, RN, FAAN
Professor and Associate Dean for Academic Affairs
University of North Carolina at Chapel Hill School of Nursing
Coinvestigator, Quality and Safety Education for Nurses (www.qsen.org)
Chapel Hill, North Carolina

STRATEGIES FOR MAXIMIZING EFFECTIVE INTERPROFESSIONAL TEAMS

The changing socialization of physicians and nurses as well as other disciplines has allowed for the formation of interprofessional teams that not only care for patients but also tackle some of the toughest problems facing health care today. In part, this change has come from changes in traditional gender roles as well as the attainment of bachelor's and master's degrees by more and more nurses. Working together, physicians and nurses have developed work processes to address quality and safety on all levels of patient care.

Methods such as **root cause analysis** (RCA) are employed to identify problems within the health care system. With RCA, teams work together to investigate serious adverse events and identify root causes or contributing factors that lead to patient injury or a negative outcome so that they can be corrected. An RCA can be conducted to identify mechanisms within the health care system that allowed for the error or near miss to occur. This reporting process allows for both individual growth and development for the nurse as well as correction within the health care system's practices to prevent future errors. RCA discovers the root of a problem by not stopping at the first answer it arrives at for its cause, but by delving deeper into why the problem occurred, asking questions until there are no more questions to ask.

Another process used to improve quality and safety is the Six Sigma method. Six Sigma is a quality assurance strategy developed in corporate America in the mid-1980s by the Motorola Corporation (Carter, 2010). Six Sigma, used to improve existing health care processes, involves five steps, also referred to as DMAIC: define; measure; analyze; improve; and control. During the define step of Six Sigma, potential teams members are identified that are knowledgeable about the health care process or service that has been identified as needing improvement. These team members must have a clear understanding of what the expectation and needs are so they know where to aim the improvement. During the measure step of Six Sigma, the problem is investigated and data is gathered to determine how, when and where the problem is occurring. The analyze step of Six Sigma allows the team to look for trends and patterns of the health care problem from the data so they can identify a root cause. During the improve step of Six Sigma, solutions are identified and implemented, and finally, during the control step of Six Sigma, control mechanisms such as retraining or monitoring systems that ensure that the problem does not occur again are put in place.

RESOURCES FOR INTERPROFESSIONAL TEAMWORK AND COLLABORATION

Nowhere is interprofessional teamwork and collaboration more important than in providing required health care to patients in need. Although all members of the interprofessional health care team possess specific expertise that would benefit the patient, if they were unable to coordinate those skills and connect vital services together, the patient may not receive optimal care. In health care, poor outcomes occur when there are breakdowns in communication, poor teamwork, or inefficient communication "handoffs" that create situations leading to errors. **Handoff** is a term used to describe the communication method that the interprofessional team uses to transfer patient care to one another between shifts or patient care units or hospitals. Effective interprofessional teams involved in direct patient care have a common goal, that is, high-quality, safe patient care. They must all work together to provide coordinated care that results in positive patient outcomes.

Interprofessional teams in health care may be focused on more long-term projects. These interprofessional teams may be assembled to address a number of concerns. These concerns may include anything from QI processes to planning for the future of the health care institution. Although the work of these types of interprofessional teams may seem slower and more deliberate, the principles that guide them are the same as teams that respond to patient emergencies. For example, a long-term goal of a hospital might be to increase the number of bachelors prepared RNs by 80% within 10 years. Collaboration between hospital administration, finance, nursing leadership, and broad representation from nursing staff would need to conduct the same steps of assessment, definition of problem, goal setting, implementation, and evaluation utilizing strategies of effective communication and collaboration.

CHARACTERISTICS OF EFFECTIVE INTERPROFESSIONAL HEALTH CARE TEAMS

Effective interprofessional teams are able to think reflectively about the situation at hand considering past experiences, contemplate options from all perspectives, and deliberate the options in an atmosphere of mutual respect. In high-functioning, successful interprofessional teams, members can voice concerns and opinions, creating a group dynamic where all members contribute and share in the decision making. Clear, focused communication, and respectful negotiation decreases the potential for misunderstandings and promotes camaraderie among the team members.

Accountability and Stages of Team Development

Forming, storming, norming, and *performing* are terms used to describe the stages experienced by teams as they progress from formation to functioning as high-performance teams (Tuckman, 1965). The forming stage is generally a short phase when team members are introduced and objectives are established. As the team moves into the storming stage, team roles become clarified and processes as well as structures for the team are established. It is within this process that the details of the approach being used to accomplish the goals or assignment are decided upon. The workload of the task becomes clear during this storming phase and can overwhelm the team members. Conflicts may arise and members build relationships with other team members as they work through conflict resolution. In this storming stage, teams will fail if the work processes and team relationships have not been well established.

In the norming stage, team members develop a stronger commitment to the team's goals and assume responsibility for the team's progress. Individuals show leadership in specific areas and team members come to respect each other's roles. As members become socialized as a team, they are able to provide constructive feedback to each other. It is important to note that teams can pass back and forth between the storming and norming stages as new tasks are assigned to the team. The performing stage is realized through achievement of the team's shared vision of the goal. At this point, teamwork feels easier and members can for the most part join and leave the team without affecting the team's performance. The progress achieved from the team's hard work establishes the team as a high-performance team.

CASE STUDY 5.1

The manager of a critical care unit wants to implement self-scheduling among his large staff. He appoints two staff members from the night shift, two staff members from the day shift, one assistant manager, and one nurse aide to a committee with the goal of developing rules to guide the self-scheduling process. The committee is scheduled to meet weekly until all self-scheduling rules are developed and the self-scheduling process can be put in place. Immediately, tensions run high in the committee as there is disagreement about the number of Fridays that must be worked by each staff member and the number of weekends that must be worked in a 6-week schedule. Through negotiation, agreement is reached on the committee regarding these issues. Just when they believe that they have all issues resolved, there is disagreement among the committee members regarding the number of schedule changes management can make to accommodate unit needs. This is a very heated topic and the negotiation for this continues for 3 weeks. Eventually it is resolved with agreement by all. It is decided that the scheduling committee will remain intact, assist with the transition for staff, and manage the scheduling process. Committee members will work together to cover the unit needs.

1. *What team stage is identified as the team begins to work to resolve the number of Fridays and weekends that will be required by each staff?*
2. *What team stage is identified when the committee decides to remain intact to assist with the transition and manage the scheduling process?*

Delegation

Willingness to assist colleagues is pivotal to interprofessional teamwork and collaboration. Teamwork requires that members can effectively delegate work to each other. In patient care, it is essential that tasks being delegated are within the scope of practice of the individual to whom the task is being delegated. For example, inserting an indwelling urinary catheter could be delegated by a nurse to another nurse. It could not be delegated to a nursing assistant. When delegating, the nurse follows four steps: assess and plan; communicate what is needed to be done; provide supervision; and evaluate effectiveness and give feedback (National Council of State Boards of Nursing, 2005).

With all delegation, clear communication of what needs to be done and confirmation of understanding from the individual being delegated to is essential to ensure patient safety. The nurse who is delegating needs to provide an opportunity for clarification and questions. If an outcome does not meet expectations, the nurse should lead the discussion with those involved to identify reasons for the unexpected outcome and determine what could be learned from the experience to improve care and to ensure a successful outcome in the future.

Crew Resource Management (CRM)

CRM refers to educating individuals that work in high-stress systems where the human aspect of operations can create an increased potential for error. Originating in the aviation industry for the cockpit crew, CRM develops communication, leadership, and decision-making safety strategies to combat the potential for human error inherent in high-stress systems and its devastating effects. The health care industry shares an interest in interprofessional teamwork and clear communication with the aviation industry to prevent catastrophic events. Health care has applied many CRM strategies to the daily interactions and continuous QI processes of the interprofessional health care team. CRM communication, leadership, and decision-making safety strategies focus on cognitive and interpersonal skills to promote situational awareness.

Situational awareness is having the right information at the right time alongside the ability to analyze that information to appropriately and effectively take action. Having this awareness, allows for all team members to be aware of the facts in any given situation. The vehicle for this awareness is effective communication between interprofessional health care team members.

TEAM*STEPPS*

Within health care, Team*STEPPS* is a program developed to provide training in effective communication techniques similar to those promoted by CRM. The program is designed to teach interprofessional teams how to communicate with each other to promote situational awareness and patient safety. Specifically Team*STEPPS* is

- A powerful solution to improving patient safety within an organization
- An evidence-based teamwork system to improve communication and teamwork skills among health care professionals
- A source for ready-to-use materials and a training curriculum to successfully integrate teamwork principles into all areas of your health care system
- Scientifically rooted in more than 20 years of research and lessons from the application of teamwork principles (Agency for Healthcare Research and Quality [AHRQ], n.d., p. 2).

Developed in collaboration with the Department of Defense, the Agency for Healthcare Research and Quality (AHRQ) initiated Team*STEPPS* to augment the effort and abilities of interprofessional teams specially to ensure the highest patient outcomes within health care institutions and systems. By focusing on a three-phased process of team development, Team*STEPPS* optimizes resources within a team, provides a framework for resolving conflict and enhancing communications, and provides the basis to effectively address potential barriers to effective patient safety and quality care.

AHRQ lists the three phases of Team*STEPPS* as assessment; planning, training, and implementation; and sustainment. Assessment involves pretraining evaluation to determine the willingness and capacity of an organization to change. Within this phase of the process, an interprofessional team is established that is made up of a cross-section of health care leaders and professionals within the organization itself. This phase also involves conducting a comprehensive site assessment that identifies areas of weakness and needs relative to teamwork. From this assessment, the second phase of Team*STEPPS* is initiated; a training program is developed to effectively overcome the deficiencies of the team as well as maximize its strengths. Once this education has occurred, the third phase of Team*STEPPS* can be initiated. The long-range goal of the third phase is to maintain and continually improve teamwork efforts throughout the organization. Through coaching, feedback, and reinforcement of strategies taught, Team*STEPPS* can be continually reinforced and built upon as applied to clinical and administrative situations identified by the organization and as opportunities for improvement.

Situation, Background, Assessment, and Recommendation (SBAR)

A framework for communication that has been implemented in many health care settings is SBAR, an acronym for the words *situation, background, assessment, and recommendation* SBAR (AHRQ, n.d.). It was developed by the military and is now applied to health care as a means to relay significant information regarding a patient's condition or to be used as patients' care is communicated and handed off from one caregiver to another (Table 5.2).

TABLE 5.2 SITUATION, BACKGROUND, ASSESSMENT, AND RECOMMENDATION

SBAR	MEANING	EXAMPLE
S	Situation: Describe what is happening with the patient	Doctor, I am calling about Mrs. Smith, your patient admitted yesterday to room 304 with respiratory distress.
B	Background: Explain the background of the patient's circumstances	She was comfortable during the evening after being placed on 2 L oxygen by nasal cannula and receiving 20 mg of Lasix intravenously, but is now complaining of shortness of breath.
A	Assessment: Identify what data you have regarding the situation	Her respiratory rate is 28. Pulse is 110/min and her oximetry measures 91%. She has crackles in the lower third of her lung fields bilaterally. She is laboring to breathe.
R	Recommendation: Identify what you think needs to be done to correct the situation	I think she may need her Lasix dose increased.

ADDITIONAL TECHNIQUES FOR EFFECTIVE COMMUNICATION WITHIN INTERPROFESSIONAL TEAMS

Clear and open communication among team members allows ideas to be shared and counteracts the potential for human errors of judgment. Techniques such as cross-monitoring require that team members listen carefully to the details being communicated and provide correction for the team if needed. **Cross-monitoring** is the process of monitoring the actions of other team members for the purpose of sharing the workload and reducing or avoiding errors (AHRQ, n.d.). An example of this technique can occur during grand rounds where interventions are discussed by a group of physicians, nurses, pharmacists, and other health care providers. Decisions verbally agreed upon can sometimes be missed as orders are articulated on paper. A nurse asking for clarification of an order he or she recalls differently is an example of cross-monitoring.

Other communication techniques can be used to bring attention to patient situations. A call out is used to communicate important information to the entire team simultaneously (AHRQ, n.d.). In a call out, the team member would call out to others for assistance. For example, during a resuscitation effort, also known as a code, a nurse monitoring the patient's blood pressure might assertively state the changing status to the medical resident. Typically, the call out is then followed by a check back, which verifies the receipt of the call out information and provides feedback and appropriate response. In this example, the resident might ask for medication to be given to stabilize the patient's blood pressure. Check back requires the receiver verbally acknowledge the message to provide opportunity for correction if needed.

The two-challenge rule states that if an individual does not believe that his or her first attempt to bring attention to a concerning patient situation has been successful, the individual is obligated to make a second attempt to make the problem known to others on the team (AHRQ, n.d.). The two-challenge rule is designed for when team member's input is ignored purposely. It is the obligation of the person to bring it forward again to make sure it is not ignored. An example of the two-challenge rule is when a nurse tells a physician about a concern she has for the patient, like a low urine output, and the physician does not address it for one reason or another. The nurse is obligated to bring it forward again.

Another tool that can be used to advocate for a patient is CUS, which is an acronym for the words *concerned, uncomfortable,* and *safety* (AHRQ, n.d.). Frequently, nurses are expected to advocate for their patients but they do not know how to do so. CUS is a tool that assists the nurse in taking an assertive stance to do what the nurse believes is needed for the patient. For example, in the case of a larger than recommended dose of medication being ordered for a patient, the nurse may approach the ordering provider and state, "I'm concerned with the dose that has been ordered. I am uncomfortable giving such a large dose to this patient because of her renal condition. I don't think it is safe."

STRATEGIES FOR EFFECTIVE COMMUNICATION WITHIN INTERPROFESSIONAL TEAMS

Timeouts are mandated in the operating room (OR) and procedure suites by The Joint Commission to help ensure patient safety (The Joint Commission, n.d.). Timeouts can also be initiated during any procedure at the bedside. The timeout is an opportunity for everyone in the room to stop and ensure that the correct patient is having the correct procedure done to the correct site. The timeout requires that everyone stop his or her clinical work and devote his or her attention to the patient. Another safety strategy the

TABLE 5.3 AVAILABLE TOPICS FOR REFERENCE AND EDUCATION ON AHRQ TEAM*STEPPS* WEBSITE

SBAR	Provides a standardized framework for communication, that is, situation, *background*, assessment, and *recommendation*
Cross-monitoring	Involves listening to other team members to identify correct and incorrect information. This allows the team to self-correct health care errors before they occur
Call out	Asks for help from other team members
Two-challenge rule	Obligates team members to make a second attempt to have a concern heard when their first attempt to bring attention to a concern is not acknowledged
CUS	Advocacy strategy using the words concerned, uncomfortable, safety
Check back/read back	Verbally calling out and repeating back information to confirm it is understood correctly.
Handoff	Transferring responsibility for a patient's care from one unit to another or from one individual to another.

team can employ is the use of safety huddles. Safety huddles allow those caring for the patient to review pertinent information and the plan of care. It is similar to a team huddle used in sports whereby team members share information to ensure everyone is aware and working toward the same goals for the patient. An example of when a huddle would facilitate effective, coordinated care is when medications need to be altered due to change in a patient's status. Responding to an allergic reaction of a patient for instance would best be handled with a focused, coordinated approach by as many of the interprofessional team members as possible.

All of the abovementioned communication strategies are developed by the AHRQ that provides reference videos for clinicians, administrators, and educators demonstrating Team*STEPPS* tools, strategies, and techniques at its website, http://www.ahrq.gov/professionals/education/curriculum-tools/teamstepps/instructor/videos/index.html (Table 5.3).

Critical Thinking 5.1

The nurse calls the physician to report that a patient has suddenly developed hives while receiving an IV dose of antibiotic. The hives are covering most of his back. The physician tells the nurse that he does not think that the antibiotic is the cause and that she should just continue to monitor the patient. The nurse is concerned that the hives may be the beginning of a serious allergic reaction.

1. What safety strategy would be most effective for the nurse to use to advocate for the patient in this situation?

Another way that team members can work to prevent errors is by reporting errors and near misses to other member of the health care team. **Near misses** are events that could have resulted in an error but were caught in time. Reporting these errors and near misses provides an opportunity for the team to learn from them. In most cases, errors and near misses are not the result of a single person's actions. They are often the result of a failure within a health care system. By reporting all errors or near misses, the need for an RCA can be evaluated more completely and effectively.

USE OF INFORMATICS FOR EFFECTIVE PROBLEM SOLVING

Minimizing the potential for errors is the goal of everyone on the health care team. Participating in behaviors that guard against error and protect patients is a fundamental part of daily health care practice. There are many available web resources funded by government agencies and national health care organizations that are designed to improve teamwork and collaboration, prevent error, promote patient safety, and improve the quality of the care that patients receive. Nurses, as well as other team members, can access these resources to learn about strategies that address quality and safety as a way to improve their practice and keep patients safe from errors (Table 5.4).

Communication and Interprofessional Teamwork in QI

All members of the interprofessional health care team have an obligation to improve patient care processes and outcomes by focusing on communication and QI. **Debriefing** is the process of reviewing performance effectiveness following challenging patient care situations. Utilizing strategies such as debriefing allows the interprofessional team to evaluate the effectiveness of their communication and teamwork and to identify areas where improvement could be made. It is during debriefing that constructive feedback is given and received. All team members should feel comfortable to participate in this process. Individuals may differ in how they provide feedback to peers, but feedback, whether

TABLE 5.4 WEB RESOURCES FOR TEAMWORK AND COLLABORATION, ERROR PREVENTION, PATIENT SAFETY, AND QI

RESOURCE	WEBSITE ADDRESS
TeamSTEPPS	http://www.ahrq.gov/professionals/education/curriculum-tools/teamstepps/instructor/videos/index.html
Patient Safety Network	http://psnet.ahrq.gov
American Nurses Association: The National Database of Nursing Quality Indicators	http://www.nursingquality.org/data.aspx
Institute for Safe Medication Practices (ISMP)	http://www.ismp.org
Institute of Medicine Future of Nursing	http://www.iom.edu/Reports/2010/The-Future-of-Nursing-Leading-Change-Advancing-Health.aspx
Quality and Safety Education for Nurses (QSEN)	http://www.qsen.org
The Joint Commission	http://www.jointcommission.org
Crew Resource Management in Health Care	http://www.saferhealthcare.com

positive or negative, should always be an unbiased reflection on what occurred, opening the door to a discussion of evidence-based practice (Clynes & Raftery, 2008). Constructive feedback should carefully detail events as they occurred and avoid opinion.

Constructive feedback recounts events, offering options for improvement. Constructive feedback is most effective when focused on a task, a process used, or on self-regulation, because that focus contributes to learning; feedback focused on the individual is less effective because it does not increase learning (Hattie & Timperley, 2007). For instance, feedback such as "It was wise to gather your supplies before you went into the patient's room" focuses on the task. Feedback such as "Your explanation to the patient before you began allowed the patient to trust you" focuses on the health care process. Feedback such as "It is good that you realized you broke sterile technique and changed your gloves" focuses on self monitoring. All of these support knowledge development. Feedback such as "You did a good job" focuses on the individual and is least effective because it doesn't add to one's understanding of what aspects of his or her practice were effective and "a good job." Although it is difficult to give and receive unflattering feedback, team members must understand that feedback is essential for growth. Feedback is the catalyst that allows one to make continual adjustments in practice. Receiving feedback is often the catalyst for change and should be viewed as an opportunity for growth. Receiving feedback that is perceived as negative challenges the team member to consider if there is validity to the comments made, including considering whether the same feedback has been provided previously by other sources. If after consideration, feedback is perceived as inaccurate, the team member can ask for examples of poor performance and focus on improvement, asking the person providing feedback how he or she feels improvement can be achieved.

Auditing Patient Care and Outcomes

Teams can work together to conduct audits and other organizational studies that measure quality, safety, and patient outcomes that can have a significant impact on the process of QI. Collecting and analyzing data regarding patient care practices and patient outcomes allows the team to document differences between the actual system's performance and the goals of the organization. By documenting differences between the two, changes can be made to bring the two closer together and improve quality of care and patient safety by the interprofessional health care team.

REFLECTION AND FEEDBACK

Communication and interprofessional teamwork skills are a huge part of the protection from injury and complications that nurses provide for patients. These skills help not only when interacting with patients and health care team members to solve problems but also when nurses reflect on patient care events and discuss ways to improve outcomes. Providing feedback to team members allows the team to identify strengths and weaknesses, make changes to the health care system, and adjust practice for individual growth and development.

Self-evaluation of one's communication and decision making is a crucial element of professional growth and strengthens one's ability to contribute to the team's decisions by employing strong clinical judgment. As discussed earlier in the chapter, reflection supports confidence in decision making and provides an opportunity for the individual to consider his or her interactions with others and determine what actions enhanced a positive outcome and what actions worked against it. Reflecting on clinical situations and their outcomes allows team members to make positive changes to improve practice.

Tanner Model of Thinking Like a Nurse

Tanner's model of Thinking Like a Nurse (2006) demonstrates how clinical judgment is developed through reflection, enhancing critical thinking skills. These skills are essential to develop as one gains expertise in protecting patients through situational awareness and mindfulness. **Mindfulness** in this context implies staying focused with the ability to see the significance of early and weak signals as well as to take strong and decisive action to prevent harm (Weick & Sutcliff, 2001). Tanner's model stems from review of approximately 200 studies focused on the nurses' development of clinical judgment. From her review, she concluded that

- Clinical judgments are more influenced by what nurses bring to the situation than the objective data about the situation at hand.
- Sound clinical judgment rests to some degree on knowing the patient and his or her typical pattern of responses, as well as an engagement with the patient and his or her concerns.
- Clinical judgments are influenced by the context in which the situation occurs and the culture of the nursing care unit.
- Nurses use a variety of reasoning patterns alone or in combination.
- Reflection on practice is often triggered by a breakdown in clinical judgment and is critical for the development of clinical knowledge and improvement in clinical reasoning (Tanner, 2006, p. 204).

EVIDENCE FROM THE LITERATURE

Citation

McBride, A. B. (2010). Toward a roadmap for interdisciplinary academic career success. *Research and Theory for Nursing Practice: An International Journal*, 24(1), 74–86.

Discussion

The complexity of today's health problems requires more than the knowledge of one provider. This necessitates an interprofessional collaborative approach. Identified by the IOM as a core competency of all health care professionals, interprofessional collaboration has different meanings to different people. Examples of interprofessional collaboration include understaffed hospital personnel working together during the night shift to ensure patient safety or nurses and physicians discussing a patient plan to decrease complications or multiple disciplines working in partnership for education and research endeavors to decrease mortality and morbidity within their institution.

One of the barriers to achieving interprofessional collaboration has been the socialization of the separate health care disciplines, which has been focused on how they differ from one another. Up until recently, each health care discipline was taught without interacting with the other health care disciplines; each establishing its own distinct body of knowledge.

(continued)

> **EVIDENCE FROM THE LITERATURE (continued)**
>
> **Implications for Nursing**
>
> Nursing has built a large body of knowledge based on scientific research. Nursing's strengths include its holistic orientation to the patient and its ability to facilitate the bridging of disciplines and boundaries, thus supporting interprofessional collaboration. The reward of interprofessional collaboration is an expanded perspective where multiple health care disciplines work together to develop new models of care, new methods of care delivery, and breakthroughs in disease management, and health promotion. Through interprofessional collaboration, knowledge obtained from research can be translated into practice for the benefit of human health. The nursing profession is in a key position to support collaboration between all health care professionals from all disciplines as they move forward to meet the core competencies identified by the IOM.

STRATEGIES TO INCLUDE THE PATIENT AS PARTNER

Communication between the health care team, the patient, and the patient's family during times of stress and illness can be challenging but it is essential to safety and a key factor in patient satisfaction. Patients and families look to the nurse to provide a personal connection with the team. In addition, many patients and families look to the nurse as a source of information. The nurse should use language that is understandable to the patient and provide patient-centered information that allows the patient to assume a role of partnership rather than dependency. The nurse plays a pivotal role in including the patient, providing explanations, and providing access for the patient to communicate with other members of the interprofessional team. To promote the patient's partnership with the interprofessional health care team, the nurse can create connections for the patient to other members of the team, such as providing information regarding when the physician usually makes rounds. The nurse can encourage the patient and family to write down their questions for the physician and put the questions in the chart so that the physician may address them.

Developing Enhanced Communication Skills

The nurse must possess strong communication skills to contribute to effective team functioning. **Communication** is the interactive process of exchanging information. Effective communication is clear, precise, and concise, with no ambiguities. Safety is enhanced when the communication sender uses the proper terminology and provides an opportunity for clarification. Ideally, in response, the receiver of the communication acknowledges the message as heard and understood.

Many barriers can interfere with communication, such as knowledge gaps, education levels, culture, language barriers, or stress. It is important for nurses to develop strategies to identify and overcome these barriers. Nonverbal cues, such as the patient's facial expression, eye contact, and body posturing, may signal a message from the patient, but when safety is a priority such as it is in health care, interpreting nonverbal cues only is not an acceptable technique for communicating. Any perception one develops from nonverbal communication must be verified verbally to maintain a safe environment.

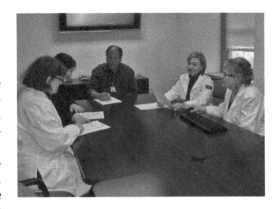

Monthly staff meeting.

Effective communication is essential to maintaining a safe and protected environment for patients. Ineffective communication has been identified as the root cause for 66% of the sentinel events reported to The Joint Commission between 1995 and 2005 (AHRQ, n.d.), which explains why improving communication has been the safety priority of the next decade. Students and nurses who are new to practice may find team interaction intimidating for several reasons, including that they do not clearly understand the culture of health care communication, they have known knowledge gaps, and they have not yet gained enough experience in the health care setting from which they can draw. Recognizing what information needs to be communicated to which individuals on the team and in what time frame is essential to developing effective communication skills. Regularly scheduled meetings of key team members help to ensure effective communications. Quality and safety in patient care are strongly influenced by the ability of the health care team to communicate clearly without uncertainty, in a timely manner, and to contribute to the health care team's productive, efficient approach to patient care.

REAL-WORLD INTERVIEW

In the OR, no one can be an individual. Everyone works as a team. We make it a team effort from the minute we meet the patient. The nurse anesthetist and the circulating nurse go together to pick up the patient. Even moving the patient onto the table is a team effort to ensure the patient's safety. Everyone has to share information and be able to communicate. The timeout procedure is a great example of team work and communication in the OR. Everyone must stop what he or she is doing and be attentive to the exchange of information to ensure the patient's safety. There is a lot of camaraderie in the OR because of the high stress associated with the work we do. Each member of the team contributes. The nurse anesthetist has to be a calming force in the room to instill confidence in the rest of the team. In the OR, there is a lot of autonomy. As an advance practice RN, I feel valued as a team member. It motivates me to communicate with everyone, go above and beyond what is required, and take pride in what I do.

Daniel Boucot, APN-A, MSN, Advance Practice Nurse-Anesthesia
Rancocas Anesthesia Associates
Kennedy Health System
Sewell, New Jersey

Strategies for Communication in Difficult Situations

Challenging patient care situations such as patient resuscitations, difficult patient procedures, rapid response efforts, or end-of-life events require extreme attention and clarity. Unnecessary conversation should cease during these situations and all communication should focus on the situation at hand without distractions. To ensure patient safety during these challenging patient care situations, communication senders and receivers should continually verify their communication using read backs or check backs. For example, during a difficult labor and delivery, the physician might assertively request many urgent medications and interventions. In this chaotic and unnerving scenario, it is essential that the nurse or other health care professional verify what was heard. In addition, documentation must be clear and accurate during these events so as to provide a written account of events. It is during these types of challenging patient care situations that communication with patients and families can sometimes be overlooked. This can be avoided by including the patient in decision making whenever possible and appointing someone on the team to provide updates to the family.

Critical Thinking 5.2

During a patient resuscitation, the nurse pulling supplies from the code cart discovers that supplies are missing. When the code has ended, the nurse reviews the documentation form to determine who stocked the cart last.

1. What would be the best approach for the nurse to initiate a discussion with coworkers about the incorrectly stocked cart?
2. What aspects should the nurse focus on during the discussion?
3. How can the nurse create a learning experience for coworkers in this instance?

Managing Conflict

It is vital to patient safety that the lines of communication remain open among all those involved in the patient's care. When there is disruption in the smooth flow of communication among team members, it is important to address it promptly before it becomes a more prolonged barrier to communication. Destructive events such as physicians who will not respond to pages, nurses who are resistant to carrying out legitimate orders, or pharmacists who do not move quickly to fill STAT prescriptions create difficult communications among health care providers that can negatively impact patient care (Table 5.5). It is important to address misunderstandings and conflicts promptly so that they do not become long-standing barriers to communication. Team members must be vigilant in fulfilling their ethical duty to work together for the patient's well-being.

Negative or difficult communication in the work environment can come from patients, families, physicians, other nurses, or any person involved in the operations of the institution. Physicians who yell, don't answer calls, and display disrespect, and condescension toward colleagues make it uncomfortable to practice. Miscommunications

TABLE 5.5 MANAGING DIFFICULT COMMUNICATIONS

HEALTH CARE PROVIDER	COMMUNICATION ISSUE	THE NURSE'S BEST COMMUNICATION APPROACH
Physician	Not answering page	Call physician's office or overhead page to solve immediate problem; later discuss with physician that the patient's needs are the primary concern and give the reason for the page.
Physician	Speaking in an angry condescending manner	Maintain calm and keep focus on the patient; state your primary concern is to solve the patient's immediate need. Identify the patient's need clearly and succinctly.
Pharmacist	Not filling STAT orders quickly	Maintain calm and explain patient's immediate need.
Unlicensed assistive personal	Not following through with delegated duties	Explore reasons for why duties were not completed. If needed, make adjustment to workload. Develop plan for future communication regarding delegated duties.
Nurse	Rolls eyes and sighs during report; indicates irritation with you	Respond in civil tone, stating that you sense there is something the nurse wants to say and that you learn when people are direct. Ask nurse to please be direct with his or her concerns.
Nurse	Does not provide assistance when needed	Explore reason for lack of assistance; develop plan for future. Offer assistance to peers when able.
Nurse	Resistant to carrying out legitimate orders	Remember to be quick to volunteer to help others so they will be just as quick to return the favor when you need help.

between the interprofessional team can put patients at risk. Stressed patients, families, and/or staff can act out frustrations and aggression.

Lateral Violence

One of the most troubling conflict for nurses is nurse-to-nurse aggression, also known as lateral violence (Griffin, 2004). **Lateral violence** is manifested as uncivil behaviors toward colleagues and may include making faces or raising eyebrows in response to a comments, making snide remarks, withholding information that interferes with a colleague's ability to perform professionally, refusing to help, or appearing not available to give help (Griffin, 2004). Scapegoating (blaming one person for all negative things that have happened), criticizing, breaking confidences, fighting among nurses, and excluding peers from dialogue and activities are all forms of lateral violence and result in injury to the dignity of another (Griffin, 2004). Nurses can experience physical consequences (loss of sleep, weight loss, irritable bowel syndrome) and/or psychological consequences (depression, anxiety, and loss of confidence) as a result of lateral violence (Becher & Visovsky, 2012). In addition, lateral violence can interfere with continuity of care and be detrimental to patients and to the institutions that provide care.

When encountering lateral violence, nurses should respond to it in a manner that focuses on consensus building rather than respond emotionally with anger. If a communication becomes angry or difficult, the nurse can refocus the interaction on the patient's safety and well-being. Refocusing on the patient's needs will take the focus off of the power struggle that occurs when people are angry. In addition to protecting one's self, nurses have an obligation to report behaviors that compromise patient safety or the well-being of coworkers to their supervisor or someone else in authority to adequately address the problem. Conflicts and negative behaviors place patients at risk because they keep nurses from communicating concerns to physicians, from asking questions when they are unsure, and from asking for help when critical situations arise.

Besides lateral violence between and among nurses themselves, nurses can experience hostile work conditions from physicians, patients, or their families. The nurse can utilize refocusing or de-escalation strategies with physicians, patients, and families as well. Again, an effective tool to de-escalate difficult or angry communication is to bring the focus of the conversation back to the patient. Refocusing the discussion back on the patient's needs takes the focus off any perceived power struggle and helps everyone to refocus on the priorities at hand. Nurses can enlist the support of more senior colleagues when conflicts arise with team members. Other useful de-escalation techniques include listening attentively to others and demonstrating concern. Nurses can reduce negative situations by identifying people that are receptive to their questions and are willing to serve as resources and by ending conversations where coworkers are being discussed in a negative manner.

New-to-practice nurses are more vulnerable to lateral violence and hostile work conditions in the health care environment due to their lack of experience. Addressing these conditions as soon as possible frequently puts an end to it. However, it is important not to be confrontational in one's approach. An effective tactic against lateral violence is to develop de-escalation strategies for these situations, which can decrease the intensity, and stress of the situation. When confronted with nonverbal innuendos such as eyebrow raising, rolling of eyes, and long sighs by peers, one can be direct and say, "I sense that there is something that you want to say to me. I learn best when people are direct. It's okay if you are direct with me" (Griffin, 2004). This type of response will directly address the lateral violence in a civil manner without aggression. This type of response indicates to the violator that his or her body language is perceived as negative and that it is preferable for the recipient to discuss the reason for it rather than ignore it. It should be said in earnest and not with anger to de-escalate the situation and open the lines of communication.

Critical Thinking 5.3

A new-to-practice nurse who is on orientation is assigned a complex patient to care for with his preceptor. During a stressful exchange, the preceptor states, "You're way too slow! You are never going to make it here if you don't pick up the pace."

1. What strategies for difficult communications would be most appropriate to use in this instance?
2. When should the new-to-practice nurse address this with the preceptor?
3. What would be the new-to-practice nurse's best communication approach with the preceptor?

Communicating With Preceptors

Preceptors are experienced nurses who provide orientation and support to the new-to-practice nurse as they learn the roles and responsibilities of a new job. Preceptors have increased responsibilities of caring for patients and providing instruction to new nurses. They are frequently chosen for this important role because of their expertise in caring for patients and because they exemplify professional behaviors. New-to-practice nurses rely heavily on their preceptors to guide them in learning how to communicate with other team members and become a productive member of the health care team. Communicating with team members requires that the nurses maintain a professional presence and act with confidence. During the orientation period, communication can be intimidating for the new nurse. It is difficult to feel like a valued member of the team when one is not sure about what is needed next. It can be a stressful time for both the preceptor and the orientee, particularly during challenging patient care situations. To diffuse any stressful communication, an honest and open exchange between the preceptor and the orientee at a quiet moment later will provide an opportunity to clarify concerns and reach an understanding about expectations. The new nurse can open the discussion by identifying his or her desire to learn and understand the situation. New nurses need to maintain realistic expectations regarding their knowledge base and expertise and seek feedback that will help them develop skill and effective clinical judgment. Accepting that he or she has knowledge gaps will allow the new nurse to ask questions without injury to self-esteem. Collaboration skills improve as the nurse develops a better understanding of the work expectation and unit routine.

Critical Thinking 5.4

The nurse is caring for a patient with an extensive burn injury. The patient has a decreased white blood cell count and is scheduled for skin grafting at the end of the week. The patient is receiving a regular diet but has a poor appetite and has not been able to eat enough to meet his required calorie intake.

1. How can the nurse involve the patient and the family to address the patient's nutrition?
2. Which members of the interprofessional team would have the expertise to address the patient's nutritional status?
3. How can the interprofessional team work together to meet the patient's nutritional needs?

REAL-WORLD INTERVIEW

Being a new nurse had its challenges. I had worked as an extern and then as a tech, but when I transitioned to an RN, I realized how much I was responsible for and had to learn quickly how to deal with the stress. The hardest part was

(continued)

REAL-WORLD INTERVIEW (continued)

knowing the right thing to do for the patient and who I could comfortably go to for questions. Even though I felt I had a good education, it took a good year to feel comfortable with my practice and confident with my knowledge and skills. I was hired at the same time as another nurse and we supported each other during orientation. My hospital also had a nurse residency program and it helped me to know that my peers on other units were having the same feelings and difficulties that I was having. In the program, we talked about communication and about working with complex patient and family situations. We supported each other a lot through my first year of nursing practice.

Katie Bicknell, RN, BSN
Children's Hospital of Pennsylvania
Philadelphia, Pennsylvania

Cognitive Rehearsal

It is most important to continually promote an environment of respect and collaboration. Nurses must challenge themselves to use respectful negotiation when disagreements occur between members of the health care team and to remain civil in the face of incivility as part of their professional development. Cognitive rehearsal is one strategy that the nurse can use when confronted with incivility from a coworker or another person. Cognitive rehearsal is a prepared response that one practices ahead of time that would address a negative comment or situation in a civil manner. It allows one to not react emotionally but to pause and respond with a rehearsed, intellectually driven, civil response. For instance, if a coworker harshly criticizes the speed with which you complete a task, rather than react emotionally and become hurt and angry, you might respond by saying, "This is different from how I learned. Can you help me to understand how you complete it so quickly?"

As mentioned earlier, reflection and the ability to gain insight into one's one actions can facilitate powerful, effective change. Specifically, reflecting on your ability to communicate with colleagues and other members of the interprofessional team provides an opportunity to consider behaviors that build consensus among colleagues and behaviors that create barriers to communication and interfere with safe patient care. During reflection, one should ask oneself, "What went well?" "What could have gone better?" "What could I have done to improve this situation?"

CASE STUDY 5.2

You and a senior colleague are assigned to the same patient room. You are caring for the patient in Bed B and she is caring for the patient in Bed A. You notice that the patient in Bed A is sleeping. On the bedside table, there is a filled medication

(continued)

syringe and an empty vial labeled heparin, 10,000 units/mL. You carry the medication syringe and heparin out to the nurse's station and state to your colleague, "These were on the bedside table." She takes them from you and states, "Yes, I have to remember to give the heparin to him when he wakes up" and returns them to the patient's bedside table.

1. *What standard is your colleague violating?*
2. *Recognizing that your colleague did not react to your implied concern for the patient's safety and the standard of practice, what communication strategy would you implement to maintain this patient's safety?*
3. *How can you address practice concerns like this from an organization's point of view to prevent this type of practice?*

Hospital and Nursing Leadership

Hospital and nursing leadership has a big influence on how teams function. Leaders can set the tone for communication, role-model effective conflict management, as well as create and foster an environment that facilitates safety and quality care. Head nurses, preceptors, and other leaders within the health care organization can support new-to-practice nurses by providing effective feedback. Nurses can approach leaders to facilitate needed change when a chain of command authority is needed. Most leaders continually assess their environment as well as the people that report to them to determine if adequate support is provided for their subordinates to do their jobs. However, leaders can miss subtle signs of trouble or inefficiency. In that case, the nurse must take it upon themselves to approach the leader to ask for help. Rules for effective communication and team building help ensure the message for requesting help or clarification will be heard.

Interprofessional teamwork and collaboration is essential to ensure quality health care for patients and maintain safety. Nurses are valued members of the interprofessional health care team. Nurses' contribution to the patient's care include knowledgeable assessments, reflective thinking, effective planning, thoughtful interventions based on evidenced-based practice, and careful evaluation of care. Nurses' communication skills play a pivotal role in team building. Nurses who communicate concerns and address problems enhance their ability to prevent errors, achieve positive patient outcomes and patient satisfaction, and improve the system in which they work.

KEY CONCEPTS

1. Interprofessional teams include physicians and nurses that provide direct patient care but also include the patient, family members and, many others who provide support services such as pharmacists, dieticians, social workers, and physical and occupational therapists.

2. All members of the interprofessional team should be valued for their contribution of a specific expertise to the plan of care for the patient.

3. Interprofessional education as well as quality and safety standards can improve the collegial interactions of members of the team.

4. Attention to quality and safety improvement have resulted in national organizations promoting the implementation of processes such as RCA, Six Sigma, and RRTs to raise the standard of care.

5. The human factors associated with providing health care contribute to the potential for errors but effective teams incorporate safety strategies to communicate, monitor each other's work, and prevent injury to patients.

6. Good communication skills for exchanging information and delegating are an essential element of successful teamwork and collaboration.

7. Giving and receiving feedback provides an opportunity for individuals and teams to identify areas for improvement and alter their practice.

8. Health care team members have an ethical duty to work together for the patient's well-being.

9. Difficult or strained communications place patients at risk because team members are afraid to ask questions or confirm practice standards.

10. Nurses can promote teamwork and prevent communication barriers by using strategies to de-escalate tense situations by framing their communications in safety language by using cognitive rehearsal and by reflecting on events to consider opportunities for building consensus.

KEY TERMS

Collaboration	Lateral violence
Communication	Mindfulness
Cross-monitoring	Near miss
Debriefing	Rapid response team
Handoff	Root cause analysis
Interprofessional education	Situational awareness

DISCUSSION OF OPENING SCENARIO

The nurse is frequently the team member who assists the patient and family to connect with other members of the health care team. The interprofessional team may consist of several physicians with specialty expertise in addition to the nurse, physical therapist, nutritionist, and others. Through the nurse's knowledge of interprofessional teamwork and collaboration, the nurse is able to connect the patient and the family to expertise provided by individual team members, as well as coordinate the overall team effort to support the patient and achieve a positive outcome.

CRITICAL THINKING ANSWERS

Critical Thinking 5.1

1. What safety strategy would be most effective for the nurse to use to advocate for the patient in this situation?

Provide constructive feedback on the process of stocking the cart. Identify that feedback is being given because of interest in the nurse's development as well as for patient safety purposes. Provide options on the best way to stock the care to ensure it is accurate.

Critical Thinking 5.2

1. What would be the best approach for the nurse to initiate a discussion with coworkers about the incorrectly stocked cart?

    Wait for a quiet moment later to discuss the situation with the preceptor.

2. What aspects should the nurse focus on during the discussion?

    Ask for examples and verbalize a desire to learn.

3. How can the nurse create a learning experience for coworkers in this instance?

    Ask for advice on increasing speed with tasks.

Critical Thinking 5.3

1. What strategies for difficult communications would be most appropriate to use in this instance?

    Utilizing de-escalation techniques, such as asking for direct feedback, can help to diffuse the tense situation.

2. When should the new-to-practice nurse address this with the preceptor?

    Wait for a quiet moment later to discuss the situation with the preceptor.

3. What would be the new-to-practice nurse's best communication approach with the preceptor?

    Ask for examples and verbalize a desire to learn. Ask for advice on increasing speed with tasks.

Critical Thinking 5.4

1. How can the nurse involve the patient and the family to address the patient's nutrition?

    Consider the patient preferences and involve the family by asking them to bring in food from home.

2. Which members of the interprofessional team would have the expertise to address the patient's nutritional status?

    Seek the assistance of the nutritionist regarding required calorie intake.

3. How can the interprofessional team work together to meet the patient's nutritional needs?

    Discuss the situation with the physician and consider a possible need for the placement of a feeding tube to supplement intake.

CASE STUDY ANSWERS

Case Study 5.1

1. What team stage is identified as the team begins to work to resolve the number of Fridays and weekends that will be required by each staff?

    The team development stage at this point is storming.

2. What team stage is identified when the committee decides to remain intact to assist with the transition and manage the scheduling process?

    The team stage at this point is performing.

Case Study 5.2

1. What standard is your colleague violating?

    The standard being violated is that the medication should not be left at the bedside. Taking it back to the nurse station to give it to the nurse that left it there does not necessarily guarantee that the nurse will understand the implied safety threat.

2. Recognizing that your colleague did not react to your implied concern for the patient's safety and the standard of practice, what communication strategy would you implement to maintain this patient's safety?

    The communication strategy that should be implemented is the CUS strategy. Using the words concerned, uncomfortable, and safety, the nurse can relay to his or her colleague direct safety information. The nurse returning the medications to the nurse station would say "I'm concerned about this medication being left at the bedside. I am uncomfortable with it sitting there unattended. I do not think it is safe." Using this strategy, the safety threat is no longer implied but is directly communicated.

3. How can you address practice concerns like this from an organization's point of view to prevent this type of practice?

    To address this from a systems view, the nurse could provide an educational program to review policy or discuss safety threats of leaving medications at the bedside with colleagues during a staff meeting.

REVIEW QUESTIONS

Please see Appendix D for answers to Review Questions.

1. A nurse receives a telephone order from a physician for specific x-ray tests. The nurse established the identity of the patient involved and the name of the ordering physician. Which of the following should the nurse do next?

    A. Write the order on the order sheet in the chart.
    B. Repeat what the physician says and then write it down on the order sheet.
    C. Ask the physician to directly place the order with the radiology department.
    D. Write the order on the order sheet and then perform a read-back to the physician to verify the order is accurate.

2. The nurse is informed that an RRT will be initiated at the hospital to better meet the needs of patients. Which of the following best describes the way in which the nurse should utilize the RRT?

   A. Provide support for medical–surgical nurses and decrease the number of patients experiencing an arrest that requires ICU admission.
   B. Rapidly move patients through the hospital system at the time of patient transfers.
   C. Notify the attending physician of the patient's deteriorating status.
   D. Provide immediate assistance to patients in the ICU.

3. The nurse is transferring a patient from the ICU to the step-down patient care unit. When the ICU nurse calls report to the receiving unit, what is the best way for the nurse to provide the handoff information?

   A. Situation, background, assessment, requirements
   B. Situation, background, assessment, recommendations
   C. Systems, background, activities, recommendations
   D. Systems, background, activities, requirements

4. The nurse pages a physician due to the patient's change in status. When the physician calls the unit, the physician yells at the nurse for interrupting dinner. Which of the following would be the nurse's best approach?

   A. Tell the physician that this interaction must be reported to the nursing supervisor.
   B. Tell the physician that the nurse is only doing the required job and it is wrong to yell.
   C. Refocus the communication on the patient and the reason for the call.
   D. Apologize for interrupting the dinner and page his partner.

5. The nurse attends an interprofessional meeting to discuss the care of a patient who is a paraplegic after an automobile accident. Which of the following best describes the purpose of assembling an interprofessional team?

   A. To provide multiple perspectives to contribute to the patient's care and well-being
   B. To divide the work appropriately among disciplines
   C. To ensure that the all disciplines support the physician's goals for the patient
   D. To provide support in difficult patient care situations

6. Following a serious medication error that resulted in patient injury, a nurse is assigned to a team assembled to investigate the cause. The nurse knows which of the following represents the best method for doing so?

   A. RCA
   B. Debriefing
   C. Six Sigma
   D. CRM

7. The nurse on the oncology unit cares for a patient who frequently comments that she would like better pain control through the night. The nurse tells the patient that a note will be placed on the front of the patient's chart alerting the physician in case the nurse misses the physician during her rounds. Which of the following represents a better process to ensure the patient's needs are met?

   A. Nursing rounds
   B. Team huddle
   C. Debriefing
   D. RCA

8. A patient's family is angry about their family member's deteriorating condition and tells the nurse that they are not satisfied with the patient's care. Which of the following would be the most appropriate action by the nurse?

   A. Notify hospital administration.
   B. Explain to the family that the patient's condition is complex and that the patient is receiving appropriate care.
   C. Convey understanding and notify members of the health care team so that a family meeting with the team can be provided.
   D. Ask the family members why they feel this way.

9. Which of the following processes would best assist the nurse to increase expertise, adjust practice, and improve self-regulation?

   A. Conduct an RCA
   B. Elicit constructive feedback from others
   C. Participate in debriefing
   D. Use the CUS technique

10. Skilled communications is essential to patient safety for which of the following reasons?

   A. Patients need to be convinced to receive specific treatments.
   B. Nurses need to explain procedures to patients.
   C. Miscommunication is responsible for many harmful events in the hospital.
   D. Poor quality of care is associated with poor communication.

REVIEW ACTIVITIES

Please see Appendix E for answers to Review Activities.

1. A patient calls the nurse into the room and complains of shortness of breath. The patient was admitted yesterday for pulmonary edema and has been successfully treated with nasal oxygen at 4 L, and furosemide (Lasix) 40 mg IV every 12 hours. The nurse determines that the patient's respiratory rate is 30, the pulse oximetry reading is 91%, and auscultation of the lungs reveals crackles half way up the back.

   Using SBAR technique, provide report to the physician regarding the above patient.

2. The nurse believes the dose of a medication ordered for a patient is too high and may be dangerous for the patient to receive. What communication strategy would the nurse implement to verbalize this? How would it be implemented?

3. The nurse receives a critical lab result via telephone from the laboratory. What safety strategy should the nurse implement to ensure safety regarding the lab value?

EXPLORING THE WEB

1. Access the web resources in Table 5.4.
2. Review the websites listed in Table 5.4. What do you identify as the consistent theme or focus of all of these websites?
3. What strategies do you see on these websites that would enhance teamwork?

REFERENCES

Agency for Healthcare Research and Quality (AHRQ). (n.d.). *TeamSTEPPS™ fundamentals course: Module 1. Introduction: Instructor's slides.* Retrieved from http://www.ahrq.gov/teamstepp-stools/instructor/fundamentals/module1/igintro.htm

Becher, J., & Visovsky, C. (2012). Horizontal violence in nursing. *Medsurg Nursing, 21*(4), 210–213.

Carter, P. (2010). Six sigma. *American Association of Occupational Health Nurses Journal, 58*(12), 508–510.

Clynes, M. P., & Raftery, S. E. C. (2008). Feedback: An essential element of student learning in clinical practice. *Nurse Education in Practice, 8*, 405–411.

Griffin, M. (2004). Teaching cognitive rehearsal as a shield for lateral violence: An intervention for newly licensed nurses. *The Journal of Continuing Education in Nursing, 3*(6), 257–263.

Hattie, J., & Timperley, H. (2007). The power of feedback. *Review of Educational Research, 77*(1), 81–112.

Institute for Health Care Improvement (IHI). (2012). *Deploy rapid response teams.* Retrieved from http://www.ihi.org/explore/RapidResponseTeams/Pages/default.aspx

Institute of Medicine (IOM). (2010). *The future of nursing: Leading change advancing health.* Retrieved from http://www.iom.edu/Reports/2010/The-Future-of-Nursing-Leading-Change-Advancing-Health.aspx

McBride, A. B. (2010). Toward a roadmap for interdisciplinary academic career success. *Research and Theory for Nursing Practice: An International Journal, 24*(1), 74–86.

National Council of State Boards of Nursing. (2005). *Working with others: A position paper.* Retrieved from https://www.ncsbn.org/Working_with_Others.pdf

Petri, L. (2010). Concept analysis of interdisciplinary collaboration. *Nursing Forum, 45*(2), 73–81.

Tanner, C. A. (2006). Thinking like a nurse: A research based model of clinical judgment in nursing. *Journal of Nursing Education, 4*(6), 204–211.

The Joint Commission. (n.d.). *The universal protocol for preventing wrong site, wrong procedure, and wrong person surgery: Guidance for health care professionals.* Retrieved from http://www.joint-commission.org/assets/1/18/UP_Poster.pdf

Tuckman, B. (1965). Developmental sequence in small groups. *Psychological Bulletin, 63*(6), 384–99. doi:10.1037/h0022100

Unknown participant. (June 2007). *Quality and safety education for nurses collaboration.* Chicago, IL.

U. S. Department of Health and Human Services. (2010a). *The registered nurse population.* Retrieved from http://bhpr.hrsa.gov/healthworkforce/rnsurveys/rnsurveyinitial2008.pdf

U. S. Department of Health and Human Services. (2010b). *The physician workforce: Projections and research into current issues affecting supply and demand.* Retrieved from http://bhpr.hrsa.gov/healthworkforce/reports/physwfissues.pdf

Weick, K. E., & Sutcliffe, K. M. (2001). *Managing the unexpected.* San Francisco, CA: Jossey-Bass.

SUGGESTED READING

Agency for Healthcare Research and Quality (AHRQ). (2011). *Preventing avoidable readmissions*. Retrieved from http://www.ahrq.gov/qual/impptdis.htm

American Nurses Association (ANA). (2001). *Code of ethics for nurses with interpretive statements*. Retrieved from http://nursingworld.org/MainMenuCategories/EthicsStandards/CodeofEthicsforNurses/Code-of-ethics.pdf

Cronenwett, L., Sherwood, G., Barnsteiner, J., Disch, J., Johnson, J., Mitchell, P.,...Warren, J. (2007). Quality and safety education for nurses. *Nursing Outlook, 55*(3), 112–131.

Halbesleben, J. R. B., Wakefield, D. S., & Wakefield, B. J. (2008). Work-arounds in the health care setting: Literature review and research agenda. *Health Care Manager Review, 33*(1), 2–12.

Institute of Medicine (IOM). (2003). *Health professions education: A bridge to quality*. Washington, DC: National Academies Press.

Kramer, M., & Schmalenberg, C. (2008). Confirmation of a healthy work environment. *Critical Care Nurse, 28*(2), 56–64.

Leach, L. S., & Mayo, A. M. (2013). Rapid response teams: Qualitative analysis of their effectiveness. *American Journal of Critical Care, 22*(3), 109–210.

6

PATIENT-CENTERED CARE

Esther Bankert, Andrea Lazarek-LaQuay,
and Joanne M. Joseph

Transforming Health Care One Nurse, One Caregiver, One Organization, At a Time. (Dr. Jean
Watson, 2012, World Caring Science Institute, watsoncaringscience.org)

Upon completion of this chapter, the reader should be able to

1. Describe characteristics of patient-centered care (PCC)
2. Identify basic components of empathetic communication and describe its importance to PCC
3. Discuss the psychosocial factors associated with the impact physical illness and injury
4. List strategies to support patient-centered health care
5. Describe the impact of legislation such as the Patient Protection and Affordable Care Act in facilitating PCC
6. Discuss discharge planning as a means of ensuring continuity of care
7. List information technologies that facilitate PCC
8. Explain the significance of patient-centered measures and monitors of quality health care
9. Describe the importance of patient satisfaction relative to measuring the accomplishment of PCC

---

*Y*ou are a clinician on a very busy medical–surgical unit. Mrs. Rodriguez is a 76-year-old patient who suffered a stroke and is being discharged within the next few days. She is a widow whose children live an hour away and her most frequent visitor is the priest from her church.

Each day, the interprofessional team completes rounds on the unit. As the contact point for Mrs. Jones and her family, you have been directed by the charge nurse to communicate the discharge plan to the patient and family/designee.

- *Before you can effectively participate in the interprofessional team rounds, what must you understand about your patient?*
- *What are some interventions that will support an effective care transition for this patient?*
- *Who will be key contact points in the family to ensure patient continuity of care posthospitalization?*

Decades ago a paradigm shift to caring within health care settings was introduced that emphasized moving from a technocratic focus to establishing caring relationships, identifying the patient as a consumer of care to recognizing the patient as a partner in care, and providing service from the perspective of the expert provider for health care services to the perspective of the collaborative partnership between patient and provider for health care services. This new paradigm embraces values, relationships, and preferences, recognizing the patient as a participant in his own care. Although this paradigm shift has taken time to be accepted within a highly technological and authoritative health care system, it has awakened the need for nursing and health care providers to support the patient's role in control of his own health care decisions.

Currently, many federal initiatives are being implemented to address the need for quality care and patient safety and are transforming health care settings into accountable, safe, patient-centered environments that respect the unique needs and values of the patient. This process of transformation within health care has evolved into providing compassionate care that recognizes the patient as an integral member of the interprofessional team. With patients central to all services, nurses and health care providers are establishing true, collaborative relationships as partners in health care service to address health care needs through the lens of the patient.

Thus, the chapter focuses on strategies and practices that support PCC that aims to improve patient safety and the quality patient care. Characteristics of PCC are discussed as are the components of communication that help to ensure it is actualized. Psychosocial factors associated with the realities of disease and illness are described within the context of how the interprofessional team can implement strategies that support patient-centered health care. Legislation impacting the ability to deliver PCC are presented. Innovations that foster PCC are discussed including how continuity of care is augmented. with effective discharge planning and use of novel technologies empowering patients to function as integral members of the interprofessional health care team. Lastly, patient-centered measures and monitors of quality health care and measurements of patient satisfaction are presented in relation to PCC.

PCC

Patient-centered care (PCC) "recognizes the patient or designee as the source of control and full partner in providing compassionate and coordinated care based on respect for patient's preferences, values, and needs" (Quality and Safety Education for Nurses, 2012, p. 1). Nurses and health care providers coordinate patient care services with compassion and respect through a collaborative partnership between the patient and interprofessional team. Today, with nurse leaders in the forefront of health care services, the Institute of Medicine (IOM) as well as other national campaigns for quality care have drawn attention to the necessity of maintaining safety, providing quality care, and keeping the patient at the center and in control of his or her care to meet his or her health needs. This attention is intended to ensure that all health care providers are accountable for quality care through centered care services, careful monitoring of patient outcomes, and validation of improvement in the patient's health. It is paramount that nurses and health care providers recognize that the patient is a full partner within the interprofessional team and that the patient is in control of his or her care. PCC is a new way of practicing and providing care through the lens of the patient with respect for his or her values, his or her meaning of health, and his or her preferences.

REAL-WORLD INTERVIEW

Our patients and families are at the center of care in the radiology department. Our main goal in the radiology department is to bring the best safe quality care to every patient and family member every time. With the patient and family at the center of care, we are able to cater to their unique needs, and preferences and work to ensure that the organization develops a relationship that is centered on the patient as a partner. We identify this relationship at our hospital as relationship-based care (RBC). RBC focuses on building caring relationships with the people of the community we serves; it helps our organizations develop great leadership through teamwork and quality outcomes. We also feel that RBC enhances our passion for the people we care for and the career we have chosen. There is no better feeling in the world then caring for someone and helping them through their time of need. We feel focusing on the patient and our relationship with the patient is a great approach to care in our organization.

Sean Whip, RT (R), CT AS
Radiology Director at Faxton/St. Luke's Health Care
Utica, New York

Advocacy

Serving as an advocate to patients is a hallmark of PCC and is an essential component of nursing and leadership within the interprofessional health care team. Advocacy refers to any activity that ultimately assists a patient in receiving the "best" care depending on the patient's needs and wishes. Florence Nightingale emphasized nurses must keep the patient central to nursing care, an obligation that remains embodied in nursing's application of values such as beneficence and fidelity (Bradshaw, 1999; Hoyt, 2010). Patient empowerment reflects a form of self-directed advocacy that enables and motivates patients to bring about changes and make decisions to manage and improve their health (Bann, Sirois, & Walsh, 2010). Through a patient-centered approach to advocacy and empowerment, a partnership between the caregiver and the patient can increase the patient's autonomy and involvement in his or her own care (Holmstrom & Roing, 2009).

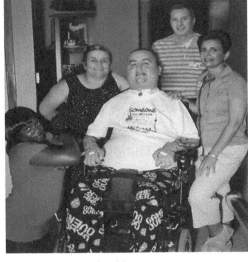

A patient with his health care team.

Critical Thinking 6.1

Consider the following situation and identify the nurse's behaviors associated with promoting the patient's sense of control over her care. Mrs. Dawes is in a subacute rehabilitation facility recovering from a knee replacement. Sue Jones is her primary nurse. Nurse Jones approaches Mrs. Dawes, introduces herself, and asks Mrs. Dawes how she would like to be addressed. She also reviews with Mrs. Dawes what she might expect from the rehabilitation program and how she might deal with the discomfort that could result from her therapy. Nurse Jones also gives Mrs. Dawes her choices of times for therapy and menus for meal selection. She answers all her questions and provides her with the list of her therapies.

1. How has Nurse Jones engaged the patient in a number of behaviors that would likely increase Mrs. Dawes's perception of her ability to impact her own health?
2. What are strategies Nurse Jones could have implemented to include with others on the interprofessional team at the onset of her meeting Mrs. Dawes to ensure advocacy and PCC?

REAL-WORLD INTERVIEW

As a practicing nurse, I encourage health promotion and empowerment for my patient and their family. I see caring as a fundamental value of nursing within a holistic and collaborative approach to nursing care. I embrace understanding the meaning of health from the perspective of the patient. I also believe to practice in a patient-centered environment, the nurse and health care team must understand the perspective of the patient and his or her family and significant others. As I practice, I see myself grow as I collaborate with the patient as a key member of the health care team. As one member of the health care team, I advocate for my patient and family to promote their health and support their wishes.

Amy Weaver, CCRN, BS
Graduate Student in Nursing Education, SUNYIT
Utica, New York

EMPATHETIC COMMUNICATION

Empathetic communication is simply the act of communicating with someone else from the vantage point of their feelings, values, perspective, and is at the foundation of establishing relationships that are consistent with PCC. When using empathetic communication, the nurse and patient enter into a relationship characterized by both empathy and a genuine sense of respect for the patient's opinions and decisions. To better understand the nature of empathetic communication, the nurse and health care provider must first recognize the difference between empathy and sympathy, be

TABLE 6.1 EMPATHETIC AND NONEMPATHETIC COMMUNICATION BEHAVIORS

EMPATHETIC COMMUNICATION	NONEMPATHETIC COMMUNICATION
Listens carefully and reflect back a summary of the patient's concerns	Interrupts patient with irrelevant information
Uses terms and vocabulary that is appropriate for the patient	Uses vocabulary that is either beneath the level of the patient or not understandable to the patient
Calls patient by patient's preferred name	Uses language that may be perceived as cajoling, patronizing, or demeaning, for example, honey
Uses respectful and professional language	Uses nonprofessional language
Asks patient what they need and responds promptly to those needs	Chastises patient
Provides helpful and informative information	Provides patient with inappropriate information
Solicits feedback from the patient	Asks questions at inappropriate times and gives patient advice inappropriately
Uses self-disclosure appropriately	Self-discloses inappropriately
Employs humor as appropriate	Preaches to the patient
Provides words of comfort when appropriate	Scolds the patient

proficient in the basic elements of communication and appreciate the major psychosocial factors associated with the role of patient.

Sympathy and Empathetic Communication

While empathy and sympathy are highly related concepts as well as integral to the provision of PCC, they are distinct and different (Decety & Michalska, 2010). Empathy involves the ability to understand and share the emotional experience observed in another person. Sympathy by contrast is defined as emotional concern for another (Kunzmann, 2011). Effective communication begins with empathy. Empathetic communication has three essential components: the ability to take the perspective of another; the ability to appreciate the emotions of another, even when they are different from your own; and the ability to communicate that understanding to the patient (Burks & Kobus, 2012; Okun & Kantrowitz, 2008). There are a number of behaviors that facilitate empathetic communication and thus PCC. Likewise, there are behaviors that hinder empathetic communication and thereby impede PCC. Table 6.1 lists a representative sample of empathetic and nonempathetic communication behaviors.

CASE STUDY 6.1

On morning rounds, a doctor and nurse enter a patient's room to assess him in preparation for his cardiac catheterization scheduled later in the day. The nurse introduces herself to the patient, "Good morning, Mr. Potter, I am Jane Smith,

(continued)

CASE STUDY 6.1 (continued)

the nurse, and I will be assisting Dr. Turk with the procedure today." Mr. Potter replies, "Okay, I hope you know what you are doing. I am already in pain and I don't need you to add to it." Mr. Potter's emotional undertones are obviously hostile and offensive.

1. *How do you think Jane Smith, the nurse, felt when listening to hostile tones in the patient's voice and remarks toward her competency?*
2. *How can you respond maintaining a respectful and open dialogue between you and the patient?*
3. *How would you respond if the doctor or another member of the interprofessional team was criticizing your skills and competency in caring for a patient?*
4. *How could you respond maintaining a respectful relationship with the health care team?*

Elements of Communication

Communication simultaneously takes place verbally and nonverbally. Verbal communication has a cognitive (what we say) and affective (emotional) component, while nonverbal communication has a behavioral (what we do) and affective (emotional) component. To communicate effectively, the listener must attend to all elements of the communication process. This is not always easy to do although particularly important to remember in terms of providing PCC.

CASE STUDY 6.2

As a senior nursing student, you are under much pressure to follow PowerPoint slides, listen to the lecture, and take notes, all at the same time! You ask a friend if you can borrow her notes from class so you can be sure you have everything you need for the next test. Your friend verbally agrees but places her notes in her book bag and immediately leaves the room. You try to contact her later that day, but she does not respond to your calls, texts, or e-mails.

1. *What are major factors underlying the communication process?*

Nonverbal Communication

Sometimes the verbal and nonverbal components of a patient's communication are incongruent and provide conflicting messages. For example, a patient might verbally indicate that nothing is bothering him or her but his or her nonverbal body language is communicating something quite different (Table 6.2). The empathetic communicator must discern

TABLE 6.2 EXAMPLES OF NONVERBAL BEHAVIOR

NONVERBAL BEHAVIOR	EXAMPLES
Eye movement and features	Either steady eye contact or inability to make eye contact, blinking, teary eyes opened or closed
Body position, movement, behavior, and stance	Tense, relaxed, jerky, fidgety, legs crossed, arms crossed, agitated, calm, use of hands, gestures
Facial expression	Grimaces, smiles, frowns, no expression or flat affect, exaggerated expression
Tone of voice	Mumbles, whispers, high pitched, quiet; rate of speech either speedy or slowed
Skin	Blushes, sweats, general pallor
General appearance	Appropriateness of dress for weather and/or event, neatness, accessories, stature

the real meaning behind the patient's verbal and nonverbal behavior. It is the nonverbal aspect of the communication that provides nurses and health care providers with the most important clues about inner feelings (Egan, 1986). For example, if your patient states he or she is not afraid to have surgery but looks away from you and or begins wringing his or her hands as you discuss his or her upcoming operation, you should think to yourself that your patient's words do not match his or her nonverbal communication.

Cultural Influences and Beliefs on Communication

Smiles, warm gestures, and welcoming words are universal signs of caring in most cultures. Nurses and other interprofessional members of the health care team, however, must also realize that expressions of caring and the interpretation of caring acts are perceived differently across cultures. Communication between the patient and provider is essential to understand the patient's needs and perspectives of healthy outcomes. However, there are many factors that can affect the quality and clarity of communications and health care providers must be proactive to address any potential barriers. For example, language barriers may be present and the use of interpreters can provide a safe space where patients can freely express their concerns and be understood through the interpreter, calming their fears and apprehensions in an unfamiliar situation and setting. While bilingual family members can be appropriately used for basic exchanges of information, communication of complex health care information may require the help of other interpreters. When bilingual family member interpreters are not available in person, health care providers can access trained interpreters through various certified telephone services, for example, CTS Language Link, which can be accessed through its website at http://www.cts-languagelink.com. Certified health care interpreters can help all parties understand

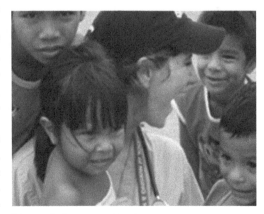

Nonverbal communication.

the strengths and needs of the patient and family. Effective patient-centered communication, even when done through an interpreter, provides an opportunity for a personal exchange between patient and provider that fosters clarity and understanding of what is needed to continue the patient's care and include the patient as an active partner in the recovery process. Patience and fortitude in understanding the patient's cultural norms and health care practices that are unique to the patient's culture must be respected.

Critical Thinking 6.2

Nurse Johnson is caring for a patient newly diagnosed with diabetes. The patient speaks English as a second language and is a recent immigrant to the United States. The patient is able to make her basic needs known but does not ask questions or speak unless prompted to do so. Nurse Johnson has been unable to determine if this patient can self-inject her insulin. The patient nods and smiles as Nurse Johnson begins teaching her about insulin and her diagnosis.

1. What strategies can Nurse Johnson employ to facilitate self-management in this patient?
2. What resources and/or services can the nurse use to ensure that the patient has understood the instruction?

PSYCHOSOCIAL FACTORS ASSOCIATED WITH THE ROLE OF THE PATIENT

Understanding how a person's life is affected by illness is essential in understanding patient reactions and emotions. This level of understanding leads to the ability to take another's perspective and is a precursor to empathetic communication, the cornerstone of PCC (Burks & Kobus, 2012). Being a patient is a role that most people find challenging. This is because illness can greatly impact a person's self-concept (Taylor, 2011). For a better understanding of the impact of illness on the patient, nurses and health care providers in PCC settings need to understand self-concept and the impact illness has on how one perceives oneself. **Self-concept** is the conception an individual holds about his or her own particular traits, aptitudes, and unique characteristics; it typically includes physical, social, and personal components (Taylor, 2011).

Physical self refers to the conception a person has of his or her physical body and physical capacities. Illness and chronic illness impact a person's physical self because it changes how an individual evaluates his or her body. Consider for example, a newly diagnosed breast cancer patient facing a mastectomy. The mastectomy has the potential of challenging her perception of herself as a woman. The mastectomy might also change the patient's conception of how she sees herself sexually. Social self involves the roles the individual holds in a social environment. In the case of the breast cancer patient, the mastectomy might affect the patient's social self as a wife and member of the community. A serious illness may change the social self the patient has in his or her family or work situation. Serious illness and injury may change the role of family breadwinner to the dependent person requiring care and assistance. Personal self embodies all the goals and dreams we have for ourselves now and in the future. Illness or injury sometimes prohibits the realization of those goals and dreams. For example, the young high school football star may have had aspirations of becoming a professional football player. A serious injury on the field may thwart those plans forever.

CASE STUDY 6.3

Mary is a 28-year-old female in the prime of her life. Mary has completed her master's degree in education and is employed as a kindergarten teacher, which she absolutely loves. She has always been independent and enjoyed being single. Mary developed generalized pain that progressively worsened over the course of 2 years. Mary also found that her general energy level was low and she could no longer concentrate for any length of time. Mary sought medical care and was diagnosed with fibromyalgia. She was forced to give up her kindergarten job and found herself not only in pain but frustrated professionally. She believes the fibromyalgia has impacted her physically and professionally.

1. *How can chronic illness impact Mary's perspective on her personal life?*
2. *Explore the web for support services that are available to her at home; what might a few services be?*

STRATEGIES TO SUPPORT PATIENT-CENTERED PRACTICE

As discussed earlier, the IOM's (2001) report identified specific aims to improve the quality and safety of health care. Among these aims, the patient-centered model of care has become a core component that ensures patient values and guides clinical decisions. Through this patient-centered model of care, the health care industry is called upon to develop innovative strategies to support patients and caregivers in becoming greater participants in their health care. Patient-centered outcomes research emphasizes decision making between the patient and provider that is collaborative, mutual, and shared. Health literacy is one major factor grounded in informed decision making. Thus, many innovative strategies exist to enhance PCC including methods for increasing health literacy.

Alleviating Barriers to Health Care Literacy

Considering a patient's health literacy is crucial to providing PCC. Ratzan and Parker's (2000) definition of **health literacy** is used in the IOM's (2004) consensus report on health literacy as "the degree to which individuals have the capacity to obtain, process, and understand basic health information and services they need to make appropriate health decisions" (p. 31). A patient's basic education and competencies in reading, writing, and mathematics are important components of his or her health literacy as well as skills such as listening and speaking. Those patients and families with limited health literacy skills and knowledge do not have the same resources, ability, or competencies to achieve optimal health services as those who are health literate. Language barriers and poorly understood cultural practices may also adversely impact health care communication. Populations vulnerable to low levels of health literacy include ethnic minority groups, recent immigrants, older adults and elderly populations, individuals living with chronic diseases, and populations of people at poverty or even lower socioeconomic class (Center for Health Care Strategies, Inc., 2010).

The issue of health literacy is very complex and requires a multidimensional approach by the interprofessional health care team to understand the impact that it has on healthy lifestyles, engagement in health promotion activities, self-efficacy, and optimizing one's potential for well-being. Nurse leaders must recognize that the health care system and the educational system, as well as social and cultural factors, all play a role on the impact of health literacy. Healthy People 2020 (U.S. Department of Health and Human Services [USDHHS], 2011c) has identified improving health literacy as one of its key goals to promoting healthy outcomes and enhancing quality of life. In the past, health literacy was considered a task of educators and viewed from the perspective of the patient's intellectual deficits. Today, health literacy is recognized as a health care system's issue.

Health literacy is ensured when nurses and the interprofessional health care team reinforce pertinent information with the patient through simple explanations that avoid medical jargon. Patients must understand their role and what it is they need to do to safely follow dietary and health care treatments. They must understand why quality of care requires adherence to prescribed medications and the importance of communicating with their provider when encountering difficulties. Health care practitioners must encourage patients to ask questions and take an active role in their education to improve care activities. Patients who are well informed and more involved in their care experience better health outcomes (USDHHS, 2010b). Patient initiatives, such as Ask Me 3 (National Patient Safety Foundation, 2011) and Questions Are the Answer (Agency for Healthcare Research and Quality [AHRQ], 2011b) are campaigns designed to promote communication and encourage patients to seek and understand the answers to common questions, that is: What is my main problem? What do I need to do? Why is it important for me to do this? Patient safety can be improved when patients understand their role in their health care.

EVIDENCE FROM THE LITERATURE

Citation

Stiles, E. (2011). Promoting health literacy in patients with diabetes. *Nursing Standard, 26*(8), 35–40.

Discussion

Patients with low health literacy may struggle with obtaining, understanding, and applying health information. Complex health care conditions such as diabetes mellitus are long-term conditions that require good patient understanding to experience positive outcomes. Strategies to help improve low health literacy include a patient-centered approach to improve communication between clinicians and patients with diabetes, providing information to patients in various formats, and improving patient access to services

(continued)

> ### Implications for Practice
>
> Nurses play a critical role in assessing and improving health literacy, especially for patients with complex chronic conditions. Culturally appropriate, individualized teaching strategies with methods such as with the use of teach back methods can reduce the impact of low health literacy, help improve PCC, and help achieve patient self-management. The "teach back" method has also been referred to as the "show me" method and is a way for nurses and other members of the interprofessional health care team to verify what was provided as education was received and understood correctly. In this technique or method of education, the patient explains to the person giving the education what was taught thus confirming or validating the information was accurately heard and comprehended.

LEGISLATION THAT SUPPORTS PATIENT-CENTERED PRACTICES

In March 2010, Congress passed the Patient Protection and Affordable Care Act (PPACA), whose legislation increases access to health insurance coverage, expands federal health insurance market requirements, and includes measures to improve the delivery and quality of car (www.innovations.cms.gov). PPACA is being implemented in a number of ways through new agency programs, grants, demonstration projects, and regulations. Under PPACA, the Centers for Medicare and Medicaid Innovation has been established to pilot payment and service delivery models driven by the need for patient-centered quality care and fiscal responsibility. Centers for Medicare and Medicaid Services (CMS, 2012) have established pilot payment and service delivery models driven by the need for patient-centered quality care and fiscal responsibility.

Patient-Centered Medical Home (PCMH)

As health care reformers seek to improve outcomes and reduce costs, the PCMH has become a major strategy in the transformation of primary care and the health care system in general (Landon, Gill, Antonelli, & Rich, 2010; Table 6.3). The Medical Homes concept includes operational characteristics of primary care that is accessible, continuous, comprehensive, family/patient centered, coordinated, compassionate, and culturally sensitive (American College of Physicians [ACP], 2006).

Patient-Centered Primary Care Collaborative (PCPCC)

In 2006, the PCPCC emerged after several large national employers sought the assistance of the ACP, the Academy of Family Physicians, and other primary care physician groups to address the issue of a failing system of comprehensive primary care. Goals of the PCPCC were to enable improvements in patient–physician relations and develop a more effective and efficient model of care delivery. The PCPCC has taken a significant interest in the development and advocacy of the PCMH model as a means to ensure the delivery of only the highest standards of effective and efficient PCC (PCPCC, 2011).

TABLE 6.3 PRINCIPLES OF THE PATIENT-CENTERED MEDICAL HOME

All patients have a personal provider of primary care	Every patient has a provider trained to deliver continuous, comprehensive care from the first patient contact throughout an ongoing patient–provider relationship.
Health care team is primary care provider directed	Under the leadership of the personal primary care provider, an interprofessional health care team takes responsibility for the ongoing care of patients.
Personal provider is responsible for all the patient's health care needs	A personal primary care provider takes the lead on providing or coordinating patient care with qualified professionals to meet all of the patient's health care needs throughout the stages of life, that is, acute care, chronic care, preventive services, and end-of-life care.
Personal provider ensures coordinated/integrated care	Across the continuum of care, the personal primary care provider implements interventions to ensure that patients receive culturally appropriate care at the right time and place (hospital, subspecialty care, home health, nursing home) for their level of need.
Personal provider pursues quality and safety of care	The personal primary care provider along with other interprofessional health care team members advocate for patients in the pursuit of optimal patient-centered outcomes guided by the use of the following principles: • Evidence-based medicine and clinical decision-support tools • Continuous quality improvement (QI) • Active patient participation in decision making and use of patient feedback to ensure expectations are being met • Information technology to support optimal patient care, performance measurement, patient education, and improved communication • Accreditation/certification of the personal primary care provider's practice to demonstrate its ability to deliver patient-centered care (PCC) consistent with the Medical Home model • Patient and family involvement in quality improvement activities
Patients have enhanced access to care	Open efforts are made to increase availability of providers as well as other members of the interprofessional health care team through flexible scheduling, extended office hours, and expanded communication options.
Proper payment to providers	Payment structure should reflect the added value provided to patients under the care of a patient-centered Medical Home.

Source: American Academy of Family Physicians (AAFP), American Academy of Pediatrics (AAP), American College of Physicians (ACP), American Osteopathic Association (AOA). (2011).

Health Home Model

The same PPACA that supports the Medical Home initiative also provides financial incentives for the development of Health Homes (CMS, 2012). Health Homes are designed to be patient-centered systems of care that enable access to and coordination of care throughout the health care continuum, that is, primary, acute, behavioral, and long-term community-based care. The Health Home model expands on the Medical Home model by moving beyond primary care to better meet the needs of patients with multiple chronic conditions. By enhancing coordination and integration of medical and behavioral health care, health homes provide comprehensive care for patients.

The Health Home model supports the CMS's approach to improving health care by improving the patient's care experience; improving the health of populations; and reducing the costs of health care (CMS, 2010). The implementation of Health Homes is expected to reduce emergency room use, reduce hospital admissions and readmissions, reduce health care costs, and become less reliant on long-term facilities, while improving overall patient satisfaction and quality outcomes.

DISCHARGE PLANNING AND CARE CONTINUITY

As health care reforms and payment structures attempt to balance the efficiency and efficacy of care, acute health care systems are facing shorter lengths of stay and rapid patient turnover. These factors can all too often contribute to fragmented patient care, for example, patients discharged while still recovering from an illness or disease exacerbation. The acuity of the patients' condition may still require continued care services and careful monitoring by his or her primary care provider and health care team. Patients transitioning between care settings and providers are at risk for potentially avoidable hospitalizations and increased health care spending (Naylor, Aiken, Kurtzman, Olds, & Hirschman, 2011). There is a call for improved patient communication handoffs to avoid common mistakes that can occur as the patient transitions from one level of care to another (Ventura, Brown, Archibald, Goroski, & Brock, 2010). Avoiding patient rehospitalization is a key priority for hospitals with higher than expected readmission rates as they will now be facing financial penalties enacted by the PPACA (Hansen, Young, Hinami, Leung, & Williams, 2011). Hospitals are implementing various initiatives and comprehensive programs such as Project BOOST (Better Outcomes for Older Adults through Safe Transitions; Society of Hospital Medicine, 2012) and Project RED (Re-Engineered Discharge; Boston University School of Medicine, 2012) to facilitate safe patient discharges that will support patients in their transition from hospital to home and prevent unnecessary readmissions to the hospital (AHRQ, 2011a). These programs also provide toolkits with various interventions and practices that can help health care providers be successful, that is, risk assessment tools and how to implement specific discharge strategies. Despite using these tools, discharge planning is complex and must be individualized to each patient.

Continuity of care is aided by the use of care transition and coordination models designed to improve the quality of care by reducing fragmentation of care and enhancing coordination and continuity of care for patients with multiple health and social needs as they receive care across the continuum (Boutwell, Griffin, Hwu, & Shannon, 2009). These models often use a number of patient-centered approaches such as patient navigators, advocates, and medication reconciliation.

Patient Navigators

Patient navigators are clinical staff members who are paired with a patient to support, educate, and facilitate their interactions throughout their experience of care within a hospital during their outpatient treatment. The concept of patient navigation has developed into a process of advocacy and engagement in the provision of high-quality PCC (Koh, Nelson, & Cook, 2011). For example, patient navigators are frequently used in oncology where patients typically need to take in a great deal of information about their diagnosis and treatment as well as coordinate care among many providers such as oncologists, their nurses, radiologists, and social workers. Patient navigation is designed to reduce patient care barriers and improve patient satisfaction and health outcomes. However, because this initiative is fairly new, more research and evaluation is needed to demonstrate the extent to which this initiative has been effective.

Patient Advocates

As discussed earlier, **patient advocacy** is a hallmark of PCC and health care professionals. In addition to advocacy that is integral to the care provided by the interprofessional team, health care organizations are making every effort to ensure patients are well informed and take an active role in their care. Some hospitals have created patient advocate positions, which provide a means to increase the flow of information to patients and staff, address patient concerns, and provide emotional support to patients and families. Patient advocates serve as a central point of contact for patients, families, physicians, nurses, and other health care staff and assist patients by responding to foreseeable or preventable breaks in service. Patient advocates are an integral part of ensuring that meaningful services are available. They enhance patient and staff communication and improve patient care services rendered. For example, a patient advocate can help a patient scheduled for surgery seeks all options to anesthesia. They can help the patient formulate the questions he or she need answers to. They can also help ensure the patient's wishes are carried out when the patient can't speak for himself or herself. The patient can also request the patient advocate accompany him or her to testing and examinations when allowed. The patient advocate can be someone supplied by the hospital and may be a nurse or social worker; however, the position does not require medical or health care training. The patient advocate may also be a friend or family member of the patient. The key to this person and/or position is that the person be someone the patients trust and someone who can effectively communicate for the patients if they are unable to speak for themselves.

EVIDENCE FROM THE LITERATURE

Citation

Buila, S. M. D., & Swanke, J. R. (2010). Patient-centered mental health care: Encouraging caregiver participation. *Care Management Journal, 11*(3), 146–150.

Discussion

Caregivers play a vital role when caring for loved ones suffering from mental illness. Viewing caregivers as partners within a patient-centered approach to care can improve the quality of care provided. Five major themes emerged from caregiver participants in the suicide prevention workshop discussed in this article. The five themes were that caregivers needed to be included in the mental health care of their family member; expressed concerns related to diagnosing process; stated a need for improved communication with professionals; articulated a desire for individualized, holistic care; and stated a need for service and resource information.

(continued)

Implications for Practice

Nurses and other members of the interprofessional team play an integral part in the treatment of mental illness, particularly in their ability to integrate caregivers into the plan of care. Supporting the perspective of caregivers and recognizing their role as partners in care services will enhance the overall care provided to patients with mental illness.

Critical Thinking 6.3

Teresa is a 10-year-old patient diagnosed with juvenile diabetes. She has been hospitalized four times in the past year for complications related to diabetic diet noncompliance. Teresa is an only child who resides with her parents and maternal grandmother of Italian immigrant decent. She and her family have been in America for 8 years; Teresa and her parents have mastered the English language; and Teresa has been a very good student. Her parents both work at the same factory on the assembly line. A number of interprofessional team members have counseled Teresa and her parents on the risks involved with diabetes and dietary noncompliance. Teresa and her parents seem to understand the importance of following her prescribed diabetic diet. As Teresa's nurse, you notice at this hospitalization that Teresa's grandmother spends a great deal of time with her and appears quite agitated by the fact that her granddaughter is "not getting better." She expresses concern to you about Teresa being readmitted to the hospital yet again.

1. Within a patient-centered environment, how would you approach Teresa's grandmother?
2. Considering Teresa and her parents seem to understand the importance of her dietary intervention, how can the interprofessional health care team collaborate in gathering potential missing information about Teresa's care to discover the cause for her multiple readmissions?

INFORMATION TECHNOLOGIES TO SUPPORT PCC

With the growing use of technology, nurses are keenly aware that the landscape for health care providers has challenged the human connection and patient relationship more than ever before. However, with PCC and collaborative relationships among the interprofessional health care team and the patient, personalized and meaningful services are provided with the patient in control of his or her care. The electronic health record (EHR) creates an opportunity for the interprofessional health care team to ensure the patients remains focal to the health care delivered as well as facilitate active collaboration between the team and the patients themselves. As patient care providers become more adept at electronic data sharing for the provision of continuity of care, many providers offer patients access to their health care record online and encourage them to take responsibility for its accuracy. For example, if a patient accesses his or her EHR online and discovers his or her list of allergies is incomplete, he or she will be expected to update and correct the list. Obviously, inaccurate patient information can lead to negative patient outcomes and health care errors.

Personal Health Record (PHR)

Several initiatives have emerged to help patients build their own PHR such as Microsoft Health Vault (Microsoft, 2012). The Josie King Foundation created a paper and electronic version of a patient journal as a tool to help patients and their families' record details of their care along with the questions to ask and important things to remember (Josie King Foundation, 2012). Hospitals can order the journals to provide patients and their families and/or patients can request a journal for themselves at the Josie King website located at http://www.josieking.org/carejournals. These initiatives are drivers of patient safety and quality care by empowering patients with specific tools to facilitate active engagement in their own health care.

Online Health Information

Patient-driven research (PDR) is an evolving phenomenon that began in the Internet's earliest days. From access to online support groups to access to world-renowned medical centers, patients have access to an incredible amount of online health information they can now use to become an active member of the care team. This access to information gives patients valuable information regarding their conditions, treatment options, best practices, as well as the health care organizations known for their clinical excellence of care delivery. Patient-driven online health care information allows interested patients to be more informed about their choices and raises their level of expectations for quality care and safety when seeking health care services.

Online Patient Communities

Online communities such as the Association of Cancer Online Resources (ACOR) offer a tool for patients to share experiences and learn about diseases and treatments (Frydman, 2009). Ferguson (2007) coined the term **"e-patient"** to identify this new breed of informed health care consumers who are *e*quipped, *e*nabled, *e*mpowered, and *e*ngaged in their health and health care decisions. Health care has responded to this trend through the development of important resources such as the Society for Participatory Medicine and Sharecare.

Participatory medicine is a model of care to support a cooperative approach by all members of the health care team, that is, patients, families, and health care professionals across the full continuum of care. Health care providers are expected to encourage and value patients and families as responsible drivers of their health and not as passengers. Providers who practice participatory medicine promote clinical transparency through the exchange of information and through support for the e-patient movement (Society for Participatory Medicine, 2011).

Sharecare (www.sharecare.org) was launched in 2010 by the founder of WebMD, Jeff Arnold, as an interactive, social question and answer platform for consumers of health care as well as health care professionals. Sharecare has enlisted the nation's leading health experts, care providers, organizations, and brands to become part of the health and wellness dialogue. Sigma Theta Tau, International Honor Society of Nursing, is one of the major content contributors for Sharecare. Users of Sharecare have free access to high-quality, relevant answers to their health questions. These answers are provided by experts, along with interactive health and wellness tools that allow patients to take action on what they have learned as an empowered, informed participant of their own care.

PATIENT-CENTERED MEASURES AND MONITORS OF QUALITY HEALTH CARE

Population-focused health care is care based on the health status and needs assessment of a target group of individuals who have one or more personal or environmental characteristic in common, such as determined by demographics or geography. Public health core functions of assessment and policy development guide the work of population focused health care. The ultimate goal of these policies is improved patient care that is more effective in treating the underlying causes of disease. By examining trends in the etiology and intervention of larger groups, population-focused health care provides information to health care providers that allow them to deliver care that is comprehensive, individualized, and ultimately more effective. The USDHHS is the lead agency responsible for providing essential human services to Americans, particularly those least able to care for themselves. Together with 12 operating divisions and over 300 programs, the USDHHS is charged with protecting the health of all Americans (USDHHS, 2011d).

Strategy for Quality Improvement (QI) in Health Care

The secretary of USDHHS has established a National Strategy for Quality Improvement in Health Care to set priorities that guide the nation to increase access to high-quality, affordable health care for all Americans (USDHHS, 2011b; Table 6.4).

TABLE 6.4 USDHHS NATIONAL STRATEGIES FOR QUALITY IMPROVEMENT IN HEALTH CARE PRIORITIES

PRIORITY	ACTIONS
1. Give safer care	• Exercise relentless effort to reduce risk for injury from care • Aim for ZERO harm to patients • Create health care systems that reliably provide high-quality care
2. Deliver patient- and family-centered care	• Give patients and families an active role in their care • Adapt care to individual and family situations, cultures, languages, disabilities, and health literacy levels
3. Promote effective communication and coordination of care	• Develop processes and use technology to provide seamless care, that is, EHR, e-prescribing, telemedicine • Eliminate health care gaps and duplication of care • Use effective care models to facilitate coordination and communication across the continuum of care
4. Promote effective prevention and treatment of leading causes of mortality: priority, cardiovascular disease	• Practice key interventions for cardiovascular disease, that is, ABCS—aspirin, blood pressure control, cholesterol reduction, and smoking cessation

(continued)

TABLE 6.4 USDHHS NATIONAL STRATEGIES FOR QUALITY IMPROVEMENT IN HEALTH CARE PRIORITIES (*continued*)

PRIORITY	ACTIONS
5. Work with communities to use best practices	• Create strong partnerships between local health care providers, public health professionals, and individuals • Provide clinical preventive services and increase adoption of evidence-based interventions
6. Provide more affordable quality care more	• Ensure the right care is provided at the right time for the right patient • Reduce health care acquired conditions • Reform payment structures, reduce waste • Establish health insurance exchanges to improve cost of insurance for individuals and small businesses

EHR, electronic health record; USDHHS, U.S. Department of Health and Human Services.
Source: USDHHS (2011b).

PATIENT SATISFACTION

Patient satisfaction has been an important aspect of feedback used by care providers for internal QI efforts. Medicare, Medicaid, and private insurance companies are beginning to place a financial value on patient satisfaction feedback. Tangible, measurable patient outcomes, such as infection rates, are an important indicator of the quality of care patients have received, patient satisfaction with the care that has been provided is now recognized as another quality indicator. This knowledge is powerful feedback regarding how respected and valued they felt as well as how engaged they were relative to their plan of care.

REAL-WORLD INTERVIEW

There are a number of health care settings implementing services with the patient in the center of all care being provided. It is not unique to nursing services. One acute care hospital where I serve on the board focuses on fostering relationships with the patient and family as they provide care to meet the patient's needs. The patient is an active participant in rounds and most staff find it very rewarding to work in a caring environment with the patient central to all services. The hospital was introduced to a relationship-based model for care and found there were many success stories from patients and families as well as the staff who embraced forming caring relationships with their patients. The hospital has developed a comprehensive program that helps ensure each service within the hospital keeps the patient central to what they do—from housekeepers to surgeons. Besides employee satisfaction, implementing a relationship-based focused of PCC has greatly influenced patient satisfaction.

Esther Bankert, Board Member
Faxton/St. Luke's Health care
Utica, New York

Hospital Consumer Assessment of Healthcare Providers and Systems (HCAHPS)

In 2005, the National Quality Forum, a national organization of health care stakeholders, consumer organizations, public and private purchasers, physicians, nurses, hospitals, accreditation/ certification bodies, supporting industries, health care researchers, and QI organizations endorsed the HCAHPS (pronounced H-CAPS) survey. The intent of this survey was to provide a standard instrument to be used by hospitals across the nation to measure the patients' satisfaction with their hospital experience. HCAHPS asks a core set of questions to assess patient satisfaction with their care by nurses, doctors, and other members of the interprofessional health care team, responsiveness of hospital staff, pain management, communication about medicines, cleanliness, and quietness of hospital environment. These standardized questions permit valid comparisons of patient care experience at hospitals locally, regionally, and nationally. The HCAHPS survey is shaped by three goals:

1. The patients' perception of care that permits objective and meaningful comparisons of hospitals on topics important to patients.
2. Public reporting of results, which provides an incentive for hospitals to improve the quality of care.
3. Public reporting, which also enhances accountability in health care by increasing transparency of the quality of the care provided (CMS, 2011a).

Since 2008, HCAHPS patient satisfaction scores have been available to the public on the CMS Hospital Compare website (www.medicare.gov/HomeHealthCompare/search.aspx).

KEY CONCEPTS

1. PCC recognizes the unique needs, values, and preferences through the lens of the patient and coordinates care services within a partnership between the patient and interprofessional team with compassion and respect.
2. Expressions of caring and the interpretation of caring acts are perceived differently across cultures.
3. Empathetic communication embodies respect for another person's feelings, values, and perspective.
4. Collaboration means to work jointly together and share expertise among experts.
5. Physical illness, disease, and injury impact a person's psychosocial self-concept.
6. Promoting health literacy is one strategy of supporting patient-centered health care.
7. The Medical Home is a result of the PPACA.
8. Continuity of care can be augmented with effective discharge planning.
9. Nurses and health care professionals can facilitate PCC by understanding their role in providing care that supports patient advocacy, continuity, and collaboration with the patient as a member of the interprofessional team across the continuum of care.

10. Nursing plays a significant role in patient satisfaction by ensuring the patient's values and preferences are incorporated into the care that is meaningful to the patient.

11. QI in health care is a major focus in America that requires an interprofessional approach to support programs and initiatives designed to develop and guide "e-patients" (equipped, enabled, empowered, and engaged) in a journey to a healthier nation.

12. Measurement of patient satisfaction can provide valuable feedback to the interprofessional team regarding the delivery of PCC.

KEY TERMS

E-patient
Empathetic communication
Health literacy
Patient advocacy
Participatory medicine

Patient-centered care
Population-focused health care
Self-concept

DISCUSSION OF OPENING SCENARIO

The primary nurse must contribute important information to the interdisciplinary team during rounds and focus on patient-specific goals to ensure the discharge transition goes smoothly. The nurse must recognize that each patient situation is unique and requires clinicians to approach care and interventions from the perspective of the patient. Through a thorough understanding of the patient, caregiver support, and community resources, the nurse can implement various strategies to support the patient and caregivers as care is transitioned along the continuum.

CRITICAL THINKING ANSWERS

Critical Thinking 6.1

1. How has Nurse Jones engaged the patient in a number of behaviors that would likely increase Mrs. Dawes's perception of her ability to impact her own health?

   Asking Mrs. Dawes how she wants to be addressed sets the tone for the conversation. By informing the patient of the likely course of therapy and instructing her on how she may handle the discomfort increases Mrs. Dawes's sense of self-efficacy, which in turn strengthens her sense of health locus of control. The nurse giving Mrs. Dawes choices for therapy times and meal selection protects Mrs. Dawes's ability to make choices and as a result increases her sense of control.

2. What are strategies Nurse Jones could have implemented to include with others on the interprofessional team at the onset of her meeting Mrs. Dawes to ensure advocacy and PCC?

   Collaboration with the health care team will facilitate a team approach to PCC. Example could be interdisciplinary daily rounding encouraging feedback and questions with the patient actively participating at the center of the discussions.

Critical Thinking 6.2

1. What strategies can Nurse Johnson employ to facilitate self-management in this patient?

   It is imperative the nurse establishes a genuine and warm, as well as trusting, relationship as a foundation to effective communication. Uses of nonverbal communication such as smiles as well as empathetic facial expressions are a thoughtful start.

2. What resources and/or services can the nurse use to ensure that the patient has understood the instruction?

   Use interpreter services to ensure that the patient understands any instruction given and is able to ask questions.

Critical Thinking 6.3

1. Within a patient-centered environment, how would you approach Teresa's grandmother?

   It would be helpful to coordinate a specific time to sit down for an unrushed conversation with Teresa's grandmother that allows the nurse to listen to all of her concerns and questions completely.

2. Considering Teresa and her parents seem to understand the importance of her dietary intervention, how can the interprofessional health care team collaborate in gathering potential missing information about Teresa's care to discover the cause for her multiple readmissions?

   It would also be helpful for the interprofessional health care team to meet with key members of Teresa's family to evaluate and brainstorm possible solutions together.

CASE STUDY ANSWERS

Case Study 6.1

1. How do you think Jane Smith, the nurse, felt when listening to hostile tones in the patient's voice and remarks toward her competency?

   The nurse could easily be influenced by the negativity expressed by Mr. Potter and defend herself and level of skills.

2. How can you respond maintaining a respectful and open dialogue between you and the patient?

   The art of empathetic communication requires Jane to first separate the cognitive content (I am in pain) from the emotional content (I am afraid that the procedure will make the pain worse).

3. How would you respond if the doctor or another member of the interprofessional team was criticizing your skills and competency in caring for a patient?

   The ability to differentiate between the two components of the verbal communication allows Jane to understand Mr. Potter's displaced anger and fear and respond to his need—not his rude behavior. This then becomes a meaningful exchange and encounter.

4. How could you respond maintaining a respectful relationship with the health care team?

The same needs to apply when communicating with health care team members.

Case Study 6.2

1. What are major factors underlying the communication process?

Verbal and nonverbal *communications occur simultaneously and are not always congruent*. In many situations, the emotional content often captures our attention and distracts us from the underlying theme of the conversation.

The exchange becomes an emotional reaction without understanding the cues behind the communication.

The listener must attend to all elements of the communication process keeping in mind the nonverbal cues provides the greatest insight to inner feelings.

Case Study 6.3

1. How can chronic illness impact Mary's perspective on her personal life?

Mary's story reveals the story of how a chronic condition such as pain affects more than the physical domain of an individual. Sometimes people can tolerate the pain but cannot accept how it might alter their professional aspirations. Personal frustration can sometimes lead to depression in some patients. Personal frustration can also lead to anger directed toward health care workers and others.

2. Explore the web for support services that are available to her at home; what might a few services be?

Community resources vary within communities but there are services to support people living alone or with limitations related to chronic conditions.

A few resources Mary might consider are support groups; home aide services as she continues to physically recover; counseling services for emotional support; and counseling services for alternative employment.

REVIEW QUESTIONS

Please see Appendix D for answers to Review Questions.

1. The nurse will attend a seminar discussing patients with family/significant others at the center for all nursing and interprofessional care services. The nurse knows that which of the following will most likely be the primary topic?

A. Primary care
B. Medical Homes
C. Interprofessional team approach
D. PCC

2. The nurse wants to use a patient-centered approach to perform patient care. Which of the following best describes the nurse's approach?

A. Developing friendships with patients as a means of providing better care
B. Creating an environment of coworkers committed to helping each other
C. Providing care through the eyes of the patient
D. Understanding the nurse's role and its relation to other care providers

3. The nurse is preparing to review discharge instructions with a patient. The nurse instructs the patient regarding her medications and wound care for her foot. What indicates to the nurse the level of understanding the patient has regarding discharge instructions?

    A. The patient signs the discharge instruction sheet.
    B. When asked by the nurse, the patient denies any questions or concerns.
    C. The patient asks for new prescriptions for the pharmacy.
    D. The nurse observes the patient changing the dressing on her foot wound.

4. When rounding, the nurse discovers that a patient on isolation has soiled the bed. Upon inquiry, the patient indicated that he did not want to bother the nurse because she was busy. The nurse tells the patient to use the call bell anytime. How can the nurse most effectively communicate that she is available to the patient?

    A. Remind the patient frequently to use the call bell.
    B. Ensure that all the patient's needs have been met before leaving the patient's room, avoid appearing rushed, and let the patient know when the nurse will return.
    C. Go in and out of patients' rooms to ensure the patients are aware that the nurse is available.
    D. Make sure the call bell is within the patient's reach every time the nurse leaves his room.

5. The nurse is caring for a patient who has multiple chronic conditions and has been hospitalized twice in the last month. The patient has a complex medication regimen, limited family support, and admits to having missed his last two physician appointments because he did not have a ride. What is the benefit of a referral to a health home for this patient?

    A. Physicians with lower rehospitalization rates operate Health Homes.
    B. Complex cases are managed through skilled nursing facilities until patients are independent again.
    C. Home care services are covered for patients regardless of ability to pay.
    D. Comprehensive care management enables access to and coordination of care.
    E. None of the above

6. A nurse is reviewing discharge instructions with a patient. The patient asks the nurse about a cardiac medication he forgot to mention to the physician because the medication is not listed on the discharge instructions. Which action by the nurse is most appropriate when reconciling discharge medications?

    A. Explain to the patient that he should follow up with his primary physician within 7 days to review the medication regimen.
    B. Contact the physician to notify him of the discrepancy and receive direction regarding the discharge instructions before discharging the patient.
    C. Instruct the patient to take only the medications listed on the discharge instructions.
    D. Advise the patient to continue taking the medication until he sees his primary physician.

7. A patient newly diagnosed with breast cancer is asking in-depth questions about her diagnosis and sharing what she has found online that has worked for other patients. The nurse recognizes that this patient represents a growing number of informed health care consumers. Which intervention by the nurse demonstrates support for the patient's involvement in her care?

   A. Caution the patient about inaccurate information that may be available on the Internet.
   B. Instruct the patient to only follow the advice of her medical provider.
   C. Advise the patient to begin building a PHR.
   D. Explain to the patient the importance of regular checkups to identify any changes in condition.
   E. All of the above

8. Which of the following actions demonstrates understanding of the role of the nurse in patient satisfaction? Select all that apply.

   A. The nurse discusses the plan of care with the patient and family.
   B. The nurse inquires about the patient's comfort with the room temperature and desire for a meal because dinner has already been served on the unit prior to arrival.
   C. At the change of shift, the nurse makes rounds with the oncoming nurse and introduces the new nurse to the patient.
   D. The nurse obtains permission for the patient's pet to visit after the nurse over-hears the patient express that she misses her dog and is afraid she will not see it again.
   E. The nurse tells the patient to fill out the patient survey she will receive after discharge and to make sure to rate her experience as excellent if the nurse met her needs.
   F. A, B, C, D
   G. None of the above

9. A non-English-speaking patient arrives in the ED and is noted to be crying quietly. Which of the following is the most important for the nurse to consider in initially providing care for this patient?

   A. Expressions and interpretations of caring may be perceived differently across cultures.
   B. Therapeutic touch is a universal communication of caring.
   C. Cultural competence includes looking patients in the eye and communicating in their language even if through an interpreter.
   D. When patients have specific cultural beliefs, nurses should consider them as part of the patient's care.

10. The nurse manager in the surgical step-down unit at a large metropolitan hospital would like to evaluate the perceived effectiveness of pain management for prior patients on the unit. The nurse knows that which of the following measures would best assist the nurse manager in understanding past patients' experiences?

    A. Home health compare data
    B. Value-based performance data
    C. HCAHPS data
    D. Sentinel events reports

REVIEW ACTIVITIES

Please see Appendix E for answers to Review Activities.

Review Activity 6.1

Review the study "The Art of Holding Hand: A Fieldwork Study Outlining the Significance of Physical Touch in Facilities for Short-Term Stay" by K. Bundgaard, E. E. Sorensen, and K. B. Nielsen (2011) in the *International Journal for Human Caring, 15*(3), 34–41.

Explain how the simple act of holding the patient's hand can instill safety and trust for the patient undergoing an invasive procedure.

What expressions would convey to you the patient is anxious or experiencing discomfort?

How can the nurse or doctor communicate reassurance to the patient while participating in the procedure?

Review Activity 6.2

To practice effective interpersonal skills within a patient-centered environment, one school tested the effects of pairing students during clinical rotations with the assignment of caring for two patients. Refer to Bartges's article, "Pairing Students in Clinical Assignments to Develop Collaboration and Communication Skills" (2012) in *Nurse Educator, 37*(1), 17–22.

Role play a scenario whereby student pairs collaborate on patient assignments and together, review the patient's records. Each student pair will round with the health care team and at the completion of the shift report out to a second pair of students who will be picking up the same assignment on the next shift.

Reflect upon your experience and describe the collaborative strategies each used to gather pertinent information about your patient.

Describe communication processes you experienced that were barriers and enhancers to effectively collaborating with the interdisciplinary team while caring for your patient.

Discuss one take-away each student learned from this experience while working with a peer–colleague.

Review Activity 6.3

Refer to the mentor–mentee program described by authors C. Latham, K. Ringl, and M. Hogan, "Professionalization and Retention Outcomes of a University: Service Mentoring Program Partnership" in the *Journal of Professional Nursing, 27*(6), 344–353.

Nurse mentors in the workplace are oftentimes sought to support new nurses or nursing students in the practice setting. Formal and informal mentoring programs are developing across academic settings to enhance their partnerships with service.

Discuss the strategies suggested in Latham et al.'s study that formalized the mentor–mentee relationship between the student nurse and staff member.

What are some of the arguments leaders of acute care organizations express in opposition to using staff to mentor student nurses in the workplace?

As a champion to mentoring programs for nursing students and new nurses, what convincing arguments would you present to nurse leaders and the health care team in your health care centers?

EXPLORING THE WEB

1. Explore the web for professional sites: Future of Nursing; Robert Wood Johnson Foundation, IOM at http://www.iom.edu/Reports/2010/The-Future-of-Nursing-Leading-Change-Advancing-Health.aspx. Identify two goals of the future of nursing in relation to PCC.

2. Browse the web for PCC at http://www.qsen.org/definition.php?id=1. Describe the attributes of PCC. Discuss how administration can support nurses and health care providers collaborate to provide PCC in acute and long-term care facilities.

3. Browse the web on any health care topic. Access the Internet and complete a basic search on the health care topic of your choice. Be sure to include sites such as WebMD and Sharecare. How can you determine if the information is valid? Evaluate if the information provided is at an appropriate level for health care consumers. Provide rationale for your answers.

REFERENCES

Agency for Healthcare Research and Quality (AHRQ). (2011a). *Preventing avoidable readmissions.* Retrieved from http://www.ahrq.gov/qual/impptdis.htm

Agency for Healthcare Research and Quality (AHRQ). (2011b). *Questions are the answer.* Retrieved from http://www.ahrq.gov/questions

American Academy of Family Physicians (AAFP), American Academy of Pediatrics (AAP), American College of Physicians (ACP), American Osteopathic Association (AOA). (2011). *Joint principles of the patient-centered medical home.* Retrieved from http://www.medical-homeinfo.org/Joint%20Statement

American College of Physicians (ACP). (2006). *The advanced medical home: A patient-centered physician-guided model of health care.* Philadelphia, PA: American College of Physicians: Position Paper (available from American College of Physicians, 190 N. Independence Mall West, Philadelphia, PA 19106).

American Medical Association, Ethical Force Program. (2006). *Improving communication-improving care.* Retrieved from http://www.ama-assn.org/ama1/pub/upload/mm/369/ef_imp_comm.pdf

American Nurses Association. (2001). *Code of ethics for nurses with interpretive statements.* Retrieved from http://nursingworld.org/MainMenuCategories/EthicsStandards/CodeofEthicsforNurses/Code-of-ethics.pdf

Balon, J., & Thomas, S. (2011). Comparison of hospital admission medication lists with primary care physician and outpatient pharmacy lists. *Journal of Nursing Scholarship, 43*(3), 292–300.

Bann, C. M., Sirois, F. M., & Walsh, E. G. (2010). Provider support in complementary and alternative medicine: Exploring the role of patient empowerment. *Journal of Alternative and Complementary Medicine, 16*(7), 745–752.

Bartges, M. (2012). Pairing students in clinical assignments to develop collaboration and communication skills. *Nurse Educator, 37*(1), 17–22.

Boston University School of Medicine. (2012). *Project RED (Re-Engineering Discharge).* Retrieved from http://www.bu.edu/fammed/projectred/index.html

Boutwell, A., Griffin, F., Hwu, S., & Shannon, D. (2009). *Effective interventions to reduce hospitalizations: A compendium of 15 promising interventions.* Cambridge, MA: Institute for Healthcare Improvement.

Bradshaw, A. (1999). The virtue of nursing: The covenant of care. *Journal of Medical Ethics, 25*(6), 477.

Buila, S. M. D., & Swanke, J. R. (2010). Patient-centered mental health care: Encouraging caregiver participation. *Care Management Journal, 11*(3), 146–150.

Bundgaard, K., Sorensen, E. E., & Nielsen, K. B. (2011). The art of holding hand: A fieldwork study outlining the significance of physical touch in facilities for short-term stay. *International Journal for Human Caring, 15*(3), 34–41.

Burks, D. J., & Kobus, A. M. (2012). The legacy of altruism in health care: The promotion of empathy, prosociality, and humanism. *Medical Education, 46*(3), 317–325.

Campbell-Yeo, M., Latimer, M., & Johnston, C. (2007). The empathetic response in nurses who treat pain: Concept analysis. *Journal of Advanced Nursing, 61*(6), 711–719.

Center for Health Care Strategies, Inc. (2010). *Health literacy implications of the Affordable Care Act.* Retrieved from http://www.chcs.org/usr_doc/Health_Literacy_Implications_of_the_Affordable_Care_Act.pdf

Centers for Medicare and Medicaid Services (CMS). (2010). *Health homes for enrollees with chronic conditions.* Retrieved from http://www.cms.gov/smdl/downloads/SMD10024.pdf

Centers for Medicare and Medicaid Services (CMS). (2011a). *HCAHPS: Hospital care quality information from the consumer perspective.* Retrieved from http://www.hcahpsonline.org/home.aspx

Centers for Medicare and Medicaid Services (CMS). (2011b). *HCAHPS: Patients' perspectives of care survey.* Retrieved from https://www.cms.gov/hospitalqualityinits/30_hospitalhcahps.asp

Centers for Medicare and Medicaid Services (CMS). (2012). *Center for medicare and Medicaid innovation.* Retrieved from http://www.innovations.cms.gov

Decety, J., & Michalska, K. J. (2010). Neurodevelopmental changes in the circuits underlying empathy and sympathy from childhood to adulthood. *Developmental Science, 13*(6), 886–899.

Egan, G. (1986). *The skilled helper: A systematic approach to effective helping.* Pacific Grove, CA: Brooks/Cole.

Ferguson, T. (2007). *E-patients: How they can help us heal health care.* Retrieved from http://www.e-patients.net

Frydman, G. (2009). Patient-driven research: Rich opportunities and real risks. *Journal of Participatory Medicine, 1*(1), e12. Retrieved from http://www.jopm.org

Hansen, L. O., Young, R. S., Hinami, K., Leung, A., & Williams, M. V. (2011). Interventions to reduce 30-day rehospitalization: A systematic review. *Annals of Internal Medicine, 155*(8), 520–528.

Holmstrom, I., & Roing, M. (2009). The relation between patient-centeredness and patient empowerment: A discussion on concepts. *Patient Education and Counseling, 79,* 167–172.

Hoyt, S. (2010). Florence Nightingale's contribution to contemporary nursing ethics. *Journal of Holistic Nursing, 28*(4), 331–332.

Institute of Medicine (IOM). (2001). *Crossing the quality chasm: A new health system for the 21st century.* Washington, DC: National Academies Press.

Institute of Medicine (IOM). (2004). *Health literacy: A prescription to end confusion.* Washington, DC: National Academies Press.

Josie King Foundation. (2012). *Josie King Foundation: Creating a culture of patient safety, together.* Retrieved from http://www.josieking.org

Kessels, R. (2003). Patients' memory for medical information. *Journal of the Royal Society of Medicine, 96*(5), 219–222.

Koh, C., Nelson, J., & Cook, P. (2011). Evaluation of a patient navigation program. *Clinical Journal of Oncology Nursing, 15*(1), 41–48.

Koh, H., Berwick, D., Clancy, C., Brach, C., Harris, L., & Zerhusen, E. (2012). New federal policy initiatives to boost health literacy can help the nation move beyond the cycle of costly 'crisis care. *Health Affairs, 31*(2), 434–443.

Kunzmann, R. (2011). Age differences in three facets of empathy: Performance-based evidence. *Psychology of Aging, 26*(11), 66–78.

Landon, B., Gill, J., Antonelli, R., & Rich, E. (2010). Using evidence to inform policy: Developing a policy-relevant research agenda for the patient-centered medical home. *Journal of General Internal Medicine, 25*(6), 581–583.

Latham, C., Ringl, K., & Hogan, M. (2011). Professionalization and retention outcomes of a university: Service mentoring program partnership. *Journal of Professional Nursing, 27*(6), 344–353.

Marks, D. F., Murray, M., Evans, B., & Estacio, E. V. (2011). *Health psychology: Theory, research, and practice.* Los Angeles, CA: Sage.

Microsoft. (2012). *Microsoft health vault.* Retrieved from http://www.microsoft.com/en-us/healthvault

National Patient Safety Foundation. (2011). *Ask me 3.* Retrieved from http://www.npsf.org/askme3

Naylor, M. D., Aiken, L. H., Kurtzman, E. T., Olds, D. M., & Hirschman, K. B. (2011). The care span: The importance of transitional care in achieving health reform. *Health Affairs, 30*(4), 746–754.

New York State Department of Health. (2011). *Medicaid health homes.* Retrieved from http://www.health.ny.gov/health_care/medicaid/program/medicaid_health_homes

Nosbusch, J., Weiss, M., & Bobay, K. (2010). An integrated review of the literature on challenges confronting the acute care staff nurse in discharge planning. *Journal of Clinical Nursing, 20,* 754–774.

Nun, B. F., & Kantrowitz, R. (2008). *Effective helping: Interviewing and counseling techniques.* Pacific Grove, CA: Brooks/Cole.

Okun, B. & Kantrowitz, R. E. (2008). *Effective helping: Interviewing and counseling techniques.* Belmont/CA: Brooks/Cole, Cengage Learning.

Patient-Centered Outcomes Research Institute. (2012). *Patient-centered outcomes research definition: Response to public input.* Retrieved from http://www.pcori.org

Patient-Centered Primary Care Collaborative (PCPCC). (2011). *History of the collaborative.* Retrieved from http://www.pcpcc.net/content/history-collaborative

Quality and Safety Education for Nurses (QSEN). (2012). *Evidence-based practice.* Retrieved from http://www.qsen.org

Ratzan, S., & Parker, R. (2000). Introduction. In C. R. Selden, M. Zorn, S. C. Ratzan, & R. M. Parker (Eds.), *National library of medicine current bibliographies in medicine: Health literacy.* NLM Pub. No. CBM 2000–1. Bethesda, MD: National Institutes of Health, U.S. Department of Health and Human Services.

Sharecare. (2011). *Sharecare.* Retrieved from http://sharecare.org

Sia, C., Tonniges, T., Osterhus, E., & Taba, S. (2004). History of the medical home concept. *Pediatrics, 113,* 1473–1478.

Society for Participatory Medicine. (2011). *Society for participatory medicine.* Retrieved from http://www.participatorymedicine.org

Society of Hospital Medicine. (2012). *Project BOOST,* Retrieved from http://www.hospitalmedicine.org/AM/Template.cfm?Section=Publications&CONTENTID=27659&TEMPLATE=/CM/HTMLDisplay.cfm

Stiles, E. (2011). Promoting health literacy in patients with diabetes. *Nursing Standard, 26*(8), 35–40.

Taylor, S. (2011). *Health psychology.* New York, NY: McGraw-Hill.

U.S. Department of Health and Human Services (USDHHS). (2010a). Agency for Healthcare Research and Quality. *National health care disparities report.* Washington, DC: Author. Retrieved from http://www.ahrq.gov/qual/nhdr10/nhdr10.pdf

U.S. Department of Health and Human Services (USDHHS). (2010b). Agency for Healthcare Research and Quality. *National health care quality report.* Washington, DC. Retrieved from http://www.ahrq.gov/qual/nhqr10/nhqr10.pdf

U.S. Department of Health and Human Services (USDHHS). (2011a). *Administration implements Affordable care act provision to improve care, lower costs.* Retrieved from http://www.hhs.gov/news/press/2011pres/04/20110429a.html

U.S. Department of Health and Human Services (USDHHS). (2011b). *National strategy for quality improvement in health care.* Washington, DC: Author. Retrieved from http://www.healthcare.gov/law/resources/reports/nationalqualitystrategy032011.pdf

U.S. Department of Health and Human Services (USDHHS). (2011c). Office of Disease Prevention and Health Promotion. *Healthy people 2020.* Washington, DC: Author. Retrieved from http://www.healthypeople.gov/2020/topicsobjectives2020/overview.aspx?topicId=18

U.S. Department of Health and Human Services (USDHHS). (2011d). *U.S. Department of Health and Human Services: About HHS.* Washington, DC: Author. Retrieved from http://www.hhs.gov/about

Ventura, T., Brown, D., Archibald, T., Goroski, A., & Brock, J. (2010). Improving care transitina and reducing hospital readmissions: Establishing the evidence for community-based implementation strategies through the care transitions theme. *The Remington Report, 18*(1), 24–30.

Watson, J. (2012, February 6). *Transforming health care one nurse, one caregiver, one organization, at a time.* World Caring Science Institute. Retrieved from www.watsoncaringscience.org

SUGGESTED READING

Brown, B. B., Stewart, M., & Weston, W. W. (2002). *Challenges and solutions in patient-centered care: A case study*. London, UK: Radcliff Publishing.

Epstein, R., Fiscella, K., Lesser, C., & Stang, K. (2012). Why the nation needs a policy push on patient-centered health care. *Health Affairs, 29*(8), 1489–1495.

Finkelman, A., & Kenner, C. (2007). *Teaching IOM: Implications of the Institute of Medicine reports for nursing education*. Silver Spring, MD: ANA.

Institute of Medicine (IOM). (2004). *Health literacy: A prescription to end confusion*. Washington, DC: National Academy of Sciences.

Jaen, C. R., Ferrer, R., Miller, W., Palmer, R., Wood, R., Davila, M.,...Stange, K. (2010). Patient outcomes at 26 months in the patient-centered medical home national demonstration project. *Annals of Family Medicine, 8*(1), S57–S67.

Koloroutis, M. (2004). *Relationship-based care: A model for transforming practice*. Minneapolis, MN: Creative Health Care Management.

Levinson, W., Lesser, C., & Epstein, R. (2010). Developing physician communication skills for patient-centered care. *Health Affairs, 29*(7), 1310–1318.

Maloney, L., & Weiss, M. (2008). Patients' perceptions of hospital discharge informational content. *Clinical Nursing Research, 17*(3), 200–219.

Manthey, M. (2002). *The practice of primary nursing*. Minneapolis, MN: Creative Health Care Management.

Rosenthal, T. (2008). The medical home: Growing evidence to support a new approach to primary care. *The Journal of the American Board of Family Medicine, 21*(5), 427–440.

7

ESSENTIALS OF QUALITY IMPROVEMENT

Cibele C. Webb, Patrick M. Webb,
Anthony L. D'Eramo, and Joanne Belviso Puckett

Undoubtedly, the most important single requisite is a commitment to quality:
an unequivocal desire and determination to dedicate oneself to the best
one is capable of, despite every obstacle. (Donabedian, 2003, p. xxix)

Upon completion of this chapter, the reader should be able to

1. Define quality improvement (QI)
2. Describe the historical evolution of QI
3. Compare and contrast QI, evidence-based practice (EBP), and research
4. Describe the different QI methodologies
5. Identify how patient satisfaction data is used in public reporting of quality care
6. Describe health care failure mode effects analysis (HFMEA) as a QI tool
7. Examine how the root cause analysis (RCA) process helps understand near miss events or sentinel events
8. Discuss the active role of the staff nurse in interprofessional QI activities

*Y*ou are a triage nurse working in a busy emergency department (ED) on the evening
shift. The waiting room is full and all beds in the ED are occupied. A middle-aged woman
arrives at triage complaining of nausea, dizziness, and pain between her shoulder blades. Her
vital signs are within normal range, but the patient appears pale and mildly distressed. You
are faced with a clinical judgment decision: Will you send this patient to the waiting room
or take her to a bed in the busy ED? Despite the inconclusive initial patient presentation,
you consider that this pain may be of cardiac origin. You know that best patient outcomes

for patients diagnosed with an acute myocardial infarction (AMI) occur when door-to-EKG time is less than 10 minutes and door-to-balloon (D2B) time is less than 90 minutes. This type of scenario is becoming increasingly common in health care institutions suffering from overcrowded EDs.

- *How will your clinical decision making affect the outcome for this patient?*
- *Why do guidelines and standards exist for door-to-EKG and D2B?*
- *What are the implications if established care standards and guidelines are not met?*

Staff nurses who provide direct patient care are best positioned to participate in the implementation of QI initiatives, thus affecting the quality of care patients receive. In such manner, it is important that nurses become familiar with QI. The purpose of this chapter is to explore the QI process as it leads to patient safety and the achievement of the best patient outcomes. QI is defined and key concepts pertaining to the history of QI are presented to showcase its interprofessional nature. Research and EBP are differentiated from the process of QI. The Donabedian model for change and Deming's Plan-Do-Study-Act (PDSA) process are introduced as tools used in QI activities that promote health and lead to health care policy change. Proactive tools such as HFMEA are presented. Reactive tools such as RCA process are discussed as an evaluation tool used to review near miss events and sentinel events and to prevent future occurrences. Implementing and sustaining a culture of safety through the delivery of evidence-based high-quality health care using an interprofessional approach is key to continuous QI. This interprofessional aspect of QI makes nurses a part of a larger team of health care professionals, in other words, interprofessionals. Therefore, it is important that nurses understand their active role in QI activities as a member of an interprofessional team.

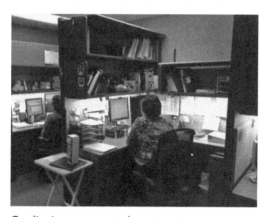

Quality improvement department.

DEFINING QI

Quality improvement (QI) is defined by the Quality and Safety Education for Nurses (QSEN) as to "use data to monitor the outcomes of care processes and use improvement methods to design and test changes to continuously improve the quality and safety of health care systems" (Cronenwett et al., 2007). QI is the process of collecting and evaluating data to discover the extent to which quality health care is being delivered according to a set standard. QI identifies the measures that need to be taken to improve care to achieve the desired outcomes. QI can be considered as both an art and a science (McLaughlin, Houston, & Harder-Mattson, 2012). Indeed, the art of QI involves asking questions and coming up with creative ideas and visionary innovations of how to approach and consider improvement interventions. The science of QI involves the ongoing process of testing improvement interventions to measure if improvements led to the intended outcomes.

A key aspect of QI includes the actions taken to decrease inconsistent patient outcomes, poor patient outcomes, patient outcomes that do not meet expectations related to EBP or regulatory standards, or do not meet the patients' needs and expectations. Such outcomes may be specific to a patient (i.e., a medication error) or groups of patients (i.e., hospital-acquired pressure ulcer rates) or they may identify a process that needs improving (i.e., patient flow from the ED to the cardiac care unit). Generally speaking, QI is an ongoing process that includes elements of prevention, recognition, and alleviation of harm as well as the ongoing search for performance excellence based on comparative benchmarks.

QI is a structured series of events that involves planning, implementing, and evaluating health care outcomes (Hughes, 2008a). There are several key steps to QI, including assembling a team, understanding the organization as a complex system, accessing and interpreting data, implementing interventions to improve outcomes, and taking actions based on performance outcomes. Certainly, it is safe to say QI focuses on improving outcomes, including those that result from practice decisions, and measuring or evaluating such outcomes compared to an established, evidence-based standard, goal, or industry benchmark.

REAL-WORLD INTERVIEW

Quality is not always the popular decision, but it is the most important decision for the patients. Quality is EBP, using the safest care, and the most up-to-date care. Quality is what I want done when I am in the hospital and when my family is in the hospital. It is what everybody deserves to have. It is our responsibility as nurses to provide it.

I am a quality review nurse. Many of my nursing peers are not familiar with what quality review nurses do. It is part of my job to oversee accrediting standards for the hospital, report to governmental and regulatory agencies, assess patient charts to ensure they are receiving high-quality care, report patient complaints to the appropriate channels, process incident reports both for nurses and physicians, refer patient cases to peer review, process patient satisfaction survey results, and participate in interprofessional disciplinary committees and taskforces. I also assist nurse managers in disseminating quality data to the units and educate staff about new standards and track their implementation. Getting staff nurses engaged in implementation and evaluation of quality measures is a key to accreditation compliance and success.

Amy Johnson, RN, CPHQ
Quality Review Specialist, Indiana University Health La Porte Hospital
La Porte, Indiana

HISTORY AND EVOLUTION OF QI IN HEALTH CARE

The history of QI in the United States dates back to the mid-1800s. During preceding centuries, the practice of medicine was largely made up of small, private, and independently functioning practices. Most medical training took place in private institutions, without a governing body or certifying organization to provide oversight to medical training or the practice of medicine as there is today. At the completion of their medical training, most physicians went into private practice. Individual physicians' training would vary a great deal between physicians and locations, as did their knowledge base and capabilities. There was no such thing as a standard of care for physicians or hospitals. Patient outcomes were not tracked or reported. QI was not a consideration.

The establishment of the American Medical Association (AMA) started in the early 20th century from the efforts of Dr. Ernest Codman. The AMA set out to create standards of care and expectations for physicians, improve medical education, and improve public health. Dr. Codman began to push for patient case review and the tracking of patients posthospitalization to ensure the care they received was effective. It was through Codman's efforts to track patient outcomes, morbidity, and mortality following hospital stays and surgical procedures that the American College of Surgeons (ACS) was born. The primary responsibility of the ACS was to act as an oversight organization to physicians and hospitals. In the early 20th century, the ACS developed five minimum standards for hospital care. To be certified by the ACS, a hospital had to

1. Organize the physicians practicing at the hospital into a medical staff
2. Limit staff membership to well-educated, competent, licensed physicians, and surgeons
3. Have rules and regulations governing regular staff meetings and clinical review
4. Keep medical records that included the history, physical exam, and results of diagnostic testing
5. Supervise diagnostic and treatment facilities such as laboratory and radiology departments (Luce, Bindman, & Lee, 1994)

For the next 40 years, meeting minimum standards for hospital care was considered the goal of QI in the United States. This QI focus began to change around the 1960s from focusing on meeting the minimum standards to identifying those findings outside the expected normal findings in medicine, also called outliers. Identifying outliers that performed below standard expectations and attempting to remedy their practice habits to improve the overall quality of care was felt to be the best avenue to achieving quality care. A common QI tool used was a peer review of patient charts. Previously, peer review was haphazard and unstructured. In the 1960s, individual physician care data were collected from patient charts and analyzed. Patient care characteristics such as readmission rates, transfers to the ICU, needs for transfusion, and antibiotic use were reviewed in an attempt to identify poorly performing physicians. Efforts could then be made to educate and support QI in physician practice through mentoring. The results of this peer-review process were then used by the hospitals in credentialing physicians. Physicians not performing up to standards or failing to correct practice deficiencies could lose their privileges to practice at an institution.

The Joint Commission on Accreditation of Hospitals (JCAHO) was founded in 1951 through the collaborative efforts of the American College of Physicians, the American Hospital Association, the AMA, and the Canadian Medical Association. JCAHO was initially charged with regulatory oversight of hospital quality (http://www.jointcommission.org/about_us/history.aspx). JCAHO, currently called The Joint Commission, also assumes regulatory oversight of nursing homes and laboratory facilities among other duties. By meeting a set of widely recognized standards and elements of performance, a health care organization demonstrates achievement of quality measure sets.

In the 1970s and 1980s, the focus of QI in health care changed again. From peer review of patient charts and identifying problem physicians, the focus of QI changed to quality assessment and improvement of overall physician performance. Instead of targeting individual problem physicians, now the focus turned to improving the performance of a group of physicians and hospitals through implementing practice guidelines. Practice guidelines are a way of standardizing care. By taking up-to-date evidence to inform the development of practice guidelines and by having physicians and hospitals follow and track their implementation, a subsequent improvement in patient outcomes, morbidity, and mortality can be expected.

As The Joint Commission matured, the focus moved from individual culpability for quality outcomes to an interprofessional focus on all health care workers in an organization. In 2002, The Joint Commission initiated the requirement that hospitals seeking accreditation report their performance on core patient quality measures (Table 7.1). These core patient quality measures are a listing of standardized evidence-based care that should be delivered to certain patient groups, for example, all patients with pneumonia should receive an antibiotic before they leave the ED or all patients with a myocardial infarction are prescribed a beta blocker. Since hospital payors (e.g., insurance companies, Centers for Medicare and Medicaid, etc.) often require proof of accreditation before they will reimburse health services, hospitals became motivated to participate in improving their performance given the financial implications. The Joint Commission patient core quality measure sets for 2012 can be viewed in Table 7.1. To learn more, go to www.jointcommission.org.

In 2003, the Centers for Medicare and Medicaid Services (CMS) implemented the **Hospital Quality Initiative** (HQI), a voluntary program where hospitals report their performance on a set of core quality measures to a public website, www.hospitalcompare.hhs.gov. This public reporting and display of data pressured hospitals to show improvement in their quality performance in order to fare well against their competitors. Furthermore, the passage of the Medicare Prescription Drug Improvement and Modernization Act (MMA) of 2003 provided financial incentives for hospitals to participate in HQI intensified the reporting of quality benchmarks to the CMS. In 2007,

TABLE 7.1 THE JOINT COMMISSION PATIENT CORE QUALITY MEASURE SETS, 2013

- Venous thromboembolism: http://www.jointcommission.org/core_measure_sets.aspx
- Heart failure: http://www.jointcommission.org/heart_failure
- Emergency department: http://www.jointcommission.org/emergency_department
- Surgical care improvement project: http://www.jointcommission.org/surgical_care_improvement_project
- Substance use: http://www.jointcommission.org/substance_use
- Tobacco treatment: http://www.jointcommission.org/tobacco_treatment
- Pneumonia measures: http://www.jointcommission.org/pneumonia
- Immunization: http://www.jointcommission.org/immunization
- Acute myocardial infarction: http://www.jointcommission.org/acute_myocardial_infarction
- Children's asthma care: http://www.jointcommission.org/childrens_asthma_care
- Hospital-based inpatient psychiatric services: http://www.jointcommission.org/hospital-based_inpatient_psychiatric_services
- Perinatal care: http://www.jointcommission.org/perinatal_care
- Stroke: http://www.jointcommission.org/stroke
- Hospital outpatient department: http://www.jointcommission.org/hospital_outpatient_department

the CMS announced that hospitals that did not participate in the reporting of quality benchmarks to CMS would have their annual payment reduced by 2% and that CMS would cease reimbursing hospitals for care resulting from medical errors. Beginning in 2013, CMS plans on implementing the **Hospital Value-Based Purchasing Program** (HVBPP), whereby incentive payments will be made by CMS to hospitals that either demonstrate improvement in performance of quality measures from a baseline period, or by how well benchmarks are achieved (CMS, 2013). Currently, the focus of QI involves reaching benchmarks that demonstrate the attainment of desirable outcomes. Reimbursement is tied to meeting these outcomes, which in turn should lead to cost containment in health care.

Today's health care organizations or systems are highly complex systems that are often multisite and provide various levels of care. Perhaps the most important element is the organizational culture and expectations regarding quality care delivery and outcomes. Such expectations involve QI work throughout the organization, from management to staff, and across many health care disciplines. A health care organization or system is responsible for supporting employees in their QI efforts. Such support includes educating employees on QI methods, providing time for QI activities, and ensuring that patients and families receive the care and services they expect when accessing an organization.

Is QI EBP or Research?

It is important to be able to differentiate QI from EBP and research. QI incorporates a data-driven systematic process in which individuals collaborate to improve specific internal processes within an organization. The key aim is the incorporation of existing information and data into QI activities. EBP is defined as a problem-solving process, which critically appraises all relevant evidence to answer a clinical, educational, or administrative question. The aim of EBP is to translate evidence into clinical, educational, or administrative practice. Research is a scientific process of generating new knowledge that influences nursing as a profession. Thus, the aim of research is to generate new knowledge by testing theories or interventions. By contrast, the intent of QI is not to generate new knowledge but rather to improve existing processes. QI outcomes are typically not generalizable, which means that the same QI process used to fix a problem at one hospital may not be applicable to other hospitals. Conducting a literature review when performing QI projects is, however, necessary when considering potential QI interventions that may be useful to improve outcomes. Therefore, QI activities will often, and should whenever possible, include the use of EBP and research findings as appropriate to help support changes in interventions or the care of patients.

When conducting research, approval and oversight by a hospital's Institutional Review Board (IRB) is a required procedure to ensure the safety of human subjects who will be participating in research studies. Although the aims of research and QI are different, the difference can be vague, especially when patients are included in the QI project. If two patient populations receive different treatments within a QI project such as when one group of patients risk for falls is assessed with one fall risk scale and another group of patients risk for falls uses a different fall risk scale, IRB approval should be sought as it constitutes human experimentation. For any QI project, where the goal of the QI team is to publish findings, it is advised that the project be presented to the IRB for their recommendations and review. Certainly, as the science of

QI expands, the rigor of QI projects will also expand. As a result, design and potential publication of QI activities that demonstrate improved patient outcomes will likely become more challenging.

QI MODELS AND METHODOLOGIES

Several QI models exist to help with improving quality of care in health care organizations. It is important to familiarize yourself with the types and workings of the models, as you will encounter them in your professional nursing practice. Some of the most common are Donabedian's structure, process, outcomes model and methodologies such as Deming's PDSA, Six Sigma's define, measure, analyze, improve, and control (DMAIC), and Lean Six Sigma.

Donabedian's Model

Over 40 years ago, Avedis Donabedian proposed a model of quality assurance that is still used today—structure, process, and outcomes (Donabedian, 2003). **Structure** refers to "the conditions under which care is provided" such as nursing staff ratios, and supplies available to provide patient care, and so on (Donabedian, 2003, p. 46). **Process** refers to "the activities that constitute health care" such as health care policies and standards of care (Donabedian, 2003, p. 46). **Outcomes** refer to the "changes (desirable or undesirable) in individuals and populations that can be attributed to health care" such as patient satisfaction results or outcomes of care (Donabedian, 2003, p. 46). It is important to understand that structure, process, and outcomes are not isolated. In fact, structures, processes, and outcomes are interdependent, that is, "specific attributes of one influence another according to the strength of the relationship" (Hughes, 2008b). Table 7.2 provides structure, process, and outcomes examples that support the delivery of high-quality patient care.

CASE STUDY 7.1

Use the questions at the end of the scenario to guide you in applying Donabedian's model of structure, process, and outcomes. A 75-year-old female patient is admitted to a medical unit with a diagnosis of pneumonia. She is alert and oriented, and her vital signs are stable. While performing rounds, the nurse finds the patient on the floor next to the bed. The patient states she did not fall, she merely slid down to the floor while getting out of bed to use the restroom. The patient could not immediately call for help after the fall because the call light was not in reach, so she decided to wait until someone checked on her.

1. *What is the definition of a fall? What factors contribute to falls?*
2. *How could this fall have been prevented?*
3. *Why must falls be reported in an incident report?*
4. *How can a QI initiative that reviews structure, process, and outcome decrease fall rates?*

TABLE 7.2 EXAMPLES OF STRUCTURE, PROCESS, AND OUTCOMES

STRUCTURE	PROCESS	OUTCOMES
Staffing (nurses, physicians, nursing assistants, advanced practice nurses)	Evidence-based guidelines	Hospital-acquired infections (e.g., catheter-associated urinary tract infections, central line associated blood stream infections, ventilator-associated pneumonia)
	Nursing process	
	Standards of care	
	Pathways	
Infection control	Policies	
Skill mix	Staff satisfaction	
Education level of staff	Core measures	
Resources (e.g., computers, library databases, etc.)	Care routines (e.g., hourly rounding)	Hospital-acquired pressure ulcers
		Fall rates
Supplies		Patient satisfaction
Technology		Medication errors
Budget		Infection rates

PDSA

Quality experts use Dr. W. Edwards Deming's **Plan-Do-Study-Act** (PDSA) model to implement QI projects. Deming incorporated knowledge of engineering, operations, and management with the goal of improving accuracy, reducing costs, increasing efficiency and safety, all leading to satisfied customers. Deming described his philosophy as "a system of profound knowledge" composed of four parts: (a) appreciation for a system, (b) understanding process variation, (c) applying theory of knowledge, and (d) using psychology (Evans, 2008). Although some refer to the cycle as Plan-Do-Check-Act (PDCA), Deming had strong beliefs that the terminology PDCA and PDSA were very different and only used the "PDSA cycle" to describe process improvement (Moen & Norman, 2009) (Figure 7.1). Deming argued that study implied more of a rigorous scientific approach to QI measurement and outcomes analysis where "check" did not have the same connotation.

The advantage of using the PDSA cycle is that it can be used cyclically on a smaller scale to perform small tests of change before implementing the change system-wide. Through use of PDSA, the relationships between changes needed in processes and outcomes are examined to establish a cause or relationship to the issue being studied. The following questions can be used during the PDSA process (Langley, Nolan, Nolan, Norman, & Provost, 2009):

1. What is the goal of the project?
2. How can it be determined that the goal of the project was reached?
3. What needs to be done in order to reach the goal?

In the "plan" stage, a plan to improve quality is developed. See Critical Thinking 7.1 for questions that can be asked during the "plan" stage. During the "do" stage, the plan is executed on a small scale initially. The plan's actual execution is evaluated during the "study" stage, and either the plan is finally implemented during the "act" stage or the plan is adjusted for further improvements. Then, the PDSA cycle restarts back to the "plan" stage again. The PDSA cycle continues until a solution is reached and implemented (Langley et al., 2009). Table 7.3 provides an overview of how the PDSA model works in an organization.

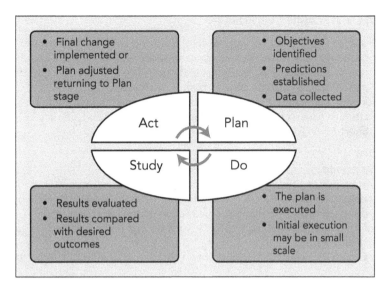

FIGURE 7.1 PDSA model.

Six Sigma and DMAIC

Six Sigma methodologies, also adopted from the business sector, encompass interventions with the goal to reduce variation in existing processes. In doing so, it often leads to new process design or redesign. In the discussion in Chapter 9 on standard deviation (SD), the upper control limits are set at 3 SD above the mean while the lower control limits are set at 3 SD below the mean. Common cause variation exists when the data points fall within the upper and lower control limits, which when added together represent six SD, or Six Sigma.

Six Sigma incorporates several problem-solving steps to reduce variation in the health care process (Evans, 2008). The steps are known as define, measure, analyze, improve and control, or DMAIC, as viewed in Table 7.4.

Lean Six Sigma

A variation of Six Sigma is **Lean Six Sigma**, the combination of Lean thinking and Six Sigma. The principles of **Lean** thinking strive to eliminate forms of waste within a process to increase efficiency while enhancing effectiveness (Shankar, 2009). There are eight identified sources of waste in organizations: unused human potential, waiting, transportation, defects, inventory, motion, overproduction, and processing (Evans, 2008). When these sources of waste occur, employees may figure out work-arounds rather than considering new processes to improve efficiency. A work-around is a nonapproved process created to accomplish a task due to all the waste associated with the approved process. For example, the nursing assistant is tasked with changing bed linens for each patient every day. To make the process quicker, the midnight shift nursing assistant collects the linens and places them in each patient's room. This action saves the day shift nursing assistant time in having to gather linens. Although

TABLE 7.3 EXAMPLE OF PDSA

Problem: Patients do not appear to understand health education provided in the hospital as evidenced by high rates of readmissions for the same diagnosis, patients not understanding medications, and not taking them as directed, and missing appointments with the physician after discharge.

Solution: Assess the patient's understanding of health information by using the Health Literacy Assessment Using the Rapid Estimate of Adult Literacy in Medicine (REALM) Short-Form Tool

Plan

We plan to

- Train nurses to use the REALM health literacy assessment tool to identify those patients with low health literacy. Patients identified as having low health literacy will have education provided at an easier to understand level.
- Implement the REALM tool for 1 week on one unit for all patient admissions to assess health literacy.
- Create an area in the computerized charting system to document the results.

Do

We found that

- Not all patients are directly admitted to the unit; therefore they did not have a health literacy assessment.
- Completing the REALM tool was time-consuming until the nurses became used to the tool.
- The findings from the use of the REALM tool were not used to individualize health education materials.

Study

We learned that

- The tool accurately identified those patients with a low health-literacy level.
- We need to create a way to use the REALM tool findings to individualized health education materials.

Act

We concluded that

- The REALM tool does identify those patients with low health-literacy.
- We need to look at what we do with the information from the REALM health-literacy assessment.
- We need to look at ways to meet the patient's individual health education needs by creating an online repository of health education materials designed for low health-literacy education.

a seemingly innocent and kind gesture, a problem arises when the original patient is discharged before the linens are used. The linens are then sent back to laundry for cleaning, causing an increase in workload for the laundry workers. Even worse, the linens might be used for the newly admitted patient, causing an increased risk of the spread of infection.

The danger of a work-around is the error that may result from creating and applying nonapproved processes. Lean interventions center on improving efficiency, reducing waste, and streamlining processes that are patient and employee centered. Lean thinking builds on the belief that it is the sum or cumulative effect of many small improvements that create the greatest impact in performance (Evans, 2008). Small, low-cost, and low-risk improvements are easily implemented with the goal to keep the project simple over a short duration of time.

TABLE 7.4 DMAIC

Define	Identifies the QI focus. Defines the team, operational definition of the variable, baseline data, and improvement aim or expected level of performance when variability is reduced, and the project timeline. Tools such as fishbone diagrams and process maps are used to define the problem.

Example: Patient satisfaction rates in the ED are lower than in any other area in the hospital at 48%. A team is assembled consisting of ED nurses, physicians, nursing assistants, department director, lab technician, registration, housekeeping, and radiology representatives. The definition of satisfaction is the number of patients who are "very satisfied" with their ED experience as rated on a hospital survey that is conducted via telephone. The team decides the goal is to achieve an 80% score within 1 year.

Measure	Includes identifying the current process, validating the variable to measure, assessing baseline performance, and selecting who will conduct measurement procedures. Tools such as Pareto charts and process control charts are often useful in this step (see Chapter 9).

Example: The team found that no current process existed to improve patient satisfaction rates in the ED. The patient satisfaction survey had been in place for the past 3 years, providing baseline data. The previous year's average for patient satisfaction was 48%. Currently, ED patient satisfaction data is sent directly to the director. The team decided that the ED director and three nurses would gather the patient satisfaction data monthly and post the findings in the staff break room.

Analyze	Rigorous analysis to understand top causes of why errors are occurring. Tools such as statistical measurements, control charts, fishbone diagrams, and hypothesis testing are often useful in this step (see Chapter 9 and the fishbone diagram in this chapter).

Example: To understand the data, the team looked at the survey questions asked of the patients to understand the origination of the problem. When broken down, the data on timeliness of care delivery was rated the lowest of all questions by patients. By taking questions relating to timeliness of care delivery out of the entire survey, the ED would have achieved an 81% patient satisfaction. The team concluded that focused efforts should be made toward improving timeliness of care delivery. The team then looked at other issues that contributed to timeliness of care delivery such as ED wait times, effectiveness of triage (deciding which patients need immediate care and which patients could wait to be seen), staffing levels, turnaround time for ED beds, time between admission orders, and transferring a patient into a hospital unit, and staff satisfaction survey data. Although there are a variety of issues that led to low patient satisfaction with timeliness of care, the team decided to focus on one issue at a time. The first problem the patient encounters relates to effectiveness of the triage system.

Improve	Brainstorming what solutions may be useful in reducing variation and conducting small-scale trials of possible solutions.

Example: When analyzing the problem with triage, the team identifies that there were several times in the past month when a newly hired nurse was assigned to triage. The ED has experienced a high turnover of nursing staff over the past year. The ED requires mandatory training for all nurses once a year on ED specific competencies that includes triaging skills. Because of the high turnover and timing of the mandatory training, very few of the current nurses had taken the training. The team decided to implement quarterly training for all ED nurses and to expand training on triage skills. The training would follow the Emergency Nurses Association's recommendations for competency skills and assessments.

(continued)

TABLE 7.4 DMAIC *(continued)*

Control	Methods to sustain improvements, such as employee education, and the process for ongoing measurement to ensure the new and improved processes are sustained over time.

Example: The new ED training program that included an expanded training on triaging skills was started within 1 month with subsequent updates and skills training occurring every 3 months. When the patient satisfaction survey scores were collected 3 months after initiating the program, the scores for timeliness of care improved from 48% to 61%. The team decided the next steps were to maintain the triage training and to examine what happens once the patient was past triage and placed in an ED bed.

Although similar, there are appreciable differences between Lean and Six Sigma. Lean addresses visible problems, for example, you can see that items in a clean utility room are orderly or in disarray. Color-coding shelves to hold specific types of equipment or supplies helps to quickly identify an item. Placing items together that are typically needed at the same time, such as an indwelling urinary catheter kit next to a clean specimen collection kit, is an example of Lean. Six Sigma on the other hand is focused on variation in performance. Also, Lean is easily taught, more intuitive, and easier to apply in practice. Six Sigma requires specialized skills and statistical tools making it a more sophisticated approach.

EVIDENCE FROM THE LITERATURE

Citation

Pocha, C. (2010). Lean six sigma in health care and the challenge of implementation of six sigma methodologies at a veterans affairs medical center. *Quality Management in Health Care, 19*(4), 312–318.

Discussion

The purpose of this improvement team was to reduce the number of portable chest x-rays in an ED. Many patients who present to an ED receive a portable chest x-ray, which may be difficult to interpret compared to the more specific posterior/anterior and lateral (PAL) x-ray. To address the problem, the team used DMAIC to work through the problem.

Define

The team hypothesized that 30% of portable chest x-rays completed in the ED would be repeated within 24 to 48 hours of admission as PAL views for improved interpretation, leading to duplication of service, and increased costs. A team of experts was gathered, including a Six Sigma consultant who served as educator and team facilitator. The team used Lean concepts of efficiency and Six Sigma

(continued)

approach to reduce variability of those patients receiving both a portable and postadmission repeated PAL x-ray.

Measure

The team collected baseline data for 6 months that demonstrated 254 patients who were admitted to medicine service through the ED had a portable chest x-ray while in the ED. Of the 254 patients, 79 (32%) received a postadmission PAL chest film.

Analyze

Many variables were assessed, for example, the cost of one portable chest x-ray was $147.98. A reduction of 30% would equate to an annual savings of $23,380, not to mention less radiation exposure, radiology technician time, and patient satisfaction.

Improve

Strict criteria for portable chest x-rays was established related to diagnosis groups, including acute coronary ischemia, pulmonary emboli, and for those patients unable to stand. After implementing this new criterion, there was a reduction in portable chest x-rays, from 32% to 23% over a 1-month period.

Control

The team will continue to monitor the percentage of patients who receive both a portable and postadmission chest x-ray.

Implications for Practice

Lean Six Sigma tools can successfully be used for the systematic implementation of an improvement process. In addition, these tools can be taught and applied by teams, leading to a high degree of success. The author describes the value of utilizing both Six Sigma and Lean within a single project. In summary, Lean incorporates a systems approach to decrease inefficiencies but does not provide the scientific rigor of Six Sigma, while Six Sigma does not offer standard solutions from a systems perspective. Interestingly, the author concludes with the criticality of the teams buy-in and willingness to change practice. Furthermore, despite an improvement project application, adaptation of new criteria by some providers did not occur. The author confirms the reality of all projects that although there may be evidence of a need to improve and a clear intervention that may be agreed upon, it does not guarantee those expected to carry out the intervention will comply. Identifying barriers and rationale for such decisions is a valuable process when analyzing outcomes.

PATIENT SATISFACTION AND QUALITY

Since 2003, the U.S. government has been collecting data on patient satisfaction with hospital care. This patient satisfaction data is published for public view online at www.hospitalcompare.hhs.gov. The Hospital Consumer Assesment of Healthcare Providers and Systems, or HCAHPS, is a government-enacted survey instrument developed to obtain standard comparative data between hospitals. HCAHPS consists of a 27-question patient satisfaction survey covering eight key areas: communication with doctors, communication with nurses, responsiveness of hospital staff, pain management, communication about medicines, discharge information, cleanliness of the hospital environment, and quietness of the hospital environment. The purpose of the HCAHPS survey is to allow (a) objective and meaningful comparisons between hospitals, (b) public reporting of data as an incentive for health care organizations to improve their care, and (c) public reporting and enhanced accountability to the public (http://www.hcahpsonline.org). HCAHPS participation is a mandatory part of participation in Medicare and Medicaid (http://www.cms.gov/Medicare/Quality-Initiatives-Patient-Assessment-Instruments/HospitalQualityInits/HospitalHCAHPS.html).

Critical Thinking 7.1

Review the HCAHPS survey questions at http://www.hcahpsonline.org/surveyinstrument.aspx. Look at questions 1 to 25. During your next clinical experience, evaluate yourself on your ability to meet the highest level of criteria during your care of the patient (e.g., "always," "strongly agree").

1. On which of the questions do nurses have the greatest impact?

One of the first patient satisfaction tools came from the Ganey Corporation of South Bend, Indiana, in 1979. This company arose out of the work of two Notre Dame professors, Dr. Irwin Press, PhD, and Dr. Rod Ganey, PhD. Dr. Press initially developed expertise in patient satisfaction and how this related to risk management. Dr. Ganey helped to develop statistical methods to measure patient satisfaction. The Press Ganey Organization is now one of the industry leaders in helping health care organizations improve their performance (http://www.pressganey.com/index.aspx).

Arbor Associates began operation around the same time as the Press Ganey Organization. Through telephone interviews, information is obtained about a patient's recent experience with the health care system. The data that are collected can then be compared to other regional hospitals and even to other similar-sized hospitals nationwide to give a comparative performance evaluation. The best performers set a "benchmark" for other organizations to emulate (Arbor Associates, Inc., 2011). Currently, in synchrony with the HCAHPS survey, Arbor has been conducting a patient expectation project with the purpose of finding out how closely patients' actual experiences match up with customer expectations in health care (Arbor Associates, Inc., 2011). The patient expectation project provides hospitals with feedback per department, giving comparative benchmarking data on how a department compares with similar departments in other hospitals.

APPROACHES TO QI PROBLEMS

The QI process is usually prompted by an adverse event, near miss, or sentinel event. To identify the actual cause of a problem and implement improvement strategies, it is important to know how the problems are identified and resulting specific actions by a QI team. Uncovering the problem can be more difficult than one might expect. Reactive strategies are those actions that occur after an event has taken place, such as peer review (discussed earlier in the chapter) and RCA. HFMEA is a proactive method to identify problems before they arise, allowing the team to fix problems before a near miss or sentinel event occurs.

Retroactive Approach: RCA

A **root cause analysis** (RCA) is an investigation of what caused a problem and why the problem occurred. The Joint Commission requires that an RCA take place whenever a sentinel event occurs (The Joint Commission, 2012). Based on the findings from an RCA, an action plan can be developed and implemented to reduce risk of a future similar sentinel event. The top reported root causes of sentinel events to The Joint Commission from 2004 to 2012 can be viewed at http://www.jointcommission.org/ assets/1/18/Root_Causes_Event_Type_2004_2Q2012.pdf.

To understand how an RCA works, we will use an example to walk through the steps. A patient with insulin-dependent diabetes is given the wrong dose of insulin. Although the patient did not experience any detrimental effects, the medication error is considered an adverse event. The quality department determined that an RCA can help determine the contributing factors to the medication error and how to prevent similar errors from occurring. An interprofessional team consisting of nurses, physicians, nursing assistants, quality department representative, central supply representative, and clinical educator is gathered to investigate the problem. To conduct an RCA, the following steps occur:

1. Identify what happened
2. Review what should have happened
3. Determine causes
4. Develop causal statements
5. Generate a list of recommended changes
6. Share findings with those who affect or are affected by the outcome

The first step, identify what happened, occurs through a dialogue among all team members. The team starts with the statement that a medication error occurred resulting in 10 times the ordered dose of insulin was given to the patient. The clear statement brings all team members to the same starting point to examine the problem.

To understand what happened, the team develops a flowchart (Figure 7.2) of the insulin preparation process. Team members use the flowchart to identify and examine factors contributing to the near miss or sentinel event. The process is mapped out to show the steps involved with insulin preparation.

The team members directly involved with the medication error provide information about steps that can highlight process problems. It is important to note here that the RCA looks at process breakdowns rather than at an individual person's error. In this scenario, the nurse is not viewed as the one who caused the error,

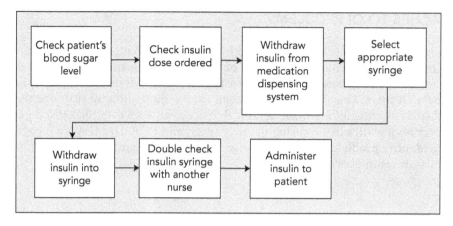

FIGURE 7.2 Flowchart of insulin preparation.

rather it is viewed as a breakdown in the process that allowed the error to occur. This encourages all participants to fully engage in identifying contributing factors.

The next step is to determine causes. A cause–effect diagram, or fishbone diagram, helps participants understand the contributing factors to the medication error. The "bones" of the fish in the diagram represent the common areas that might contribute to the problem and include at minimum task factors, patient characteristics, work environment, and staff factors (Institute for Healthcare Improvement [IHI], 2012). An example of a cause–effect diagram, or fishbone diagram, can be viewed in Figure 7.3. It is important to note that the categories, or bones of the fish, may have different labels depending on what template is used. The IHI describes seven categories, whereas Taxonomy of Error, Root Cause Analysis and Practice-Responsibility (TERCAP) identifies five core areas (https://www.ncsbn.org/441. htm). Both methods get at the cause of the problem.

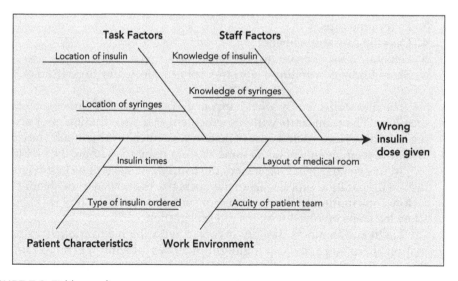

FIGURE 7.3 Fishbone diagram.

Each area is discussed by team members and examined in terms of what happened during the near miss or sentinel event that contributed to the outcome. During this process, an effective method to get at the core causes of the problem is to ask "why" five times. Asking "why" five times helps the team dig deeper into the actual process issues that caused the problem.

Critical Thinking 7.2

Consider a problem you are now facing, or have faced in the past. Ask yourself "why" five times. Be honest with your responses. Your problem could be finding time to study for a big exam, preparing for clinicals, or needing to give a presentation to your class. Write down your responses.

1. Did the fifth "why" question provide information on the root of your problem?

During the creation of the flowchart, the team identified that the nurse reached for a syringe from a drawer labeled "insulin syringes" but instead, the drawer was stocked with tuberculin syringes. This resulted in the nurse giving 10 times the ordered dose of insulin. Another misstep occurred when the nurse asked another nurse to double check the dose of insulin. The second nurse glanced at the syringe and agreed the dose was correct.

CASE STUDY 7.2

A patient arrives in the ED at 6:30 a.m., nearing the end of the night shift, complaining of chest pain. The electrocardiogram shows an acute myocardial infarction (AMI) in progress and orders morphine sulfate 2 mg, nitroglycerine drip IV, and oxygen. The nurse goes to the medication dispensing unit, removes a syringe of morphine sulphate 2 mg, and administers the medication IV push as ordered. Within 3 minutes the patient stops breathing, going into anaphylaxis shock. The nurse calls a code. The patient survives despite being allergic to morphine sulphate. The nurse feels terrible about this human error, which resulted in a sentinel event. The nurse fills out an incident report and also alerts the nursing supervisor.

1. *Name the factors that contributed to this medication error.*
2. *How could this sentinel event have been prevented?*
3. *Name safety guards that can be implemented to prevent future similar sentinel events.*

Based on findings from the flowchart and cause–effect diagram, a list of causal statements and recommended changes is created (Table 7.5).

TABLE 7.5 CAUSAL STATEMENTS AND RECOMMENDED CHANGES

CAUSAL STATEMENTS	RECOMMENDED CHANGES
Tuberculin syringes were inappropriately stocked in the insulin syringe drawer	Move tuberculin syringes to a different location
Tuberculin and insulin syringes both have orange caps and black markings on the syringe	Check with other vendors about the availability of different colored syringes
Verifying the insulin dose with another nurse did not catch the medication error	Double checks with another nurse's need to include specific steps such as looking at the type of syringe, the amount of medication in the syringe, and the dose ordered

RCAs generally focus on system problems rather than placing individual blame for any problems or sentinel events. Nevertheless, if the sentinel event occurred due to human error or a breach in standards of care and/or policy, the health care provider in question is usually given an opportunity to respond to the accusations. The provider's response is reviewed, and the peer-review committee then makes a formal ruling. Conclusions from the RCA investigation may result in remedial education, a change in a policy or a care pathway, or a change in a work process. In the rare situation when negligence with irresponsibility, negligent intent, or personal neglect is found, punishment of the health care provider may occur, including suspension or termination. In the case of physicians, this may include losing privileges at the health care institution for a period of time or even permanently. Furthermore, any quality complaints against a particular physician are reviewed at the time of any reapplication for medical staff privileges at an institution. If enough quality concerns were identified, this would prevent future membership to the medical staff at that hospital.

REAL-WORLD INTERVIEW

In years past, QI peer review for physicians occurred in the following manner. A clinical department would set the expected standards of quality care. If the physician's standard of care provided did not meet these set standards, the patient's chart was sent for peer review. The peer-review committee was responsible for determining if (a) the care was fine, (b) the care was fine but it could be improved by____(a percentage), or (c) the care was not fine. When the latter two conclusions were reached, the chart would then go back to the physician for his or her comment. The physician and the peer-review committee were expected to reach an accord about the situation and follow any recommendations to improve care. If an accord could not be reached, the case would then be sent to the physician's clinical department for a resolution.

Presently, QI efforts continue as above in a retrospective manner to address cases of substandard care delivery. Additionally, efforts are in place for physicians to deliver care that is evidence based, meets set benchmarks, and results in best outcomes. Payors, such as Medicare, have begun not reimbursing physicians and hospitals for care not delivered according to this new set of standards.

(continued)

The goal of this new movement is to both improve patient outcomes and contain health care costs.

The future looks at incorporating informatics into everyday care. Through evidence-based computerized charting, the health care provider receives prompts to provide thorough, comprehensive health care, thus decreasing the margin of human error and oversight. Communication between hospital care and outpatient primary settings should be improved with electronic systems.

Dr. G. Larson Kneller, MD
Medical Director, Memorial Medical Group
La Porte, Indiana

Proactive Approach: HFMEA

Failure mode and effects analysis (FMEA) is a proactive method used to assess high-risk processes. FMEA has its roots in the aviation industry, where steps are taken to ensure that an accident does not occur. Health care organizations adopted this approach calling it **HFMEA**. HFMEA involves a comprehensive risk assessment of select processes that the organization identifies as high risk (http://www.ihi.org/knowledge/Pages/Tools/FailureModesandEffectsAnalysisTool.aspx). Three questions are the focus of an HFMEA:

1. Failure modes (what could go wrong?)
2. Failure causes (why would the failure happen?)
3. Failure effects (what would be the consequences of each failure?)

The goal of the team is to improve the safety of a known complex, high-risk health care processes before they result in adverse events by identifying and eliminating high-risk aspects of the process. Both flow mapping and fishbone diagrams are commonly used tools by HFMEA teams. For example, the administration of a heparin infusion, a high-risk medication, involves many complex steps including calculating the patient's weight in kilograms, ensuring the correct amount of heparin is in the solution, changing doses, and administering boluses based on laboratory studies. Consider the role of the provider who must order the heparin correctly, the pharmacist who may prepare or deliver the heparin, all of which are processes that may lead to errors. HFMEA allows the team to assess potential risks of each step before an error occurs. Teams prioritize actions based on a severity of risk rating scale. Five steps are completed during an HFMEA (http://www.patientsafety.gov/CogAids/HFMEA, including:

1. Mapping the process
2. Identifying failure modes through brainstorming
3. Apply a scoring methodology to prioritize risk
4. Identifying causes
5. Implementing strategies to prevent the causes

HFMEA improvement strategies commonly involve redesigning processes to eliminate identified risks. Of consideration, nurses can identify high-risk processes that may serve well for an HFMEA. Nurses may participate or lead HFMEA teams as many of the high-risk processes that occur involve nursing judgment and oversight.

Critical Thinking 7.3

Go to http://app.ihi.org/Workspace/tools/fmea/AllTools.aspx and select a tool that interests you from the list. Select one of the topics and view the report. Explore the failure mode, causes, and effects listed.

1. How do the actions listed on the right-side column affect the failure mode, cause, and effect listed?
2. How are the failure modes, causes, and effects ranked?

THE ROLE OF THE NURSE IN QI

Traditionally, nurses are taught to collect and analyze patient data early in their student experiences, which is an important aspect of the nursing and QI process. This analysis leads to prioritizing nursing interventions that are implemented and evaluated over time. Nurses must assess the impact of their interventions and determine the need to eliminate or implement new interventions based on observed patient outcomes.

In today's complex health care organizations, it is the responsibility of both novice and expert nurses to improve practice (Painter, 2010). Increasingly, nurses are taking the lead in QI initiatives. It is intuitive to nurses to want to improve and focus on enhanced patient outcomes (Berwick, 2011). Asking questions is an important aspect of QI. Nurses are expected to have the knowledge, skills, and attitudes (KSAs) to assess, analyze, intervene, and evaluate not just patient outcomes, but outcomes that reflect individual and interprofessional practice. The optimal goal of nurses caring for patients is to improve health, improve the processes and systems that contribute to positive outcomes, and reduce harm. Nurses approach the processes and systems of care they use every day as variables that constantly need evaluation, recognizing processes that may enhance care or lead to errors, and recognizing how such processes can be improved to promote patient safety and performance excellence.

As a novice-nurse QI participant, you can assume a variety of roles required when conducting QI activities, such as data collection, assisting with literature reviews, or helping to implement an improvement intervention. Advanced practice and experienced nurse experts are expected to lead QI teams and serve as a resource to the team members, contributing to the organization, service, unit, and patients. It is important to know how to access data, what staff resources are available to assist with the acquisition of existing data, and who are the QI experts available within the organization for consultation.

Leadership Support

A supportive and empowering hospital culture and leadership is necessary for optimal QI. Given the ramifications of quality outcome performance for hospital reimbursement, it is imperative that the hospital, nursing, and medical staff have leadership's full support for improving hospital processes. Leaders who round on patient care units and directly talk to staff about quality and safety concerns tend to be more effective in identifying areas of improvement and involving staff in the pursuit of a solution.

Effective leaders partner with their employees by empowering them to ask questions, seek new ways of doing business, and try new ideas that may improve organizational performance. Lindberg and Kimberlain (2008) note that if the intent of every health care worker is to provide quality care, then the responsibility of executives is to create a culture for that to occur.

Hospital leaders support QI activities by providing a set of clear expectations and ongoing and meaningful feedback. When hospital leadership is involved initially with QI projects from the top down, it sends the message that quality is a shared team responsibility. By the same token, nurses, physicians, and the entire health care team must actively engage in QI efforts by bringing issues to leadership's attention from the ground up. By actively engaging staff and promoting an interprofessional health care team partnership, results of a QI project tend to be meaningful with sustained improvements. The interprofessional health care team partnership supports a collective brainstorming of solutions to quality problems by using peer pressure on their respective peer groups and soliciting participation, support, and compliance.

Feedback and dissemination of the results of QI projects is essential for improvement. Hospitals use a variety of mechanisms including newsletters, new employee orientation, e-mail communication, staff training, staff meetings, and unit-based communication boards. One method of sharing QI data is to use scorecards or dashboards that use a quick-look approach to show where the current standing is on a quality issue in relation to benchmarks. Dashboards and scorecards are detailed in Chapter 8.

Quality information tends to be most effectively disseminated at the departmental level; in other words where direct patient care is given, so nurses can readily implement changes. Nurse managers and leaders must use caution, however, on the amount of information shared, as large quantities of shared information can become difficult to understand and less meaningful for staff. It is best to share concise information that highlights how a quality process was improved or how a quality benchmark was met (Lindberg & Kimberlain, 2008).

Overcoming Barriers

Although it is the goal of many health care facilities to engage the health care team in QI initiatives, many barriers to QI exist. Most QI initiatives are started and led by leadership staff. Having adequate nursing staff to allow for the participation of nurses in meetings and QI task forces can pose a challenge. Nurses may feel obligated to participate but may lack the education necessary to function in QI initiatives. Leadership needs to provide education and training for staff nurses to assist them in understanding QI processes. These challenges can be overcome with a style of leadership called shared governance.

Shared governance is a professional practice model, founded on the cornerstone principles of partnership, equity, accountability, and ownership that form a culturally sensitive and empowering framework, enabling sustainable, and accountability-based decisions to support an interprofessional design for excellent patient care (Porter O'Grady, 2008). It is the shared control over nursing practice and clinical decision making that empowers staff nurses and managers to work together for successful QI projects. Shared governance embodies four principles: partnership, accountability, equity, and ownership (Anthony, 2004). When frontline staff nurses actively participate in QI and take control over their practice, the expected result is a better work environment, better staff satisfaction, improved staff retention, and better patient outcomes.

Critical Thinking 7.4

Magnet™ hospitals possess formal shared governance structures that empower nurses to actively participate in QI activities, evaluating their own practice for opportunities for QI, and better outcomes. According to the American Nurses Credentialing Center (ANCC), the Magnet Recognition Program® requires organizations to advance, propagate, and enculturate evidence-based criteria that promote quality care practices and a positive work environment. Furthermore, the Magnet Recognition Program provides a framework for QI, as Magnet facilities must attain and maintain a certain level of benchmark achievement in nurse-sensitive quality indicators.

1. Can an organization achieve Magnet status without having a formal shared governance structure?
2. How does QI support the bedside nurse? The pharmacist? The physician? The social worker?

Leaders at all levels of the organization are responsible for the creation and over-sight of a quality culture, safe environment, and high-quality patient outcomes. QI education and training is clearly necessary for this process as is the leadership commitment of both patients and staff.

It is truly an exciting time for nurses and those participating in and leading QI activities. The ability to contribute to improving care and services empowers nurses to make decisions that impact the quality and safety of their patients' care. To successfully contribute to QI efforts, nurses must be prepared to understand and utilize a broad array of QI tools. Identifying new, improved ways to provide care and services is only one part of the QI equation. Disseminating outcomes from QI projects to other health care organizations helps others to improve their own practices.

KEY CONCEPTS

1. QI is defined as to "use data to monitor the outcomes of care processes and use improvement methods to design and test changes to continuously improve the quality and safety of health care systems" (Cronenwett et al., 2007).
2. QI began with the work of the AMA in the early 1900s. Over time, QI changed from standardizing care to include measurements of the process of care and health care outcomes in response to accreditation standards of The Joint Commission. The current focus of QI continues to evolve in response to the CMS programs such as hospital value-based purchasing.
3. QI is the incorporation of existing information and data into QI activities. EBP focuses on to translating evidence into clinical, educational, or administrative practice. The aim of research is to generate new knowledge by testing theories or interventions.
4. Donabedian's model looks at three areas for QI: structure, process, and outcomes. Deming's model prescribes how QI takes place in a cyclical manner using PDSA.

Six Sigma prescribes five steps for QI to reduce variation in performance: DMAIC. Lean interventions focus on improving efficiency, reducing waste, and streamlining processes through the cumulative effect of small improvements.

5. Patient satisfaction data is collected and reported to the CMS. CMS makes the patient satisfaction data publicly available on their website. The data allows consumers to make an informed decision about where to seek health care.

6. An RCA is conducted after a near miss or sentinel event has occurred. An RCA is an investigation of what caused a problem and why the problem occurred. The Joint Commission requires that an RCA take place whenever a sentinel event occurs.

7. Examine how the RCA process helps understand near-miss events or sentinel events.

8. HFMEA is a QI tool that looks at a health care process to determine the potential for risk. The goal of an HFMEA is to improve the safety of a complex, high-risk health care process before an adverse event occurs by identifying and eliminating high-risk aspects of the process.

9. Nurses, both experienced and novice, are expected to have the KSAs to assess, analyze, intervene, and evaluate not just patient outcomes, but outcomes that reflect individual and interprofessional practice. Nurses approach the processes and systems of care they use every day as variables that constantly need evaluation; recognizing processes that may enhance care or lead to errors, and recognizing how such processes can be improved to promote patient safety and performance excellence.

KEY TERMS

Health care failure mode effects analysis
Hospital Quality Initiative
Hospital Value-Based Purchasing
  Program
Lean
Lean Six Sigma
Outcomes
Plan-Do-Study-Act

Process
Quality
Quality improvement
Root cause analysis
Shared governance
Structure

DISCUSSION OF OPENING SCENARIO

1. How will your clinical decision making affect the outcome for this patient?

   Clinical decisions made while caring for a patient directly affects patient outcomes. Every decision, both minor (should I ambulate my patient at 2 p.m. or 4 p.m.) and major (should I refer this patient to the ED) will have consequences on patient outcomes. In addition, every clinical decision has an effect upon the next step of care (e.g., ambulating the patient at 4 p.m. may interfere with the meal time, medication time, or a family visit, or referring the patient to the ED has an effect on wait times, timing of treatment, and/or delay in treatment). It is essential that the decisions are based on sound clinical data and reflect the care required for the patient.

2. Why do guidelines exist for door-to-EKG and D2B?

   Guidelines, also known as clinical guidelines, are based on evidence and reflect valid and reliable steps to direct the care for patients. When guidelines are followed, there is a predictable sequence to care delivery that optimizes patient care outcomes. Guidelines exist for door-to-EKG and D2B to improve efficiency of care delivery as well as support effective care decisions. The guidelines help to predict the outcomes from care when they are followed.

3. What are the implications if established care standards are not met?

When care standards are not met, the desired outcomes are less likely to be achieved. The patient does not receive the best care possible. Economic implications include reduced reimbursements for not meeting measurable outcomes. In addition, there are legal ramifications to the individuals who do not follow standards of care. This constitutes a deviation in practice.

CRITICAL THINKING ANSWERS

Critical Thinking 7.1

1. On which of the questions do nurses have the greatest impact?

Nurses should be aware of the questions on the HCAHP survey. Because the survey measures patient satisfaction and is tied to hospital reimbursement, it falls on all health care professionals to know the questions in order to improve patient satisfaction. Nurses have the greatest impact on those questions that relate to direct patient care. It is important to understand that as the patient advocate, it is the nurse's responsibility to coordinate patient care, to respond to patient requests, ensure a safe and quiet environment, and to regard the patient as the central focus for care provided while he or she is in the hospital.

Critical Thinking 7.2

1. Did the fifth "why" question provide information on the root of your problem?

To fully understand influences on a problem, it is necessary to ask "why" five times. By the time you answer the fifth "why," you should have a good understanding of the root cause of a problem.

Critical Thinking 7.3

1. How do the actions listed on the right-side column affect the failure mode, cause, and effect listed?

Examples of completed health care failure modes, causes, and effects are provided in the website to allow an actual example of how the health care failure modes, causes, and effects worked.

2. How are the failure modes, causes, and effects ranked?

The ability to understand how the actions taken affected the potential outcomes help to illustrate the usefulness of the HFMEA process.

Critical Thinking 7.4

1. Can an organization achieve Magnet status without having a formal shared governance structure?

To achieve Magnet status, hospitals must demonstrate that nurses are involved in decisions that affect nursing practice. In theory, an organization can achieve Magnet status without a formal shared governance structure but there must be a venue for nurses to participate in decisions affecting nursing practice.

2. How does QI support the bedside nurse? The pharmacist? The physician? The social worker?

Quality improvement is a process that is not discipline specific. All health care professionals benefit from examining structure, process, and outcomes of care data. These data help identify areas of opportunity to improve.

CASE STUDY ANSWERS

Case Study 7.1

1. What is the definition of a fall? What factors contribute to falls?

Falls can be defined as an unplanned descent to the floor (or extension of the floor, for example, trash can or other equipment) with or without injury to the patient, resulting from a physiological or environmental reason. Assisted falls, such as when a staff member attempts to minimize the impact of the fall, are also considered a fall (www.ana.nursingworld.org/qualitynetwork/patientfallsreduction.pdf).

Factors contributing to falls include such things as the bed not in the locked position, water on the floor, personal items outside of the patient's reach, call lights not being answered, not wearing nonskid slippers, recent administration of a narcotic or sleep aid, or the patient's need to get up out of bed to use the toilet.

2. How could this fall have been prevented?

Using a fall risk assessment on every patient can help minimize falls. In addition, health care providers should be aware of factors affecting the risk for falls (see response to question 1) and take steps to minimize these factors. For example, hourly rounding on every patient by the nursing assistant or the nurse with attention to toileting the patient, asking if they have everything they need, monitoring the effects of narcotics or sleep aids, making sure the area is free from hazards (water, fluids, cords, etc.), and communicating the risk of falling with the patient and family.

3. Why must falls be reported in an incident report?

Reporting falls allows an investigation into the situation, usually conducted by the quality department or QI team. By examining the factors that existed when the patient fell, the QI team can understand what occurred and take actions to minimize future falls.

4. How can a QI initiative that reviews structure, process, and outcome decrease fall rates?

Assessing whether the patient is at risk for falls should be the first step. Many facilities use existing evidence-based fall assessment scales, such as the Morse scale. Once fall risk is identified, a number of interventions can be implemented to decrease falls (www.ana.nursingworld.org/qualitynetwork/patientfallsreduction. pdf). Below is a suggested list, although not all inclusive:

a. Placing one star decal on the patient's door with a Morse score greater than 25
b. Placing two falling star decals on the patient's door for a patient who experienced a fall during his or her current hospital stay
c. Placing a yellow wristband on the patient to alert to fall risk
d. Placing the patient in a room near the nurse's station
e. Use of a sitter if necessary
f. Involving the patient's family in the care
g. Frequent nursing rounds to ensure the patient has a call light and personal belongings in reach

h. Adequate lighting

i. Offering to take the patient to the restroom on a regular schedule, such as every 2 hours

j. Discussing fall risk status in change of shift report

According to the ANA, nurse-sensitive quality indicators are those from which the quality of nursing care impacts the outcomes. Falls are considered a nurse-sensitive quality indicator. The nurse can assess the fall risk, give it a nursing diagnosis, plan and implement fall prevention measures, and evaluate their effectiveness.

Case Study 7.2

1. Name the factors that contributed to this medication error.

Many factors contribute to medication errors in general: noise, lighting, interruptions, and so on. In this particular scenario, the nurse may have been tired because it was the end of the night shift. The critical nature of the situation, and the lack of a second nurse to assist the primary nurse in the scenario, may also have played a role. In addition, it is not known if the patient stated an allergy to morphine sulfate, didn't know about the allergy, or wasn't asked.

2. How could this sentinel event have been prevented?

Documentation should include the initial admission assessment of allergies prior to any medication being given.

3. Name safety guards that can be implemented to prevent future similar sentinel events.

The complex interactions of the health care environment contribute to human errors and unanticipated outcomes. In order to prevent similar events of this type, an interprofessional team should be formed to look at current processes not only in the ED, but also throughout the hospital, and determine how these processes can be improved. This may result in a change in physician order sheets, clinical pathways, the environment, and established safety nets. The physicians, nurses, pharmacists, and other affected clinicians will need to receive additional education on the situation, the change implemented, and how it will be evaluated. This would be a good instance to use the PDSA cycle.

REVIEW QUESTIONS

Please see Appendix D for answers to Review Questions.

1. The definition of QI includes which of the following actions. Select all that apply.

A. Using data to look at health care processes

B. Improving processes to efficiently provide care

C. Monitoring the outcomes from health care processes

D. Selecting appropriate QI methods

E. Collecting data on changes made to health care processes

F. Focusing on data from improvement efforts

G. Using data to design changes to the organization

H. Testing changes made to identify if improvement occurred

I. Providing data to nurses and interprofessional personnel annually

2. Which of the following is a primary goal of QI?

   A. Improve patient outcomes
   B. Improve data reported to external regulatory agencies
   C. Improve cost-effectiveness of care delivery
   D. Improve reimbursement rates by insurers

3. Many initiatives shaped how QI is viewed today. Which of the following options did not historically influence the current status of quality health care delivery in health care organizations?

   A. Conducting peer reviews of care provided
   B. Outlier identification
   C. Publicly reporting of data
   D. Value-based purchasing

4. A group of nurses on a medical–surgical unit identified that patients were readmitted to the hospital based on a lack of understanding of discharge instructions. They decided to look at how they could assess every patient's health literacy level (understanding of health information). The group identifies three tools commonly found in the literature and systematically searched for evidence and evaluated each tool. They decide on one tool that is appropriate for their medical–surgical population of patients. To implement the tool, they teach the nurses how to use it and document the patient's literacy level score in the chart. Is this considered research, QI, or EBP?

   A. It is research since the nurses research each tool to find evidence.
   B. It is QI since the goal was to improve the quality of patient care.
   C. It is EBP since the nurses evaluated the evidence and selected the most appropriate tool for their patient population.
   D. It is none of the above since the nurses only wanted to find out the patient's literacy level.

5. Which of the following processes demonstrates the use of Deming's PDSA method for QI?

   A. Collect baseline data, evaluate the improvement, measure outcomes, and redesign the plan
   B. Collect baseline data, use small-scale trials for change, collect data and compare against desired outcomes, and adjust the plan
   C. Implement small-scale change, collect data, disseminate the data, and sustain the improvement
   D. Implement changes, evaluate effects from change, identify data, and readjust the plan

6. Many organizations are combining Lean and Six Sigma concepts within their QI efforts. What option below best explains why this combination may be successful?

   A. Lean focuses on optimizing existing processes for cost reduction and efficiency while Six-Sigma focuses on minimizing variability to eliminate defects.
   B. Lean focuses on variability reduction over time while Six Sigma focuses on efficiency in the current existing process.
   C. Lean, emphasizing efficiency, and Six Sigma, emphasizing increasing variability, are seldom combined as they both focus on separate improvement methods.
   D. Lean focuses on eliminating existing processes to reduce costs while Six Sigma focuses on eliminating defects to increase variability over time.

7. Which option below is true about a fishbone diagram?

    A. It is a useful data analysis tool in determining variability over time.
    B. It visually represents a process from beginning to end.
    C. It is commonly used to study cause and effect relationships.
    D. It is a QI tool to identify relationship between possible factors.

8. HFMEA is different from an RCA because of which of the following?

    A. HFMEA is a proactive process to assess and eliminate complex, hazardous processes before they result in adverse events. RCA is a retrospective analysis of an event that has already occurred.
    B. HFMEA is a proactive process of an event that has already occurred. RCA is a retrospective process to identify the most appropriate intervention when developing a PDSA.
    C. HFMEA is an adverse events documentation system commonly employed by organizations to track sentinel events. RCA is an improvement tool that must be done annually on one significant event that occurred within the organization.
    D. HFMEA is one single process used to enhance the quality culture within the organization. RCA is a part of every PDSA and is documented as part of the D ("Do") phase.

9. Which of the following types of problems would prompt the initiation of an RCA? Select all that apply.

    A. A suicidal patient signs out AMA in the ED (against medical advice).
    B. An adult dose of heparin is given to an infant.
    C. Surgery was performed on the wrong leg.
    D. Failure to resuscitate a patient after an inadvertent morphine overdose in the hospital.
    E. A patient with an order for full ambulation by self-falls.
    F. Readmission of a patient within 24 hours for the same medical diagnosis.

10. How can a new nurse participate in QI activities?

    A. Conduct data collection and share information with others.
    B. Assemble a team to look at a quality problem.
    C. Conduct reviews of the literature and use analytical tools to synthesize evidence.
    D. Lead a QI team in identifying a problem and developing a practice guideline.

REVIEW ACTIVITIES

Please see Appendix E for answers to Review Activities.

1. Go to the IHI website at http://www.ihi.org. Select IHI Open School. Select Courses and Certificates. Select course number PS 104 (Root Cause and Systems Analysis) and complete the course.
2. Try conducting a HFMEA on a current clinical process. Use the template provided at http://app.ihi.org/Workspace/tools/fmea/CreateTool.aspx. You will need to register on the website before being able to access the tool.

3. Go to the Agency for Healthcare Research and Quality website and select the QI Toolkit at http://www.ahrq.gov/qual/qitoolkit. Access the Toolkit Roadmap link. Access section A.3. "Getting Ready for Change Self-Assessment." Complete the self-assessment.

4. Use the survey in the pdf file (http://www.ahrq.gov/qual/qitoolkit/a3_selfassessment.pdf) to interview a nurse about the organization's readiness for QI. Discuss your findings with a classmate. Think about what this tells you about the organization's readiness for QI initiatives.

EXPLORING THE WEB

1. Agency for Healthcare Research and Quality: www.ahrq.gov
2. Magnet Recognition Model: http://www.nursecredentialing.org/Magnet/ProgramOverview/New-Magnet-Model
3. National Committee for Quality Assurance (NCQA): www.ncqa.org/tabid/142/Default.aspx
4. Patient Safety Measure Tools & Resources (Agency for Healthcare Research and Quality): www.ahrq.gov/professionals/quality-patient-safety/patient-safety-resources/index.html
5. Quality Improvement Methodology: http://www.hrsa.gov/quality/toolbox/methodology/index.html
6. Quality Measures and Resources: www.ahrq.gov/professionals/quality-patient-safety/quality-resources/tools/index.html

REFERENCES

Anthony, M. (January 31, 2004). Shared governance models: The theory, practice, and evidence. *The Online Journal of Issues in Nursing, 9*(1), manuscript 4. Retrieved from www.nursingworld.org/MainMenuCategories/ANAMarketplace/ANAPeriodicals/OJIN/TableofContents/Volume92004/No1Jan04/SharedGovernanceModels.aspx; www.ana.nursingworld.org/qualitynetwork/patientfallsreduction.pdf

Arbor Associates, Inc. (2011). *Arbor specializes in telephone mode patient satisfaction surveys.* Retrieved from http://www.arbor-associates.com

Berwick, D. M. (2011). Preparing nurses for participation in and leadership of continual improvement. *Journal of Nursing Education, 50*(6), 322–327. doi:10.3928/0148483420110519–05

Centers for Medicare and Medicaid (2013). *Hospital quality initiative: Value-based purchasing.* Retrieved from www.cms.gove/Medicare/Quality-Initiatives-Patient-Assessment-Instruments/HospitalQualityInits/index.html?redirect=/HospitalQUALITYINITS/30_HOSPITALHCAHPS.ASP

Cronenwett, L., Sherwood, G., Barnsteiner J., Disch, J., Johnson, J., Mitchell, P., Sullivan, D., & Warren, J. (2007). Quality and safety education for nurses. *Nursing Outlook, 55*(3),122–131

Donabedian, A. (2003). *An introduction to quality assurance in health care.* New York, NY: Oxford University Press.

Evans, J. R. (2008). *Quality & performance excellence: Management, organization, and strategy* (5th ed.). Mason, OH: Thompson South-Western.

Hughes, R. G. (2008a). Tools and strategies for quality improvement and patient safety. In R.Hughes (Ed.), *Patient safety and quality: An evidence-based handbook for nurses.* Chapter 44. AHRQ Publication No. 08–0043. Rockville, MD: Agency for Healthcare Research and Quality. Retrieved from http://www.ahrq.gov/qual/nurseshdbk

Hughes, R. G. (2008b). Nurses at the "sharp end" of patient care. In R. Hughes (Ed.), *Patient safetyand quality: An evidence-based handbook for nurses.* Chapter 2. AHRQ Publication No.

08–0043. Rockville, MD: Agency for Healthcare Research and Quality. Retrieved from http://www. ahrq.gov/qual/nurseshdbk

Langley, G. L., Nolan, K. M., Nolan, T. W., Norman, C. L., & Provost, L. P. (2009). *The improvement guide: A practical approach to enhancing organizational performance* (2nd ed.). San Francisco, CA: Jossey Bass. Retrieved from http://www.institute.nhs.uk/quality_and_service_improvement_tools/quality_and_service_improvement_tools/plan_do_study_act.html

Lindberg, L., & Kimberlain, J. (2008). Engage employees to improve staff and patient satisfaction. *Hospitals & Health Networks, 82*(1), 28–29. Retrieved from http://www. hhnmag.com/hhn-mag/jsp/articledisplay.jsp?dcrpath=HHNMAG/Article/data/01JAN2008/0801HHN_FEA_QualityUpDate&domain=HHNMAG

Luce, J. M., Bindman, A., & Lee, P. R. (1994). A brief history of health care quality assessment and improvement in the United States. *The Western Journal of Medicine, 160*, 263–268. Retrieved from http://www.ncbi.nlm.nih.gov/pmc/articles/PMC1022402

McLaughlin, M., Houston, K., & Harder-Mattson, E. (2012). Managing outcomes using an organizational quality improvement model. In P. Kelly (Ed.), *Nursing leadership & management* (3rd ed., pp. 474–496). Clifton Park, NY: Delmar.

Moen, R., & Norman, C. (2009). *Evolution of the PDCA cycle*. Associates in process improvement. Retrieved from http://pkpinc.com/files/NA01_Moen_Norman_fullpaper.pdf

Painter, D. R. (2010). Nurse's responsibility to improve practice (editorial). *Nephrology Nursing Journal, 37*(3), 227.

Pocha, C. (2010). Lean six sigma in health care and the challenge of implementation of six sigma methodologies at a veterans affairs medical center. *Quality Management in Health Care, 19*(4), 312–318.

Porter O'Grady, T. (2008). *Implementing shared governance: Creating a professional organization.* Retrieved November 25, 2012, from http://www.tpogassociates.com/SharedGovernance.Htm

Shankar R. (2009). *Process improvement using six sigma.* Milwaukee, WI: ASQ Quality Press.

The Joint Commission (September 30, 2012). *Summary data of sentinel events reviewed by The Joint Commission.* Retrieved from http://www.jointcommission.org/sentinel_event.aspx

SUGGESTED READING

Burhans, L. M., & Alligood, M. R. (2010). Quality nursing care in the words of nurses. *Journal of Advanced Nursing, 66*(8), 1689–1697. doi:10.1111/j.1365–2648.2010.05344.x

Draper, D. A., Felland, L. E., Liebhaber, A., & Melichar, L. (March, 2008). *The role of nurses in hospital quality improvement.* Research Brief Number 3. Center for Studying Health System Brief. Retrieved from http://www.rwjf.org/pr/product.jsp?id=27532

Kohn, L. T., Corrigan, J., & Donaldson, M. S. (1999). *To err is human: Building a safer health system.* A report of the committee on quality of health care in America, Institute of Medicine. Washington, DC: National Academy Press.

BENCHMARKING QUALITY PERFORMANCE

Beth A. Vottero, Michelle E. Block, and Lindsay Bonaventura

Be a yardstick of quality. Some people aren't used to an environment where excellence is expected.—*Steve Jobs* (Young, 2009)

Upon completion of this chapter, the reader should be able to

1. Describe the use of benchmarking in health care
2. Apply the systematic steps of benchmarking to a health care issue
3. Describe appropriate internal and external sources for benchmarking
4. Understand the benefits and limitations of benchmarking performance

---

*Y*ou are the department director of a medical unit. You recently received the monthly report on your unit's 30-day readmission rates for patients with heart failure (HF). You see that the readmission rates improved from the previous 3 months, but you are just not convinced that the rates are as good as everyone says. A group of physicians and pharmacists created a patient discharge protocol that was put into place 6 months ago. Many of the nurses and physicians are still not aware of the protocol and its use is haphazard. Not all charts of patients with HF have the protocol included. The nurses on the unit are asking why the protocol isn't computerized and put into their documentation. You still have questions that you want to find answers to, for example:

- *How do you know how well your unit performed?*
- *Who do you need to include on a team to work on decreasing the 30-day readmission rates for patients with HF?*
- *How can you determine, and help set goals for, excellence in patient care to minimize or prevent unwanted outcomes?*

*T*he provision of health care is a team effort that requires coordination of interprofessionals to ensure that health care meets quality standards. Each profession contributes to the delivery of high-quality patient care and has its own measures of quality. Measuring the quality of care provided is critical to ensuring that each patient experiences the best possible outcome from his or her health care encounter. A frame of reference is necessary to understand findings from quality measures. Benchmarks can help an organization, unit, or team evaluate performance, identify opportunities for improvement, and focus resources on specific quality issues.

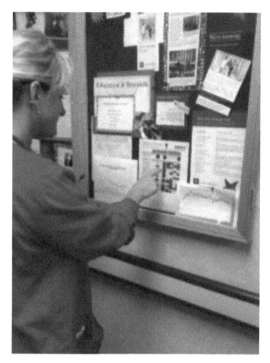

Nurses reviewing quality data.

This chapter provides an overview of how benchmarking is used in health care with definitions and practical applications. Benchmarking is explored as a quality improvement (QI) tool using a systematic process. An examination of internal and external sources of benchmarks, benefits, and limitations of using benchmarks, and the purpose and value of benchmarking performance is included. The application of benchmarks to current nursing practice is explored, including actions taken to improve health care processes and care outcomes based on benchmarked results.

BENCHMARKING IN HEALTH CARE

The Institute of Medicine's (IOM) report, *To Err Is Human* (IOM, 1999) highlighted the need to provide high-quality care to every patient every time. To do so, hospitals need to carefully examine and measure current patient care processes and outcomes, then select appropriate benchmarks for comparison. Following a clinical practice guideline that includes turning a patient who is bedridden every 2 hours to prevent skin breakdown is an example of patient care processes. **Benchmarking** is defined as "the continual and collaborative discipline of measuring and comparing the results of key work processes with those of the best performers in evaluating organizational performance" (Hughes, 2008). The Agency for Healthcare Research and Quality (AHRQ) define benchmarking as "an attribute or achievement that serves as a standard for other providers or institutions to emulate" (AHRQ, 2012).

Benchmarking begins with identifying what to measure, commonly known as the quality indicator. Indicators are generally classified as structure, process, or outcome indicators, and reflect standards of care. **Structure indicators** include attributes in the environment where care is delivered and often consist of materials, people, and the structure of the organization (IOM, 2006). Availability of technology such as MRI at the organization, clinical guidelines updated every 2 years, or nurse-to-patient ratios are examples of structural indicators. **Process of care indicators** include the

TABLE 8.1 EXAMPLES OF STRUCTURE, PROCESS, AND OUTCOME INDICATORS

STRUCTURE	PROCESS	OUTCOME
• Location of the unit, storage, medication room, supplies, and so on • Skill, education, experience, and certification of nurses	• Frequency of assessments • Turning patients every 2 hours • Indwelling urinary catheter removed within 24 hours after surgery • Medications administered within one-half hour before and one-half hour after the dose is due	• Falls/falls with injury • Hospital-acquired pressure ulcer • Catheter-associated urinary tract infection • Medication error

evidence-based steps (interventions, actions, or tasks) that when performed help to meet desired outcomes (www.qualitymeasures.ahrq.gov/tutorial/ProcessMeasure.aspx). Compliance rates with hand hygiene standard or the proportion of patients whose care follows clinical guidelines are examples of process of care indicators. **Outcome indicators** include the end result from the delivery of care, for example, the presence of falls, pressure ulcers, hospital-acquired infections, patient satisfaction, or readmission to the hospital (www.qualitymeasures.ahrq.gov/tutorial/ProcessMeasure.aspx). Examples of structure, process, and outcome indicators can be found in Table 8.1.

For additional examples of structure, process, and outcome indicators, go to http://patientsafetyed.duhs.duke.edu and select "A. What is Quality Improvement?" by clicking on the "begin" button. On the left side, select "Measurement: Process and Outcome Indicators." For this chapter, we focus on process of care and outcome indicators that are typically benchmarked.

CASE STUDY 8.1

A hospital measures surgical-site infection rates every quarter and benchmarks them at zero. Last quarter, their rate of infection was 12. The previous year their average rate of infection was 4. The quality department director convened a QI team consisting of surgeons, surgical technicians, nurses, laboratory, radiology, and administration to address the rise in their infection rates. Because surgical-site infections can be related to a variety of issues, the team decided to first tackle the preoperative site preparation issue. Current practice on the medical–surgical units is to have the patient take an antiseptic shower the night prior to surgery. When indicated, the nurse removes the patient's hair using a razor. The committee decided to standardize preoperative care throughout the hospital by identifying best practices for preparing skin to reduce surgical-site infections. They begin by reviewing the evidence related to preoperative preparation of surgical patients:

- Clipping of hair should be done as close to surgical time as possible. Shaving hair and the use of depilatory lotions are not recommended.
- Antiseptic bathing does not alter the rate of postoperative surgical-site infections. It also does not contribute to surgical-site infections.

(continued)

CASE STUDY 8.1 (continued)

1. *Create two indicators based on the information provided. One process of care indicator and one outcome indicator.*
2. *How will you measure the indicators?*
3. *Create one benchmark for the scenario.*
4. *Who should be responsible for measuring the indicators and evaluating performance toward the benchmark?*

Benchmarking incorporates QI principles of using a systematic method to identify a problem, select best practices, determine how the best practice fits with the organization, initiate a change process, and evaluate outcomes. Data is produced from measuring patient processes of care or outcomes. The data is compared against other data to determine performance levels. In Chapter 9, data collection is explored in detail. Once a patient process of care or outcome is measured, it becomes necessary to evaluate this measurement against a reference benchmark point to determine if performance is good or bad. By comparing your outcomes against a benchmark, you can then determine if a process requires improvement.

Critical Thinking 8.1

Based on recent internal trended data, your hospital's clinical staff believes they are doing very well with measures regarding venous thromboembolism (VTE) prophylaxis. You have just finished learning about benchmarks and you notice that there are no benchmarks provided for VTE prophylaxis. Use the information from the National Guidelines Clearinghouse website, http://www.guideline.gov/content.aspx?id=39350, to help answer the following questions:

1. How do you identify an appropriate benchmark?
2. What VTE process of care benchmarks would be appropriate for pharmacists? For physicians? For nurses?
3. How would you explain the need for and value of benchmarking to your colleagues?

Dashboards

To be worthwhile, data need to be turned into usable information. A **dashboard** is a useful tool that provides a way of displaying quality data over time. Data is visually displayed in a systematic manner that allows users to quickly understand the meaning. Dashboards can include color graphics and highlights to help users see the data, identify trends or patterns, extract meaning, and clarify implications. Table 8.2 is an

TABLE 8.2 HAND HYGIENE COMPLIANCE DASHBOARD

	JANUARY	FEBRUARY	MARCH	APRIL	MAY	JUNE	TARGET	BENCHMARK
Unit A	**91%**	80%	87%	86%	73%	69%	90%	100%
Unit B	40%	45%	44%	54%	79%	59%	90%	100%
Unit C	87%	88%	84%	88%	**90%**	**93%**	90%	100%

Note: Values in bold meet target.

example of a dashboard that illustrates hand hygiene compliance rates for 6 months on three different units. The dashboard includes the target of 90% compliance with hand hygiene, which is determined by the organization as to be the acceptable rate for hand hygiene compliance. The benchmark established by the top performers in hand hygiene compliance is 100%. The units and months that achieved the target of 90% are bolded. By using bold for the data meeting the target of 90%, the data become information on trends and patterns regarding hand hygiene compliance for the units. You can quickly identify that Unit B did not meet the target or benchmark for any of the 6 months. Unit A did meet the target for January but demonstrated a decrease in hand hygiene compliance during the 6-month period. Unit C show hand hygiene compliance rates rose during the time period to meet the target of 90%. This example illustrates how a dashboard takes isolated bits of data (each month's hand hygiene compliance percentage for each unit) and brings the data together to make usable information through trends on a unit, comparisons between units, and comparisons against the target, goal, and benchmark for hand hygiene compliance.

Critical Thinking 8.2

The North Carolina Quality Center created a website that represents data from all hospitals in the state in a standardized dashboard. Go to http://www.nchospitalquality. org and select "quality dashboards" on the lower right. Select a hospital from the drop down list. Examine how the color coding helps the viewer to understand the data displayed.

1. Examine the use of color coding to represent the quality of care. How do the colors help in understanding the care provided at the hospital?
2. How do the findings from the hospital you selected compare with the hospital where you have clinicals or where you work?

Small tests of change are appropriate when an intervention is applied then measured to see if it affected the compliance rates. For example, posting reminders to follow hand hygiene compliance then collecting data to see if the reminders caused a change in compliance rates. Since hand hygiene compliance rates are measured and reported monthly, any change in compliance rates may be a reflection of the intervention. This is especially important if a unit is significantly underperforming, such as Unit B in Table 8.1. For Unit B, a target of 90% is overwhelming when their compliance rates with hand hygiene are low. In this case, it is acceptable to set a target at an achievable rate and increase the target percentage rate over time.

Balanced Scorecard

A similar, yet slightly different tool used to evaluate quality measurement findings against benchmarks is called a balanced scorecard. A balanced scorecard helps the hospital translate their strategic goals into a set of performance measures. The performance measures help the hospital administrators understand how well they are doing in terms of their strategic goals. The "balanced" part of the name represents the ideal, in that the scorecard should include measures from all aspects of the hospital and include both long- and short-term indicators. Similar to the dashboard, each of the indicators includes a target or benchmark to identify excellent performance as well as color coding of red, yellow, and green. If an indicator is not reaching the target or benchmark, an action plan is created. We discuss action plans in the systematic problem assessment section.

Critical Thinking 8.3

Perform a Google Image search for "hospital balanced scorecard." Examine the various formats, types, and displays of the different balanced scorecards.

1. Which of the balanced scorecards is easiest for you to understand? Explain why.
2. Do the balanced scorecards you found compare performance measures against benchmarks or targets? Why is this important?

SYSTEMATIC STEPS IN BENCHMARKING A CURRENT ISSUE

To understand how benchmarking can support quality health care, an example of a current health care quality issue provides the framework for discussion. Readmission rates for patients with HF are a current quality measure required for all inpatient hospitals as mandated by the Centers for Medicare and Medicaid Services (CMS, 2012). Readmission within 30 days of discharge is considered high cost, preventable and, in most cases, an adverse event for the patient (Lacker, 2011). For example, an inpatient unit discharges 20 patients with HF during the past month. Four of the patients return within 30 days of their discharge with similar HF symptoms, resulting in a 20% readmission rate. It is difficult to determine if this is a good or a bad number unless there is a benchmark for comparison.

Having a database, or repository, from many hospitals can strengthen benchmark comparisons. Comparing a hospital's performance against one organization's data is one thing; comparing it against a database of hundreds of hospitals makes the comparison stronger. If the national average for patient readmission rates is 53%, a hospital's achievement of a 20% rate seems relatively good in comparison. Keep in mind, the lower the rate, the better it is, since a higher rate means more patients are readmitted to the hospital. However, if the best-performing hospitals reported a readmission rate of 5%, then the hospital would want to look at their processes for care delivery. Remember, when comparing numbers, it is essential to compare or benchmark against those hospitals that are leaders in the delivery of care to patients with HF. In this scenario, the hospital may want to set their benchmark at zero readmissions, aiming for excellence in care.

EVIDENCE FROM THE LITERATURE

Citation

Nielsen, G. A., Bartely, A., Coleman, E., Resar, R., Rutherford, P., Souw, D., & Taylor, J. (2008). *Transforming care at the bedside how-to guide: Creating an ideal transition home for patients with heart failure*. Cambridge, MA: Institute for Healthcare Improvement. Retrieved from www.IHI.org

Discussion

Approximately 5 million people have HF in the United States. A diagnosis of HF involves a significant effect on quality of life and is the leading cause of rehospitalization among older adults. The economic toll on the individual and the health care system is staggering, costing an estimated $29.6 billion annually. Implementing evidence-based interventions that prepare the adult patient with HF for discharge can significantly impact patient readmission rates. Such interventions include admission assessment clarification of postdischarge needs, enhanced teaching, patient- and family-centered handoff communication between health care providers and patient follow-up after discharge. The authors described the need to include a variety of health care disciplines in the formation of a team to decrease patient readmissions.

Implications for Practice

To decrease readmission rates for patients with HF, a focused interprofessional team approach is critical.

Systematic Problem Assessment

The process of benchmarking involves a series of steps or stages that begins with identifying a problem. Problems are usually identified from triggers. A **trigger** is an event or change that requires subsequent action (Institute for Healthcare Improvement [IHI], 2012). For example, triggers may include downward changes or trends in data such as hand hygiene compliance dropping from 93% to 70% in a given time frame. Another trigger is a negative comparison to industry standards such as hand hygiene compliance required at 90% and a health care organization demonstrating 70% compliance. Triggers can also come from changes to regulatory requirements, such as hand hygiene compliance for a health care organization currently at 93%, The Joint Commission changes their ruling for compliance to 95% making performance on this measure below required levels. Once a problem is identified, the organization uses a series of steps, similar to the nursing process, to address the issue: assess the current problem, diagnose the problem, develop a plan for change, implement the plan, and evaluate and monitor outcomes.

Using readmission rates for patients with HF, we will look at how these steps can be applied in a health care organization. It is important to note that benchmarks for HF readmission rates are subject to change. The current national 30-day HF readmission rate is 24.7% (https://data.medicare.gov/Hospital-Compare/Hospital-Outcome-Of-Care-Measures-National-Average/i2h8–79qx).

Step 1: Assess the Current Problem

At a local hospital, a trigger is identified from data collected on readmission rates. The HF readmission rates for the hospital are 28.6%. Data on the highest performing hospitals used as a national benchmark are reported at 9%. The national average for patients with HF readmission rates is 20.7%. Based on the data, the hospital's readmission rate of 28.6% is higher than the national average of 20.7% and significantly higher than the top-performing hospital's rate of 9%, constituting a trigger. Another trigger for change comes from reimbursement adjustments made by the CMS for patients with HF readmitted within 30 days of discharge for the same diagnosis. As the organization already monitors readmission rates for HF, it is able to quickly identify that a problem exists.

Before going further, it is essential to assemble an interprofessional team to perform the systematic problem assessment. The interprofessional team should include all stakeholders—those individuals and roles that affect and are affected by the process under investigation. Including stakeholders allows insights into parts of the process that only they may know about. For example, a pharmacist on the team provides valuable information on medications, the ability to provide access to necessary medications, timing of dosing, potential interactions, and educational resources for teaching patients about their medications for home use. Including stakeholders also allows an understanding of how each person's role affects the care of the patient while hospitalized and after discharge. Table 8.3 describes the stakeholders, their roles, and the rationale for including them on the team.

The QI team begins by assessing the current health care process, from admission through discharge. In this case, outcome indicator measurements include the patient with HF 30-day readmission rates. Process of care indicator measurements can include the use of evidence-based interventions designed to support the patient with HF such as discharge teaching that includes specific elements such as educating the patient on the medications and signs and symptoms of worsening HF, prescribing certain medications such as an angiotensin-converting enzyme (ACE) inhibitor or angiotensin receptor blocker (ARB) for left ventricular end diastolic dysfunction, smoking cessation counseling, and assessment of left ventricular heart function (LVHF) using an echocardiogram with documentation of findings in the chart (Heidenreich et al., 2012). Examination of current health care processes involves reviewing all related policies, protocols, and guidelines, as well as the chart of a patient with HF from admission through discharge to develop a full understanding.

Critical Thinking 8.4

One of the benchmarking measures for patients with HF is smoking cessation education. The evidence supports smoking cessation education as directly affecting patients' functional outcomes and reducing both ED visits and future hospitalizations. To meet the benchmarking measure, a hospital has a checklist for patient discharge that

(continued)

includes smoking cessation education. When checking the list, the health care worker checks off that the patient has received both a packet of preprinted smoking cessation education and face-to-face counseling.

1. Does the checklist capture the quality of the smoking cessation education and counseling? Why or why not?
2. Is the checklist method effective in capturing the outcome of smoking cessation education and face-to-face counseling on patient readmission rates?
3. Develop alternate ways of capturing the quality of the smoking cessation education and face-to-face counseling.

TABLE 8.3 HEART FAILURE READMISSION COMMITTEE COMPOSITION

STAKEHOLDER/ROLE	RATIONALE
Bedside nurse	The bedside nurse understands the needs of the patient at discharge, including education, home support, and health care needs.
Case manager	The case manager identifies community resources available to assist the patient.
Physician	The physician brings the medical perspective to the patient's care. This includes information on the patient's office visits and the need for continuity of care.
Pharmacy	The pharmacist helps to coordinate the medication needs of the patient, from the hospital to home; including the availability of resources to help the underserved access any needed medications.
QI representative	The QI representative collects and represents data using graphs, charts, and other visual aids to assist other health care workers in understanding the data. This includes data on patient readmission rates and comparisons to benchmarks.
Laboratory	The laboratory helps identify both inpatient and outpatient laboratory resources.
Patient education representative	The patient education representative develops and coordinates educational materials for the patient with HF.
Nurse for patients with HF	In some organizations there is a dedicated nursing position with the sole focus on patients with HF. This nurse coordinates care in the hospital and assists with community outpatient services.
Social services	The social worker brings knowledge about community resources for the patient with HF. These resources may include information on coordinating home health services.
Finance	A representative from the finance department of the hospital brings the economic impact perspective to the committee.
Informatics	The informatics specialist helps make sure the appropriate documentation is captured for the specified patient population and can suggest or make changes to the electronic charting system.
Pastoral care	A pastoral care representative brings the holistic aspect of body–mind–spirit needs to the discussion.

QI, quality improvement. HF, heart failure.

Step 2: Diagnose the Problem

After establishing a knowledge base of current best practices, the QI team identifies those areas in need of change. **Performance gaps** describe the difference between current practice and the recommended standard of care (AHRQ, 2010). For example, the standard of care is that all patients with HF who smoke receive smoking cessation counseling. If a hospital does not provide smoking cessation counseling for all patients with HF that currently smoke, it is considered a performance gap. The QI team starts by evaluating their current practices against the best practices of high performers. There are several places to look for information on best practices, for example, the IHI (www.ihi.org), the AHRQ (www.ahrq.gov), and The Joint Commission (www.jointcommission.org). The National Guidelines Clearinghouse (www.guidelines.gov) is a repository of clinical practice guidelines on a wide variety of topics. Evidence from the literature such as systematic reviews also provide guidance in crafting policies, protocols, and guidelines for care of many types of patients, including the patient with HF. Some high-performing organizations are willing to share their practices, including pathways, protocols, and guidelines, often providing information upon request.

Step 3: Develop a Plan for Change

The QI team develops a plan for implementation that specifies the type of indicator, actions that need to be completed, person(s) responsible, date for completion, current data, and the benchmark. Table 8.4 illustrates a sample action plan to address a smoking cessation counseling process of care indicator.

The plan should be specific and clear so that every team member knows his or her responsibilities. For example, if a revision of the current care pathway is necessary, a temporary team can be formed from the larger QI team to work on a revision of the care process. The temporary team may include a variety of interprofessional disciplines whose role relates to the specific issue for which the team is formed.

Step 4: Implement and Educate

The implementation plan for the new care process should require that all who will work with the process are educated about changes. Based on the composition of the team, members must develop a strategy for teaching the new care process to the staff of their respective departments. Although this appears simple, it is at this point that many projects fail. Dissemination of all changes must be clear and include how the changes should proceed and the expectations for performance. For example, if the team is created to focus on the prescribing of ACE inhibitors, then a physician must be on the team and would take the changes to the physician quality committee for approval. Once approved, a dissemination method may include a handout explaining the care process changes, given to all physicians in their mailbox, sending an e-mail, and posting notices in the physician lounge. This step-by-step change strategy helps disseminate the information.

Step 5: Evaluate and Monitor Outcomes

Once education is completed for all stakeholders and departments, evaluation data on compliance rates with the change are collected and analyzed. Postimplementation data is collected and compared against preimplementation data. Stating who is responsible for data collection, what data is collected, who holds the data, and when to bring

TABLE 8.4 SAMPLE ACTION PLAN

PROCESS OF CARE INDICATOR	ACTIONS	PERSON(S) RESPONSIBLE	DATE FOR COMPLETION	CURRENT DATA	BENCHMARK
Smoking cessation counselling completed for all patients with HF	Define who is responsible for smoking cessation counselling	QI team	2 weeks	15% compliance	100% of all patients with HF who smoke will have smoking cessation counselling
	Define where and when the smoking cessation counselling will occur	QI team	1 month		
	Create an area to document counseling provided	Informatics representative and nursing representative	1–2 months		
	Define who will collect the data	QI team	2 weeks		

QI, quality improvement. HF, heart failure.

the data back to the team is essential. The anticipated result of data collection is the identification of adherence to changes in practice as measured through process of care indicators. Earlier we identified the process of care indicators as discharge teaching, prescribing an ACE inhibitor or ARB for left ventricular end diastolic function, smoking cessation counseling, and documentation of LVHF. Ideally, when the process of care indicators is followed, identified by data collection on the indicators, there is a reduction in the associated outcome indicator, readmission rates of patients with HF within 30 days of discharge.

CASE STUDY 8.2

A surgical unit experiences a rise in the number of catheter-associated urinary tract infections over the last quarter. In looking at its data, the unit notes that it has had the same number of postsurgical patients with catheters each month over the past year. To follow benchmarking principles, the nurses decide to look at their processes of care including the insertion of catheters and the care of patients with catheters. They review evidence on best practices for care of patients with catheters. The current practice for the care of postsurgical patients with catheters is to cleanse the perineal area daily with betadine, ensure patency of the catheter tubing, maintain the drainage bag at a level below the patient for gravity drainage, and remove the catheter per established standards of care on Day 3 postinsertion of the urinary catheter.

(continued)

> ### CASE STUDY 8.2 (continued)
>
> 1. *Who should be included on a team to look at the practice of urinary catheter care and removal?*
> 2. *Perform a web search on the topic of care of patients with urinary catheters. What are the best practices for care? How do the current practices in the case study compare with your findings?*
> 3. *What process of care indicators should be monitored?*

INTERNAL AND EXTERNAL BENCHMARKING

Internal benchmarking is using data from within the health care organization as a comparison (Hughes, 2008). For example, outcome data collected from Unit A shows inpatient fall rates of 25/1,000 patient days. Unit B's outcome data show inpatient fall rates of 3/1,000 patient days. Unit A could decide to benchmark its performance against Unit B. To have the same outcome as Unit A, Unit B would also need to examine Unit A's process of care indicators, what Unit A is doing to prevent patient falls, and the type of patient on each unit. One concern with internal benchmarking involves the small comparison. Unit B is only benchmarking their performance using single measures from a unit within the same organization. Internal benchmarking can work when there are multiple departments or units to compare against, such as nursing units throughout a health care organization. For other disciplines such as radiology or laboratory, internal benchmarking is difficult if not impossible due to the lack of comparisons. For example, the radiology department could not benchmark the amount of dye usage for imaging since it is the only department using dye for imaging.

External benchmarking compares what you are doing against what others are doing (Hughes, 2008). The value of external benchmarking is the strength in numbers. Using the inpatient falls example, health care organizations report their fall rates to the CMS which, in turn, posts the results on its public website (www.hospitalcompare.gov). Using external benchmarking provides information on top performers from across the country. Unit A can choose to benchmark against the highest performing hospital with 0.5 falls per 1,000 patient days. In this case, the fall rate is much lower than if it used internal benchmarking. In addition, external benchmarking provides a wide variety of indicators for all disciplines. For example, the radiology department could benchmark its dye usage against other health care organizations. The radiology department can benchmark against the national average for dye usage or against levels of safe dye administration for a patient as determined by its standards of practice. Table 8.5 lists the major quality benchmark sources and access information.

External Benchmarking in Nursing

Many nursing organizations provide frameworks and standards for clinical practice. For example, the Association of periOperative Registered Nurses (AORN) has formulated a way to integrate data into an existing health record system to organize and structure clinical data to increase safety while providing patient care. Perioperative nursing is a specialty area that uses terms, vocabulary, and standards that are unique to perioperative care. The AORN worked closely with electronic medical record developers

TABLE 8.5 MAJOR SOURCES OF QUALITY BENCHMARKS

ORGANIZATION	FOCUS	WEBSITE/SOURCE
National Database for Nursing Quality Indicators (NDNQI)	Information on unit level data with comparison across participating hospitals	http://www.nursingquality.org
Centers for Medicare and Medicaid Services (CMS)	Information on Medicare and Medicaid services, health outcomes	http://www.cms.gov
The Joint Commission (TJC) Accountability Measures	Information on top-performing hospitals	http://www.jointcommission.org (type "accountability measures" in the upper right hand text box)
The Joint Commission ORYX Measures	Information on core clinical process and outcome measures	http://www.jointcommission.org (type "core clinical process and outcome measures" in the upper right hand text box)
Consumer Assessment of Healthcare Providers and Systems (CAHPS)	Information on outpatient satisfaction with health care	http://www.cahps.ahrq.gov
Hospital Consumer Assessment of Healthcare Providers and Systems (HCAHPS)	Information on inpatient's satisfaction with health care	http://www.hcahpsonline.org
American Customer Service Index	Information on all private and government industries performance	http://www.theacsi.org
Bureau of Labor Statistics, Department of Labor	Information on all industries occupational health/illnesses and injuries, lost time claims rate, top quartiles for performance	http://www.bls.gov

to create a unique documentation system for perioperative nursing care provided. The AORN framework provides a nursing data set, the Perioperative Nursing Data Set (PNDS), which standardizes a perioperative nursing vocabulary. In addition, the AORN provides regularly updated recommended best practices, invites comments related to proposed recommended best practices, furnishes guidance on implementation of recommended best practices, and expands knowledge of standards and recommended best practices through their *Independent Study Guide Based on Perioperative Standards and Recommended Practices* (AORN, 2012). Each of the framework provisions is web based and allow for external benchmarking of perioperative nursing practices.

The American Association of Critical-Care Nurses (AACN) provides standards, which are defined as "authoritative statements that describe the level of care or performance common to the profession of nursing by which the quality of nursing practice can be judged" (AACN, 2012). These standards include standards of practice for acute and critical care nurses, clinical nurse specialists, and nurse practitioners, as well as standards for establishing and sustaining a healthy work environment reference. In other words, the AACN has devised standards for the practice of acute and critical care nurses, which can be used to compare the practice of these nurses to the practice of nurses in other facilities.

Similar to the AORN, the Emergency Nurses Association has devised a web-based computer application for benchmarking with external agencies. The web-based computer application functions with various types of electronic health records and allows subscribers to make self-selected peer comparisons with ED nursing care provided in other agencies and provides timely, monthly reporting on ED key performance indicators (Emergency Nurses Association, 2012). This web-based computer application reviews three categories of patient care, that is, specific quality measures related to ED nursing care, throughput or the speed in which patients are registered, provided care, and either discharged or admitted, and productivity measures of ED care. It allows users to analyze trends, compare their performance with peers, assemble benchmarking reports, and analyze data to support evidence-based decision making.

The American Nurses Association (ANA) initiated the National Database of Nursing Quality Indicators (NDNQI, www.nursingquality.org). The NDNQI provides the registered nurse with research-based national comparative data on nursing care and its relationship to patient outcomes (NDNQI, 2012). The NDNQI serves as an archive for nursing-sensitive indicators, which are those outcomes from patient care that reflect the nursing care provided. The NDNQI gathers and reports comparisons of data compiled at the nursing unit level. In essence, the NDNQI provides key external benchmarking information on a local, state, and national basis. Examples of some of the nursing-sensitive indicators include patient falls, hospital-acquired pressure ulcers, nursing hours per patient day, restraints prevalence, and central line–associated blood stream infections. Reports allow for comparison of hospital type, staffed bed size, teaching status (teaching hospital vs. nonteaching hospital), location (metropolitan, state, census division), Magnet™ status, and case mix index (type of patients that use the hospital facility). Unit types include both adult and pediatric units of critical care, step-down, medical, surgical, medical–surgical combined, bone marrow transplant, high acuity, moderate acuity, blended acuity, burn unit, and universal bed (adults only). As of January 2012, there were 1,834 hospitals within the United States participating in the NDNQI. Reporting is voluntary but a fee applies to participate in the program.

REAL-WORLD INTERVIEW

Hospital participation in the NDNQI database is voluntary. The NDNQI database correlates closely with the National Quality Forum standards (Montalvo, 2007). The NDNQI database provides participating hospitals with important numbers that show how a hospital compares with others of similar size. In Magnet facilities, data is collected and reported to NDNQI. Staying at or above set benchmarks is one important component needed for Magnet redesignation. Therefore, using NDNQI data to drive and implement change to achieve benchmarks is necessary. This process empowers nurses to work in interprofessional teams to find solutions to problem areas. NDNQI benchmarking becomes a tool for implementation of evidence-based practice (EBP) that leads to best outcomes and results in policy changes.

Pat Larson, MSN, RN
Clinical and Professional Development Coordinator
Indiana University Health La Porte Hospital
La Porte, Indiana

Interprofessional Benchmarking

Interprofessional benchmarking with other health care organizations is a relatively recent endeavor. Interprofessional benchmarking includes the definition of comparing against the highest performers but includes consideration that some benchmarks require an interprofessional focus due to the multifaceted basis of quality issues. Interprofessional benchmarking reflects the understanding that patient care and patient outcomes are a result of care provided by a variety of health care professionals working together. Such benchmarks are set by organizations such as AHRQ, CMS, The Joint Commission, National Quality Forum, and others. Each agency identifies specific core measures, or those indicators that are central to providing quality patient care. Table 8.6 shows the major core measures resources.

Critical Thinking 8.5

Why Not the Best (http://www.whynotthebest.org) is a nonprofit website that gathers publicly available data and allows the user to examine the data in different ways. You can view the data from hospitals across the country and compare them against benchmarks, compare different size and types of hospitals, or examine total performance data by region. You can find out if the core measures in one region are better or worse than another region. Select your state on the map and click on your region. Take note of the outcomes. Select another state and click on a region. Compare the data on the core measures between the two regions.

1. *What makes one region better or worse than the other in terms of data from the core measures? Consider factors such as location, demographics, proximity to larger cities, and so on. Go to the Census website (http://www.census.gov/compendia/statab) and learn more about the area.*
2. *Do disparities between the outcomes of care on the core measures exist? Why or why not?*

TABLE 8.6 CORE MEASURES RESOURCES

Agency for Healthcare Research and Quality (AHRQ)	http://www.ahrq.gov/research/findings/nhqrdr/nhdr09/Core.html
Centers for Medicare and Medicaid Services (CMS)	https://www.federalregister.gov (type "initial core set of quality measures" in the search box, top right of screen)
The Joint Commission (TJC)	http://www.jointcommission.org/core_measure_sets.aspx
National Quality Forum	http://www.qualityforum.org/Measures_List.aspx

---

CASE STUDY 8.3

A patient is seen by a physician in the physician's office for lower back pain. The patient tells the physician that the pain is so severe that walking causes problems. The physician examines the patient, finding no lower extremity weakness, but finding significant problems with mobility due to the pain. The physician decides that the pain is related to a back muscle strain rather than a disc herniation. The patient and the physician discuss the treatment plan consisting of chiropractic care, physical therapy, and medications such as anti-inflammatories and muscle relaxers. The patient insists on having an MRI of the lower back to assist with diagnosis, stating, "I just know it's a disc, my father had a herniated disc, my sister had surgery on her back, and this is just like what they had." After consulting with a radiologist, the physician decides to follow the original treatment plan and not order an MRI. The radiology department's current MRI numbers are slightly above the national average for lower back MRIs.

1. *Is the physician correct in requiring treatment consisting of chiropractic care, physical therapy, and muscle relaxers?*
2. *Do you think the physician decided not to order the MRI because the current radiology use of MRIs for lower back pain is currently higher than national benchmarks? Defend your reasoning.*
3. *Does the patient have a voice in his or her treatment plan when what he or she wants is contrary to standards of practice?*

Benchmarking in Uncommon Areas

Nurses work in a variety of areas within a health care organization. Areas such as intensive care, medical, surgical, and other inpatient units have a vast array of recognized national benchmarks established. Other areas where nurse's work may not have nationally recognized benchmarks established. Some of these areas include cardiology, infusion centers, radiology, informatics, or outpatient cardiac rehabilitation.

An example of an area without nationally established benchmarks is the heart catheterization lab. In the heart catheterization lab, specific quality indicators are used to measure the quality of care provided. One of the indicators for quality and safety is monitoring exposure to radiation given to a patient during the procedure. The nurses closely monitor the exposure to radiation to ensure that the patient only receives the recommended exposure. This data is documented as part of the procedural record. It should also be noted that, in addition, personnel in the heart catheterization lab are also monitored for radiation exposure via radiation dosimeter badges. Exposure data is collected, recorded, and tracked for trending patterns. Data is compared on a quarterly basis (every 3 months) with data from previous quarters. To determine best practices, however, outside sources are sought to help establish benchmarks.

Sources for determining best practice and benchmarking for radiation exposure may come from professional organizations, such as the Alliance of Cardiovascular Professionals (http://www.acp-online.org) and the Society for Cardiovascular

Angiography and Interventions (http://www.scai.org). The composition of both of these organizations is interprofessional and include nurses, physicians, hospital management, and radiology technicians. Membership in these organizations offers professionals relevant information on care related to invasive and noninvasive cardiology, including the topic of radiation exposure. Such organizations set recommended limits for exposure for both patients and heart catheterization lab personnel through written guidelines and protocols, which can then be translated into policies and guidelines that drive safe practices in the clinical setting (Chambers et al., 2011). In effect, these guidelines act as a model to set benchmarking thresholds and drive the quality process.

BENEFITS AND LIMITATIONS FOR BENCHMARKING

The primary goal of health care delivery is to provide quality care to all patients during every encounter that supports positive outcomes for patients. The organization benefits from providing quality care to patients by receiving higher reimbursement rates from insurers and the CMS that support the economic stability of a health care organization. An additional benefit is improving the quality of health care provided for the community. Ideally, when using health care services from an organization that monitors care processes and compares itself against the industry leaders, the patient is the one who benefits as the recipient of high-quality health care. The public reporting of quality data in relation to benchmarks allows consumers to make informed choices for health care services. Health care organizations that focus on quality outcomes and meeting benchmarks enjoy a competitive advantage in the health care market. In a perfect scenario, all staff members are involved in benchmarking and providing quality care. This builds a culture of quality for all patients.

The use of benchmarking can create a culture where innovation or new ideas about care processes result from a continual analysis of health care processes. When an organization identifies a problem, the process of working through the issue lends itself to creativity and brainstorming for new and improved care delivery. Sustaining this creativity and levels of excellence requires an organization-wide commitment to maintaining quality outcomes as a priority from all health care workers.

REAL-WORLD INTERVIEW

Traditionally, performance in pharmacy, especially in a community pharmacy, has been measured primarily around prescription volume and percentage of medications dispensed as generics. All other things being equal, the busier your pharmacy was and the more generic medications you dispensed, the more successful you were. However, the profession of pharmacy, like the profession of medicine, is steadily moving to one in which our performance and reimbursement will be determined more by the quality, that is, clinical and economic outcomes, than by the volume of our services. There are a number of challenges inherent in this transition. One of the major challenges is determining what our performance is today versus what is a realistic expectation of what it should/could be based on industry best practices and benchmarking.

(continued)

Limitations of Benchmarking

Although beneficial, benchmarking can pose difficulties. First, it is difficult to consistently measure outcomes in the same way within an organization, as well as among multiple organizations, as measures among health care provider organizations may vary. For instance, similarities and differences in data collection methods, interpretation of data, and reporting can be found within and among organizations. This lack of consensus on the way data is measured between and among organizations leads to possible inconsistencies. Chapter 9 describes the importance of quality data being collected in a standardized manner and efforts taken to ensure accuracy of reporting.

Differences in resources available to organizations can also lead to over- or underreporting of data. For instance, having a dedicated data collection person enables the organization to focus education and training on data collection and reporting on specific individuals to help ensure accuracy of data collection. Technical resources of an organization can also affect data reporting. Having electronic data collection resources can speed up the data collection and reporting process and allow quicker analysis than hand collecting using paper and pencil. In addition, not all organizations have the same resources and database-building capabilities, which may affect data collection and reporting.

Another issue is that outcomes of care are not typically related to one care component; they are usually a result of multiple phases of care delivery. For example, part of the benchmark for 30-day readmission rates for patients with HF includes documentation of left ventricular end diastolic function. The ability of the cardiology department to provide services such as an echocardiogram at a specific point in time, having the physician interpret the findings from the echocardiogram, having a medical transcriptionist type the report, and inserting the documentation of the echocardiogram into the chart takes coordination between several departments. If each point in the process does not line up, the ability to meet the outcome benchmark of documentation of left ventricular end diastolic function is affected.

KEY CONCEPTS

- The use of benchmarking in health care is to measure the quality of the process of care and outcomes of care against the best performers on the quality indicator. Findings help the health care organization understand its performance on quality of care measures.
- Benchmarking incorporates QI principles of using a systematic method to assess a problem, diagnose what needs to be done, create a plan of action that incorporates best practice, implement a change, and evaluate outcomes.
- Benchmarking allows the organization to examine its product or services against excellence to identify areas of opportunity for improvement.
- External or comparative benchmarking provides a way to compare an organization's quality outcomes with those from an outside organization.
- Benefits of benchmarking include the ability of an organization to receive the highest level of reimbursement from insurers and the CMS, provide quality care to patients, and allows consumers of care to make informed decisions.
- Limitations of benchmarking include the possibility of inaccurate data reported for benchmarks, lack of consistency in measuring performance, and that the outcomes of care represent interprofessional contributions rather than one single care provider, making it difficult to separate out any one aspect of care.

KEY TERMS

Benchmarking
Dashboard
External benchmarking
Internal benchmarking
Outcome indicators

Performance gaps
Process of care indicator
Structure indicators
Trigger

DISCUSSION OF OPENING SCENARIO

1. How do you know how well your unit performed?

   One would need to be able to compare the data collected against a benchmark, or against data from top performers on this topic, to get a true understanding of how the unit performed. Without a comparison, the data do not mean anything. When compared to top performers, you would have a better understanding of how your data stack up against others.

2. Who do you need to include on a team to work on decreasing the 30-day readmission rates for patients with HF?

   The team would include professionals from all departments that affect the rates or work with the patient population: lab, radiology, cardiology, nursing, physician, nursing assistant, ED, case management, pastoral care, pharmacy, quality department, education department, community health, outpatient, and others listed in the table in the chapter.

3. How can you determine, and help set goals for, excellence in patient care to minimize or prevent unwanted outcomes?

This would require a team effort with interprofessional collaboration. The entire team needs to work together to set goals and coordinate care that supports excellence.

CRITICAL THINKING ANSWERS

Critical Thinking 8.1

1. How would you identify an appropriate benchmark?

The students should be able to identify a benchmark that is from a high-quality source, reflects the best practices in VTE prophylaxis, and reflects the same process of care.

2. What VTE process of care benchmarks would be appropriate for pharmacists? For physicians? For nurses?

To identify interprofessional measures, the benchmark may include actions taken by other disciplines in the measurement. For VTE, it is important to include pharmacists because they stock anticoagulants and assist the nurse in calculating dosages when required. The physician must be aware of laboratory values for clotting to order the correct medication and the correct dose. In addition, since this is a process of care benchmark, there may be a specific benchmark from the discipline's professional organization.

3. How would you explain the need for and value of benchmarking to your colleagues?

The need and value of comparing against top performers can be explained by looking at their data without a comparison. They cannot determine how well or poorly they are performing unless a comparison is available that reflects best practices.

Critical Thinking 8.2

1. Examine the use of color coding to represent the quality of care. How do the colors help in understanding the care provided at the hospital?

Students should identify that color coding helps to quickly identify areas of high and low performance. Guide students to examine the codes at the bottom of the table on the website. Information on data presentation, comparison methods, and determining color coding can be found in this area.

2. How do the findings from the hospital you selected compare with the hospital where you have clinicals or work?

Not all hospitals have the same quality outcomes from care provided. Consider the variances in quality data between the hospital selected and a hospital that is familiar to you. Think about the quality factors that influence the outcomes.

Critical Thinking 8.3

1. Which of the balanced scorecards is easiest for you to understand? Explain why.

    Students should consider the ability to understand the meaning of the scorecard, the use of colors to clarify areas of excellence, and opportunities for improvement, and defend why they selected the scorecard. Students should be able to explain their rationale clearly and in terms of how the scorecard clearly summarizes the organization's standing against benchmarks.

2. Do the balanced scorecards you found compare performance measures against benchmarks or targets? Why is this important?

    Benchmarks and/or targets should be clearly shown on the scorecard. This is important to evaluate the organization's current performance on the selected indicators.

Critical Thinking 8.4

1. Does the checklist capture the quality of the smoking cessation education and counseling? Why or why not?

    The checklist does not assess the quality of the education, only that the education has been delivered. An audit of smoking cessation education content would provide valuable information on the quality of the content and asking the patient about the effect of the education would identify impact of teaching.

2. Is the checklist method effective in capturing the outcome of smoking cessation education and face-to-face counseling on patient readmission rates?

    The checklist does not address the effect of the education on the patient. This would need a separate assessment. Discussion can include what content should be included to assess the effect of education on the patient's smoking cessation plan with follow-up.

3. Develop alternate ways of capturing the quality of the smoking cessation education and face-to-face counseling.

    The students should develop a set of questions to ask the patient regarding the effect of the education on their plans to stop smoking. It should include any behavioral changes as well as a follow-up to be performed over time to capture long-term effects.

Critical Thinking 8.5

1. What makes one region better or worse than the other in terms of data from the core measures? Consider factors such as location, demographics, proximity to larger cities, and so on. Go to the Census website (http://www.census.gov/compendia/statab) and learn more about the area.

    Students should consider factors such as location, demographics, proximity to larger cities, and so on in the response. To better understand the factors making one region better than another, use demographic websites such as the Census website. The demographic information helps to develop an awareness of the patient population and the influence on core measure outcomes. Students should understand that core measure outcome data is influenced by more than care provided. The data is also related to the type of patient population, socioeconomic factors, and demographics as well as quality processes in place in the health care organization.

2. Do disparities between the outcomes of care on the core measures exist? Why or why not?

Students should be able to compare the outcomes of care on the core measures, taking into account the location, services available in the area, and so on from the Census report. Students can compare their home region against another location, whether it is one they are familiar with from a vacation or where the student previously lived to examine if any disparities between the two regions exist.

CASE STUDY ANSWERS

Case Study 8.1

1. Create two indicators based on the information provided. One process of care indicator and one outcome indicator.

Process of care indicator can include clipping of hair (when indicated), not using razors to remove hair, and the use of antiseptic agents to cleanse the skin.

Outcome indicator is the absence of surgical-site infections.

2. How will you measure the indicators?

The process of care indicator can be measured by performing chart audits on the topic, looking at documentation of hair removal methods or the use of antiseptic skin preparation. The outcome indicator can be measured by performing chart audits on the presence of surgical-site infections.

3. Create one benchmark for the scenario.

Surgical-site infections of 0
100% compliance with hair removal clipping
100% compliance with antiseptic skin preparation

4. Who should be responsible for measuring the indicators and evaluating performance toward the benchmark?

At the unit level, a nurse can be assigned to audit charts and report to both the unit staff members and the quality department.

Case Study 8.2

1. Who should be included on a team to look at the practice of urinary catheter care and removal?

Members should include bedside nurses, physician, laboratory representative, central storage representative (for supplies), a unit manager, quality department representative, and a clinical educator representative at minimum.

2. Perform a web search on the topic of care of patients with urinary catheters. What are the best practices for care? How do the current practices in the case study compare with your findings?

Students should be able to compare their findings of care for patients with urinary catheters against the practices in the case study. Best practices for caring for patients with urinary catheters can and do change; therefore, there may be discrepancies between the two. The student should be able to identify resources that are reliable such as guidelines from www.guidelines.gov or from a repository of systematic reviews (Cochrane or Joanna Briggs Institute for EBP).

3. What process of care indicators should be monitored?
   • Cleansing of the perineal area is done daily with betadine
   • Checking the patency of the catheter tubing
   • Maintaining the drainage bag at a level below the patient for gravity drainage
   • Removing the catheter per the physician's preference on Day 3 postinsertion of the urinary catheter.

Case Study 8.3

1. Is the physician correct in requiring treatment consisting of chiropractic care, physical therapy, and muscle relaxers?
   Yes, the physician is correct and is following the standards of care based on the patient's symptom presentation.

2. Do you think the physician decided not to order the MRI because the current radiology use of MRIs for lower back pain is currently higher than national benchmarks? Defend your reasoning.
   The decision to not order an MRI was based on the standards of care for patients presenting with back pain. Although the current radiology use of MRIs for lower back pain are higher than the benchmarks, it is not the rationale for the type of care prescribed by the physician.

3. Does the patient have a voice in his or her treatment plan when what he or she wants is contrary to standards of practice?
   Yes, the patient can request a change in treatment plans but the physician is the final authority as to whether or not to deviate from the standard of care. If the physician deviates from the standard of care, there must be compelling documentation to support why the deviation was necessary.

REVIEW QUESTIONS

Please see Appendix D for answers to Review Questions.

1. A key element of benchmarking is to do which of the following?

   A. Provide the organization with a goal for improvement.
   B. Measure and compare the results of key work processes with those of the best performers in evaluating organizational performance.
   C. Identify key clinical areas in need of improvement.
   D. Determine the organization's ability to collaborate on initiatives to meet key standards for excellence.

2. In which of the following situations is internal benchmarking useful?

   A. When a health care organization wants to measure its performance against a nationally recognized standard
   B. When a health care organization seeks to improve a process that historically resulted in poor outcomes
   C. When a health care organization determines a need to evaluate a process that currently has no standardized benchmarks
   D. When a health care organization does not want to compare itself against different sized organizations

3. Which of the following would not be considered a trigger for process improvement?

   A. First quarter fall rate for a unit was 2, second quarter was 1. The previous year's average fall rate was 4.
   B. The hospital initiates a chest pain clinic with an average wait time for health care services at 12 minutes. The previous wait times in the ED were 23 minutes.
   C. Compliance with pneumococcal vaccinations upon discharge is 70%. The national average is 89%.
   D. Patient satisfaction with care is up 17% for the first quarter, from 80% to 97% for the intensive care unit (ICU).

4. A checklist of specific steps to follow when caring for a patient on a ventilator is instituted in the ICU. The goal is to eliminate ventilator-acquired pneumonia. The checklist is based on evidence-based guidelines. This is an example of what type of indicator?

   A. Outcome
   B. Quality
   C. Clinical care
   D. Process of care

5. Handoff reports between the ED and the admitting unit have resulted in long wait times for the admitting of patients. At times, the report is incomplete and other times the ED nurse has to wait until the admitting unit nurse is able to take report. Which of the following individuals absolutely must be included on a team formed to look at the problems?

   A. Nurses from units admitting patients from the ED
   B. ED nurses
   C. Radiologist
   D. Transcriptionist
   E. ED physician
   F. Unit secretary

6. At what point in the systematic problem assessment do most QI plans fail?

   A. During education and dissemination of changes because of the lack of clarity on how the new care process will affect staff and expectations for performance
   B. During analysis of the problem because many times the teams focus shifts to other problems that emerge
   C. During evaluation of outcomes because most plans do not include a system for monitoring the outcome data
   D. During planning because creating a specific timetable was not done

7. The NDNQI was created to provide access to measurements from different types of hospitals on specific quality indicators. Which of the following statements best describes the benefits of using nationally standardized benchmarks from the NDNQI?

   A. Comparing against national benchmarks shows a snapshot of how other clinical units are performing on any type of quality indicator from a variety of health care professions.
   B. Comparing against national benchmarks shows a clinical unit how to fix its quality indicators that are underperforming.
   C. Comparing against national benchmarks allows a clinical unit to evaluate its performance on a quality indicator against a large database of other similar units.
   D. Comparing against national benchmarks allows a clinical unit to evaluate its standing on quality indicators against others in the local area.

8. The National Quality Forum is a repository of clinical indicators. The clinical indicators are tested and validated before being released to the public. As of 2011, how many quality health care indicators does the National Quality Forum endorse?

   A. 300
   B. 400
   C. 500
   D. 600+

9. Informatics nursing is an uncommon area for benchmarking quality indicators. What would be an appropriate source for a nurse informaticist to look for quality indicators and benchmarks?

   A. National Association for Nurse Informaticists
   B. American Medical Association
   C. Computers and Technology Engineers Society
   D. Computers in Nursing

10. Limitations to benchmarking can affect the entire QI process. Which of the following is an example of a limitation to benchmarking?

   A. Health care organizations having similar resources and measurement styles
   B. Differences in the types of benchmarks selected among organizations
   C. Health care organizations having similar populations and demographics of the communities they serve
   D. Differences in understanding data collection techniques

REVIEW ACTIVITIES

Please see Appendix E for answers to Review Activities.

1. Explore the National Library of Medicine/National Institute of Health's Health Services Research Information Central website at http://www.nlm.nih.gov/hsrinfo/quality.html. The website is a repository of quality information, resources, and research related to all aspects of health care quality.
2. Create a scorecard for your region using the website http://datacenter.commonwealthfund.org/#ind=529/sc=38. Compare your findings against another region of your choice.

3. Review the Department of Health and Human Services resources for comparing hospitals at www.hospitalcompare.gov and comparing providers at www.providercompare.gov. Compare the outcomes from two hospitals and two providers in your area on an indicator of your choice.

4. The National Guideline Clearinghouse at http://www.guideline.gov provides guidelines based on the best evidence for care. Select a guideline from the site and compare it against a current guideline in your clinical setting.

5. The Registered Nurses Association of Ontario provides a repository of free to access clinical practice guidelines at http://rnao.ca/bpg. Review the available guidelines. Consider what it means to nursing practice to have best practice guidelines available at no cost.

6. Read about falls and benchmarking databases at http://www.ahrq.gov/professionals/clinicians-providers/resources/nursing/resources/nurseshdbk. Why is it difficult to benchmark falls according to the author of Chapter 10? What can be done to decrease falls? How do other disciplines affect fall rates?

7. Use the AHRQ website (http://www.ahrq.gov/news/press/pr2011/tfosteopr.htm) to develop criteria for osteoporosis screening. Describe how this would be measured including the responsible person(s) for collecting and reporting the data.

8. Go to the IHI website at www.ihi.org/knowledge and select "Improvement Stories" from the list on the left. Read about how hospitals have improved their quality using benchmarks for performance.

9. Register for the free subscription to the National Quality Forum (www.qualityforum.org). Enter the site and click on performance measures. Search for NQF# 0048, Osteoporosis: Management Following Fracture. Review the performance indicators paying particular attention to those that require an interprofessional approach.

EXPLORING THE WEB

1. AHRQ (www.ahrq.gov)
2. NDNQI (www.ndnqi.org)
3. CMS (http://www.cms.gov/Research-Statistics-Data-and-Systems/Research-Statistics-Data-and-Systems.html)

REFERENCES

Agency for Healthcare Research and Quality (AHRQ). (2010). *2010 National healthcare quality and disparities reports*. Retrieved from http://www.ahrq.gov/qual/qrdr10

Agency for Healthcare Research and Quality (AHRQ). (2012). *Patient safety network glossary*. Retrieved from http://www.psnet.ahrq.gov/popup_glossary.aspx?name=benchmark

American Association of Critical-Care Nurses (AACN). (2012). *Standards*. Retrieved from http://www.aacn.org/wd/practice/content/standards.pcms?menu=practice

Association of periOperative Registered Nurses (AORN). (2012). *EHR periperative syntegrity-framework*. Retrieved from http://www.aorn.org/syntegrity

Centers for Medicare and Medicaid Services (CMS). (2012). *Readmissions reduction program*. Retrieved from http://cms.gov/Medicare/Medicare-Fee-for-Service-Payment/AcuteInpatientPPS/Readmissions-Reduction-Program.html

Chambers, C. E., Fetterly, K. A., Holzer, R., Lin, P., Blankenship, J. C., Balter, S. & Laskey, W. K. (2011). Radiation safety program for the cardiac catheterization laboratory. *Catheterization and Cardiovascular Interventions, 77*(4), 546–556.

Emergency Nurses Association. (2012). *Emergency department benchmarks and advanced analytics support key ED performance initiatives.* Retrieved from http://sites.mckesson.com/edbc/home.htm

Heidenreich, P. A., Hernandez, A. F., Yancy, C. W., Liang, L., Peterson, E. D., & Fonarow, G. C. (2012). Get with the guidelines program participation, process of care, and outcome for Medicare patients hospitalized with heart failure. *Circulation Cardiovascular Quality Outcomes, 5*(1), 37–43.

Hughes, R. (2008). Tools and strategies for quality improvement and patient safety. In R. Hughes (Ed.), *Patient safety and quality: An evidence-based handbook for nurses.* Chapter 44. AHRQ Publication No. 08–0043. Rockville, MD: Agency for Healthcare Research and Quality. Retrieved from http://www.ahrq.gov/qual/nurseshdbk

Institute for Health Care Improvement (IHI). (2012). *Global trigger tool.* Retrieved from http://www.ihi.org/knowledge/Pages/Tools/IHIGlobalTriggerToolforMeasuringAEs.aspx

Institute of Medicine (1999). *To err is human: Building a safer health system.* In L.T. Kohn, J.M. Corrigan, & M.S. Donaldson (Eds.). Washington, D.C.: National Academies Press. Retrieved from books.nap.edu/openbook.php?record_id=9728

Institute of Medicine (IOM). (2006). *Appendix E methodology and analytic frameworks. Performance measurement: Accelerating improvement (pathways to quality health care series).* Washington, DC: The National Academies Press.

Lacker, C. (2011). Decreasing 30-day readmission rates. *American Journal of Nursing, 111*(11), 65–69. ISSN: 1538–7488.

Montalvo, I. (2007). The national database of nursing quality indicators (NDNQI). *The Online Journal of Issues in Nursing, 12*(3). Retrieved from http://gm6.nursingworld.org/MainMenuCategories/ANAMarketplace/ANAPeriodicals/OJIN/TableofContents/Volume122007/No3Sept07/NursingQualityIndicators.aspx

National Database of Nursing Quality Indicators (NDNQI). (2012). *NDNQI transforming data into quality care.* Retrieved from https://www.nursingquality.org

Nielsen, G. A., Bartely, A., Coleman, E., Resar, R., Rutherford, P., Souw, D., & Taylor, J. (2008). *Transforming care at the bedside how-to guide: Creating an ideal transition home for patients with heart failure.* Cambridge, MA: Institute for Healthcare Improvement. Available at www. IHI. org

Young, S. (2009). *12 Rules of success in The Journey is the Reward.* Glenview, IL: Scott, Foresman.

SUGGESTED READING

Brown, D., Donaldson, N., Bolton, L. B., & Aydin, C. E. (2010). Nursing-sensitive benchmarks for hospitals to gauge high-reliability performance. *Journal for Healthcare Quality, 32*(6), 9–17.

Center for Health Policy/Center for Primary Care and Outcomes Research and Battelle Memorial Institute. (2011, May). *Quality indicator measure development, implementation, maintenance, and retirement* (Prepared by Battelle, under Contract No. 290–04-0020). Rockville, MD: Agency for Healthcare Research and Quality. Retrieved from http://www.qualityindicators.ahrq.gov

Chassin, M. R., Loeb, J. M., Schmaltz, S. P., & Wachter, R. M. (2010, August). Accountability measures: Using measurement to promote quality improvement. *New England Journal of Medicine, 363,* 683–688. Retrieved from http://www.nejm.org/doi/full/10.1056/NEJMsb1002320

Haines, S., & Warren, T. (2011, May). Staff and patient involvement in benchmarking to improve care. *Nursing Management, 18*(2), 22–25.

National Database of Nursing Quality Indicators (NDNQI). (2012). *Frequently asked questions.* Retrieved from http://www.nursingquality.org/FAQs

The Joint Commission. (2011). *Benchmarking in health care* (2nd ed.). Oakbrook Terrace, IL: Joint Commission Resources.

Zrelak, P. A., Utter, G. H., Sadeghi, B., Cuny, J., Baron, R., & Romano, P. S. (2012, April-June). Using the Agency for Healthcare Research and Quality patient safety indicators for targeting nursing quality improvement. *Journal of Nursing Care Quality, 27*(2), 99–108. doi:10.1097/NCQ.0b013e318237e0e3

TOOLS OF QUALITY IMPROVEMENT

Anthony L. D'Eramo and Joanne Belviso Puckett

Modern health care demands continual system improvement to better meet social needs for safety, effectiveness, patient centeredness, timeliness, efficiency, and equity. Nurses, like all other health professionals, need skills and support to participate effectively in that endeavor, and, often, to lead it. (Berwick, 1991)

Upon completion of this chapter, the reader should be able to

1. Define data as used to measure quality
2. Differentiate the various types of data and the methods used to display data
3. Identify the value of using basic statistics in quality improvement (QI) work
4. Differentiate common cause variation from special cause variation
5. Discuss the tools used by QI teams

*A*s a day shift nurse on a patient care unit, you perform assessments on your patients at the beginning of the shift. The first patient that you assess is an 85-year-old male admitted yesterday with pneumonia. During shift report, the night nurse stated that the patient had a fever on admission but that the patient's temperature was normal during the night shift. The patient had an elevated white blood cell count of 12.4 K/cmm on admission and received three doses of IV antibiotics since admission. As you assess the patient's vital signs, you find the patient has a temperature of 101.1° F (38.4 °C). The patient offered no complaints other than shortness of breath. You noted the patient is flushed with a respiratory rate of 20 and a pulse oximeter reading of 95% on 1.5 L of oxygen delivered through a nasal cannula. His repeat white blood cell count on the *morning of your care is 13.2 K/cmm. Prior to your assessment, the health care team enters the patient's room. The physician asks, "Is he improving?"*

- *How will you respond to the physician?*
- *What questions should you have asked during the handoff shift report when it was reported that the patient had a normal temperature during the night shift?*
- *Is a temperature finding of 101.1 or a white blood cell count of 13.2 an improvement?*

Quality is whatever patients and family members define it to be. Beyond the prevention, reduction, or elimination of harm is the search for innovations and breakthrough improvements that contribute to quality outcomes. With innovative improvements comes the opportunity to advance good performance to excellence in performance. Such innovations occur with visionary thinking of what can be, what health care processes can be changed to enhance patient and staff satisfaction, and by understanding, and applying improvement methods into our daily clinical practice. This chapter focuses on the science and process of QI.

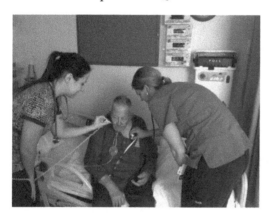

Nurses assessing a patient.

Quality improvement (QI) was developed based on the Quality and Safety Education for Nurses (QSEN) definition: "Use data to monitor the outcomes of care processes and use improvement methods to design and test changes to continuously improve the quality and safety of health care systems" (Cronenwett et al., 2007). This chapter includes basic tools and methods used by most QI teams. We explore the types and uses of data for QI including how data is displayed for analysis and how data is analyzed to identify both the need for improvement or if improvement occurred. When indicated, interprofessional teams may conduct QI activities. The teams have a variety of improvement tools and methods they can employ. The most basic and effective processes used by teams will be described.

WHAT ARE DATA

Nursing practice decisions and organizational health care processes all produce outcome data that can be measured, displayed, and compared. So what are data? **Data** is the raw numbers or results collected to measure processes within a health care organization. Data can also be results provided by outside health care–related sources. Data is used to determine if health care performance meets the expected goal (e.g., the number of patients with blood pressure in control). Data is used to measure performance quality that is valued by purchasers of care, accreditation agencies, governing bodies, the general public, and providers of health care (Carey, 2003). The following questions put data measurement in context: What is the measureable goal? Why was that selected as the goal? Are we striving to meet a defined requirement; a minimum standard, or a long-term goal?

By itself, data are not actionable. Consider the following: a heart rate of 60 is an isolated piece of datum from one assessment finding. By itself, the heart rate datum looks good. As health care workers, we do not base any changes on one piece of data. If we look at heart rate readings over time (e.g., the heart rate is taken twice a shift for 1 day providing six pieces of data), we can see if a trend exists. A trend looks at changes in data over time. If the six heart rate readings were 110, 100, 90, 80, 70, and 60, we would have information. **Information** is the collected and analyzed data, such as the trend in blood pressure, which is used to take action. With the heart rate example, the trend provides information that the heart rate has steadily fallen over three shifts. We may choose to take action such as informing the physician of the trend, review medications or changes in medications over the past three shifts, or monitor the patient closely to watch for any other assessment changes.

In health care practice, patients provide both subjective and objective data. **Subjective** patient **data** may include the patient's description of how he or she feels. For example, the patient may state that he or she feels dizzy, hot, or lightheaded. **Objective data** may include what the health care worker can see or measure, such as the patient's blood pressure or glucose results. Both subjective and objective types of data is collected and analyzed to make conclusions about whether the patient is getting better, worse, or if the data require physician notification.

Sources of Data for QI

Nurses in complex health care systems are inundated with data representing unit or organization performance outcomes. **Internal data** is data found within a health care organization and is generated by staff, such as falls and medication errors. **External data** is data provided from outside sources (e.g., state quality review organizations). **Baseline data** is the preintervention data measurement that usually identifies a quality problem. **Postintervention data** confirms the success or failure of the intervention. For example, a team is working to decrease hospital-acquired pressure ulcers (HAPU). The average HAPU were six/month for the last 3 months, which represents the baseline data that triggered the QI intervention. After the QI intervention, the average HAPU was three/month, or a reduction of 50% in HAPUs over a 3-month period. This finding is the postintervention data measurement and helps determine the subsequent next actions.

When data is collected internally, it is important to distinguish between incidence and prevalence measures. Incidence and prevalence both typically use a quarterly time frame. A quarter is 3 months, represented as first quarter (January, February, and March), second quarter (April, May, and June), third quarter (July, August, and September), and fourth quarter (October, November, and December). **Incidence measures** are the actual counts of every event that occurred during a specific time frame. For example, counting the number of falls that occurred on a medical–surgical unit for one quarter. **Prevalence measures** are a snapshot of the problem during 1 day. For example, counting the number of falls that occurred on one specific day during the quarter. To illustrate further, suppose the prevalence rate was measured on one specific day and no fall occurred on the specific date of measurement, the prevalence rate would be zero. Now suppose over the same 3-month period, the actual incidences of falls were 11. Based on how the data were collected, either incidence or prevalence, it can result in dramatically different outcomes. It is important to understand the difference between incidence and prevalence as some organizations may use these terms depending on where the quality data is reported. For example, the National Database of Nursing Quality Indicators (NDNQI) requires reporting of pressure ulcers as incidence and prevalence data.

Aggregate Data

When collecting data, it is important to ensure that no patient identifiers are captured linking outcomes to specific patients, families, or staff to ensure privacy and confidentiality of information. QI projects generally use **aggregate data**, which is grouped data without patient identifiers; this aggregate data may be grouped by time, cause, diagnosis, or the variables being studied. An example of a variable can include the timing and number of physical therapy treatments for a hip replacement. Aggregate data is commonly presented in a table format. In Table 9.1, nursing hand hygiene compliance data is reported in aggregate form that compares three units over a 9-month period. Notice that there is no ability to identify which staff were in or out of compliance during measurement based on the aggregate data.

The use of bolding (met the target) and shading (did not meet the target) in Table 9.1 helps to quickly identify areas needing improvement when looking at large numbers of aggregate data. While data sources are endless, accessing the data may be challenging. Leadership and local experts (e.g., the QI department, business office, utilization management, and patient safety) may be helpful in identifying sources of internal and external data.

Operational Definitions

An essential part of looking at any data is to have a clear definition of what is being measured to ensure that everyone is measuring the same thing. An **operational definition** describes in detail what is being measured, how it is being measured, and when measurement should occur. Let's say that you are asked to collect data on the number of classmates who like candy. The term "candy" is ambiguous, meaning it can be interpreted in different ways. One student may think that chocolate is not candy and answer negatively even though he or she loves chocolate. Another student may think of candy as lollipops, which the student does not like and responds negatively. In both cases, the responses did not accurately reflect the person's position. Had the term "candy" been clearly defined, the problems with the collected data might have been avoided.

It is important to know how the data for QI activities are collected and defined using operational definitions. Having one clear operational definition ensures that the data is collected and measured the same way, regardless of where the data is collected or who collects the data. For example, in Table 9.1 we looked at aggregated data on hand hygiene compliance from three different units. To make sure the data is collected and measured the same way on all units, we would need to state the following in the operational definition: the definition for hand hygiene, who is to collect the data, when the data is to be collected, the number of hand hygiene observations expected, and when the results are to be reported and to whom.

Hand hygiene is defined as compliance with the Centers for Disease Control (CDC) hand hygiene guidelines. Each unit will identify a "secret" observer for each shift, who will monitor that unit on the 1st day of each month. Each observer will assess at least 10 individual staff on the unit by observing their interactions with patients. Results of

TABLE 9.1 PERCENTAGE COMPLIANCE WITH CDC HAND HYGIENE GUIDELINES USING OBSERVATIONS (3-MEDICAL–SURGICAL UNITS)

	JANUARY	FEBRUARY	MARCH	APRIL	MAY	JUNE	JULY	AUGUST	SEPTEMBER
Unit A	**91%**	80%	87%	86%	73%	69%	80%	77%	79%
Unit B	40%	45%	44%	54%	79%	59%	50%	50%	61%
Unit C	87%	88%	84%	88%	**90%**	**93%**	**90%**	79%	89%

Note: Compliance goal is set at 90%. Bolded, meeting 90% compliance goal; shaded, not meeting 90% compliance goal.

compliance with CDC guidelines will be reported to the infection control staff within 48 hours of observation and will be aggregated as follows:

> Numerator: Number of hand hygiene observations that were completed using CDC guidelines
> Denominator: Total number of observations requiring hand hygiene
> Example: 39 hand hygiene observations were correct out of 45 hand hygiene observations (87% compliance)

There is a clear numerator and denominator for reliable measurement. It can be challenging to develop a clear operational definition to guide a sustainable, consistent process for data collection among the observers.

Critical Thinking 9.1

Select the best operational definition for a fall and explain why you selected the option.

1. *A "fall" is defined as the number of patients who fall and for which an incident report is completed. The patient safety officer will collect the data and report it to the unit practice council annually using a control chart.*
2. *A "fall" is defined as the number of patients admitted to the unit who fall and who suffer no injuries, whether minor (e.g., a laceration) or major (e.g., fractured hip). All such incidents will be reported using electronic incident reporting procedures per policy 101–5.*
3. *A "fall" is defined as any patient who falls that results in no injury, a fall that results in a minor injury (laceration), or a fall that results in a major injury (fractured hip). All such incidents will be reported using electronic incident reporting procedures per policy 101–5. The fall numerator is the number of falls and the fall denominator is the total number of patients on the unit during the measurement time period.*

Data Collection

Data is only useful when collected rigorously, meaning that collection tools are valid (measures what it is supposed to measure) and reliable (consistently measuring what it is supposed to measure). To illustrate, in the hand hygiene compliance example, although all staff are expected and taught to follow hand hygiene compliance, every "secret" observer should complete additional training on the CDC guidelines and demonstrate competency in hand hygiene compliance before monitoring and observing other staff. The additional training can help the observer accurately measure if hand hygiene compliance occurred according to the CDC guidelines (validity). Another trained observer may review the findings. By doing this, the second observer is helping to establish reliability of data collected by the first observer on hand hygiene compliance. **Interrater reliability** (IRR) is a process that provides evidence that those collecting data are following the same data collection procedures. When IRR exists, the data is considered reliable because data is collected in a consistent manner. Additional education and testing prior to data collection can help prevent data collection errors. One type of data collection error is identifying that a problem exists when in fact there is not a problem. For example, hand hygiene compliance may include both hand sanitizer and soap-and-water hand washing when nothing is touched in a room. If the observer misunderstood the definition of hand hygiene compliance and only counted the instances where the health care worker used soap and water, the findings would be in error. In this case, the number of health care workers who used the hand sanitizer was not counted causing a decrease in the percentage of compliance. If you read the findings, you might think that hand hygiene compliance is a bigger problem than it really is.

An opposite error can also occur. Let's say the observer misunderstood the hand hygiene guidelines, as the only time the health care worker had to use the hand sanitizer or wash his or her hands was if he or she touched the patient. The observer would only count compliance when the patient was touched and hand hygiene was completed, missing the fact that hand hygiene should be completed every time the health care worker enters and leaves the room. The compliance rates would miss the problem needing improvement. In both cases, establishing IRR allows the identification of the observer's misunderstanding and fixing the issue before it becomes a problem.

CASE STUDY 9.1

Two nurses have agreed to collect data on a QI project to decrease the number of patients who cancel their clinic appointments at two different surgical clinics. These patients are called clinic no-shows. The nurse manager over both clinics asks the two nurses to ensure IRR. Not being familiar with the concept of IRR, the nurses look to the literature and discover that this term refers to those who are collecting data are following the same data collection procedures. The nurse manager requests a written plan to ensure IRR between both nurses at the two clinics.

1. *How would you write this plan and ensure both nurses are measuring their clinic no-shows consistently?*

DESCRIPTIVE (SUMMARY) STATISTICS

Statistics are tools used to analyze and summarize relationships among variables. Statistics can identify significance within the data and relationships between variables (Nelson et al., 2007). **Descriptive statistics** are used to define and describe a set of data. For aggregate data, basic descriptive statistics are commonly calculated and include mean, median, mode, range, and standard deviation (SD) of a set of data. Table 9.1 data is used to illustrate how these statistics are applied. Beginning with the **mean**, or average of a set of numbers, add all the numbers together and then divide by the total number of observations. In looking at hand hygiene compliance for Unit A, note that there are 9 months of hand hygiene compliance percentages reported. The mean compliance for Unit A is calculated by adding all findings and dividing by 9, the number of months. Table 9.2 demonstrates the calculation of mean for Unit A. The mean is often abbreviated when used in tables and figures as X bar, x, or the Greek letter μ.

TABLE 9.2 UNIT A DESCRIPTIVE STATISTICS

SUMMARY STATISTIC	ILLUSTRATION
Mean	91+80+87+86+73+69+80+77+79 = 722 722 divided by 9 (months) = 80.22
Median	91, 80, 87, 86, **73**, 69, 80, 77, 79 73 is the middle point
Mode	91, **80**, 87, 86, 73, 69, **80**, 77, 79 80 is repeated
Range	91, 80, 87, 86, 73, 69, 80, 77, 79 69 (lowest value) to 91 (highest value)

An example of a mean that may be familiar is grade point average (GPA). A common GPA scale: A = 4 points, B = 3 points, C = 2 points, D = 1 points, and F = 0 points. If you took all of your grades earned in each class over the time spent in college and converted the grades to point values as described, you could calculate your GPA using the illustration from Table 9.2.

The **median** of a set of data is determined by listing the findings from lowest to highest values. Once listed, the median is the value at the separation point. Here are five values arranged from lowest to highest: 4, 6, 11, 13, and 15. The median is 11 or the middle number of the set, as there are two results before and after it. When there is an even number of results, the median is the average of the two middle results. For example, if the values were 4, 6, 7, 11, 13, and 15, the median would be 9, the average of 7 and 11, or 18÷/2 = 9. Table 9.2 illustrates the mode for Unit A. The median is used less frequently than the mean in QI.

In QI activities, the mode is of less use compared to the other descriptive statistics but it may be included in analyses, therefore it is necessary to define. The **mode** is simply the value that is repeated most frequently in a set of data or the "typical" value observed. To illustrate this, refer to Table 9.2.

Variability refers to the differences among the range of numbers in a data set. A simple measure of variability can be determined by observing the range of the data set. The **range** represents the lowest and highest values in the data. In discussing the median, we used the following set of data: 4, 6, 7, 11, 13, and 15. The range of these five data points is the lowest value or 4 and the highest value or 15. Using range is a quick measure of variability. Table 9.2 illustrates the range of values for Unit A. Knowing the variability helps you to identify just how far apart the data is. Consider this: You are working on a QI project to reduce falls. Over 12 months (1 year), one unit has a high number of 13 falls and a low number of zero falls. The variability shows you that the unit is not consistent in reducing falls.

The most common method used to describe variation of a data set is the **standard deviation** (SD) that reflects how "tightly" the data points cluster around the mean as seen in Figure 9.1. SD is often abbreviated as the Greek letter sigma (σ). In a "normal" distribution of a data set, most measures hover around the mean while a few measures tend to be at opposite extremes from the mean. In an SD curve, the mean is located at the center of the graph and is represented as 0 in Figure 9.1. In a normal distribution, it is expected that 68.3% of outcomes will fall within 1 SD above or below the mean (+1/−1). Another 27.1% of outcomes should fall within 2 SDs from the mean (+2/−2) accounting for 95.4% of all expected outcomes. An additional 4.2% of outcomes should fall within 3 SDs from the mean (+3/−3), which accounts for 99.8% of all outcomes. Recall and apply

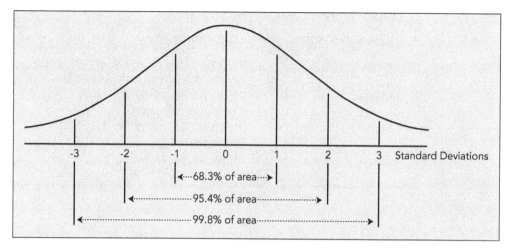

FIGURE 9.1 A normal distribution standard deviation curve.

From Pelletier and Beaudin (2012, p. 79). Copyright ©2012 by the National Association for Healthcare Quality, reprinted with permission.

what you have learned about the mean value or average of a data set. If 20 students completed a test with a mean score of 80%, it is expected that most of those students (68.3%) would hover around an 80% score. Less would fall within 2 SDs of 80% and even fewer would fall 3 SDs from the mean. SD of a set of data can be easily calculated using software, such as Microsoft Excel.

As seen in Figure 9.1, outcomes (99.8%) are expected to fall within 3 SDs of the mean. Outcomes that do fall within 3 SDs are expected, a common finding. There are, however, data points that are not expected or considered special findings, known as **outliers**. When a data point falls above or below 3 SDs; a few students who excel or do not may score extremely high or low falling beyond the expected 3 SDs. Variability in a data set is an important concept in QI activities and is further examined with statistical process control later in the chapter. For practice calculating basic descriptive statistics refer to Case Study 9.2.

CASE STUDY 9.2

You have just completed data collection on a QI project to reduce call-offs on your unit. To obtain call-off baseline data, you have been asked to document the number of call-offs over a 3-week period to identify the number of call-offs more prominently for each shift. Your results are listed below:

Week 1: (Days) 3	(Evenings) 1	(Nights) 1
Week 2: (Days) 4	(Evenings) 2	(Nights) 2
Week 3: (Days) 1	(Evenings) 3	(Nights) 1

1. *Now that you have your outcomes, calculate the mean, median, mode, and range of these results.*

DATA DISPLAY

Data is visible in all health care settings. It is difficult to walk onto an inpatient or outpatient area without seeing data. It is necessary however, to analyze and interpret data into usable information. **Data display** refers to a visual picture or graphing of data that best depicts the story you want that data to exhibit. Data should be displayed in ways that staff, patients, and families can understand. Figures, graphs, and tables are acceptable methods of displaying data. Whatever the format, data must include a clear title of what is being presented, including the use of footnotes to clarify aspects of the table or figure (Nelson et al., 2007). For example, footnotes may be useful to define a column title, or to refer the reader to the operational definition of a specific value. Recall Table 9.1, hand hygiene compliance for three nursing units. For easier interpretation, those months meeting the targeted goal of 90% were highlighted while those not meeting were shaded. Specialized software is available for creating data display from a variety of sources.

Data alone does not always offer guidance regarding improvement priorities. For example, looking at Table 9.1, Unit B lists outcomes for May (79%) and June (59%), respectively. Does this decrease in compliance require immediate attention? A "yes" response may be premature. In fact, the answer to that question should not be determined by comparing two results alone. Fortunately, more sophisticated methods are available to better inform improvement decisions. As you will learn, visually displaying data over time is useful when assessing outcomes to better inform if interventions are needed, if improvement occurred, or was sustained.

Data is generated from QI activities but must be interpreted as meaningful information before improvement interventions are identified. For example, in Table 9.1, if Unit B wanted to improve their hand hygiene compliance rate (mean = 40% over 12 months), some change or intervention must be implemented. The 40% or baseline measure will be compared to the postintervention percentage compliance to determine if the intervention worked. Recall that QI projects are data driven. At this point, we have only discussed data. We will now look at how data is displayed in various graphical formats. Our discussion will focus on commonly used formats including a histogram, scatter plot diagram, and Pareto charts, as well as run and control charts. Note that when data is plotted within a graph, the horizontal axis of the graph is referred to as the X-axis and the vertical axis of the graph as the Y-axis.

Histograms

A **histogram,** as seen in Figure 9.2, is a bar graph that displays the data. Data displayed using a histogram allows for easier visualization of large, aggregate data that may originate from a table. To understand a histogram, it is important to know the Y-axis and X-axis. The Y-axis is the vertical line and is easily remembered as "Y to the sky." The X-axis is the horizontal line and can be remembered as "X to the left." Histograms are useful in determining patterns within historical data or displaying baseline data. In Figure 9.2, the histogram uses a bar to display the length of stay for the last 50 admissions.

The number of admissions is located on the vertical Y-axis. The variable along the horizontal X-axis (number of days of length of stay) is sequential starting with the shortest to the longest length of stay. The most frequent average length of stay (15 observations) is between 3 and 4 days. Histograms are easily made with or without software and quickly depict the distribution of a set of data or outcomes.

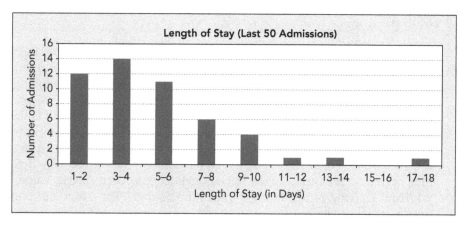

FIGURE 9.2 The histogram.

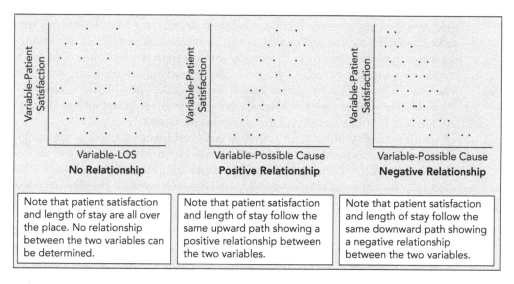

FIGURE 9.3 Basic scatter plot patterns.

Scatter Plot Diagrams

Scatter plot diagrams display relationships between two variables by providing a visual means to test the strength of the relationship between the two variables. The design of the plots within the diagram is used for interpretation. Although several designs can be realized, three are most common, a positive, negative, or no relationship design. Examples of each design are depicted in Figure 9.3. The scatter plot looks at two variables, or issues, that you want to look at. A relationship between two variables does not indicate that one variable caused the other. The scatter plot only allows for determining if a relationship exists.

Consider the length of stay data displayed in the histogram in Figure 9.2. The relationship between the variable of length of stay could be compared to another variable, such as patient satisfaction using a scatter plot (Figure 9.3).

The scatter plot diagram in Figure 9.4 illustrates the relationship between length of stay (in days) and patient satisfaction scores using a Likert-type scale ranging from 5.1, where 5 is most satisfied, 3 is neutral, and 1 is least satisfied. In Figure 9.4, the design

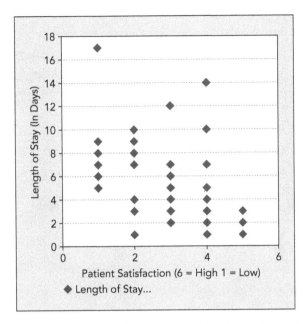

FIGURE 9.4 Scatter plot diagram (variables patient satisfaction and length of stay).

of the scatter plots indicates there is no relationship between length of stay and patient satisfaction for the 50 patients in this sample.

Pareto Charts

The **Pareto chart** is another type of bar graph. It is similar to the histogram because it depicts how often data represent a particular value. The difference between a histogram and a Pareto chart is that the Pareto chart orders findings in a descending order from high to low with the most frequent issue contributing to the results furthest to the left of the X-axis. Visualizing results from high to low allows prioritizing, or identifying, what data most impact the variable in question. One benefit of the Pareto chart is in demonstrating the Pareto principle that 80% of the problem comes from 20% of the causes. When the causes are ranked in order of effect on the QI problem, you can clearly identify those having the greatest effect. The Pareto chart in Figure 9.5 illustrates that tardiness, furthest to the left, is the most common cause of unit overtime during a 1-month time period.

In Figure 9.5, the four most common causes of overtime are ranked from high to low as you read from left to right. These four causes represent 81% of the problems leading to overtime. You can look above the column labeled "staffing patterns" and see where the line marks 81% of the problems. These four causes will serve as target problems needing improvement to reduce overtime costs. The manager can easily visualize, prioritize causes, and plan improvement interventions to reduce overtime usage. Appreciate that the leading cause of a problem may not be the focus of improvement. In this example, if meeting with the employee health department was the greatest cause of overtime, it may not be feasible to address since the manager of the unit may have little control over employees appropriately seeking employee health services.

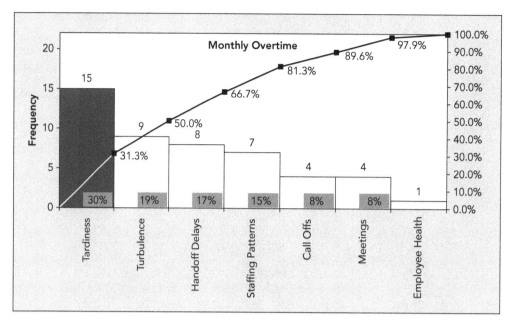

FIGURE 9.5 Pareto chart on causes of overtime for 1 month.

Statistical Process Control

Thus far, we have discussed graphics and charts commonly used to analyze and represent data. In the Pareto chart depicted in Figure 9.5, although tardiness is the most significant cause leading to overtime, was that a change from previous months? Were call-offs once the most frequent cause of overtime but are now reduced? Are these causes of overtime changing month to month? The Pareto chart categorizes factors leading to specific outcomes, however, this data is static (remains the same); mainly a snapshot of what existed at the time the data were collected (Grube, 2008). More scientific or statistical approaches exist that depict trends over time, which is referred to as a time series design, allowing for improved decision making and prioritization. **Statistical process control** (SPC) is an approach for analyzing data adding science to QI decision making (Nelson et al., 2007). SPC uses statistical methods to monitor and control quality processes to reduce or eliminate waste. Although statistics are a high-level function, we will only introduce you to and cover the basics as they apply to QI projects.

SPC applies science by adding the ability to identify variation within processes (Evans, 2008). In Figure 9.5, after identifying tardiness the major contributing factor to overtime, it would be valuable to apply principles of SPC to assess variability and need for change. For example, 15 causes of overtime were from tardiness. Is this new? Was tardiness noted only twice last month and suddenly increased? Is this a priority to fix and why? SPC depicts processes variability, the degree to which the process is stable or unstable over time. Think about the hand hygiene data in Table 9.1. The change in the percentage of hand hygiene compliance from 1 month to the next month is variability. In Table 9.1 data is presented in a time series, from January through September. What we do not know is if the differences in numbers are stable, meaning they are consistent even if they vary, or unstable, meaning they fluctuate unpredictably from high to low.

On any given day, your lunchtime may vary anytime between 11 a.m. and 1 p.m. This is an expected variation, referred to as **common cause variation** or "noise," the inherent variability seen in stable "in control" processes (Carey, 2003). If an emergency prevented you from eating lunch until 3 p.m., that time point is very different from your expected lunchtime. When a data point varies in an unpredictable or unexpected manner, it is referred to as **special cause variation**, which signals that something happened that changed the process for better or worse and that the process is "out-of-control" (Carey, 2003).

Assessing for common and special cause variability captures the essence of SPC, or being able to look at data over time to determine the type of variability that exists. Both common and special cause variation require further interpretation. When special cause variation is found, efforts should focus on identifying what occurred that resulted in the process being out of control? This can be either a problem or an improvement, both of which stand out from the norm. If the process exhibits common cause variation, it may not need improvement. It may also mean that the process may not be performing at an acceptable level, which could lead to a QI activity. In this case, the improvement focus should be on stabilizing the process itself with the goal of decreasing variation (Carey, 2003). In SPC, assessing variability requires use of formats such as the run chart or Shewhart control chart. As the goal is to reduce variation within processes and to sustain that over time, there is considerable movement in health care to use SPC as a QI methodology when analyzing outcome data (Mohammed, Worthington, & Woodall, 2008).

The Run Chart

The **run chart** depicts data in a time series format. Recall that a time series format refers to the representation of data over consecutive months. It can be used for any type of data, including measurement and count data created by hand or using software. Characteristic of all time series charts, X-axis (vertical) represents the time period and the Y-axis (horizontal) represents the variable being studied (Figure 9.6).

The run charts depicted in Figure 9.6 show how the data is organized. The time frame being shown is 12 months (X-axis) in chronological order. The outcome variable, percentage compliance of pain reassessment is seen on the Y-axis. When using SPC, the range of percentages will vary by unit based on the range of each Unit's outcomes. In Figure 9.6, Unit A has a range between 48% and 75% (lowest point and highest point) and Unit B has a range between 30% and 71% (lowest point and highest point). You may choose to include a table of the raw data within the run chart for additional detail. Expert opinions vary, but generally, 12 to 16 time points are adequate for statistical differentiation. In addition, more than 25 data points will not increase the statistical power (Carey, 2003). The median of the data set is used as the centerline on run charts because it is not sensitive to outliers, like the mean may be. For the purpose of this discussion, an outlier is an "astronomical" finding significantly distant from the median centerline. When using the median, half the outcomes are above and half are below the median point. If we used averages, we would have to include all numbers, including the outliers in the equation, which would affect our numbers. In Figure 9.6 Unit C, the median center line is at 49%, which was determined by the raw compliance percentages in chronological order from low to high: 43, 43, 44, 44, 44, 47, 51, 55, 55, 60, 60, and 62. Because we have an even number of data points, the two middle points (47 and 51) are averaged (47 + 51 = 98/2 = 49%).

SPC can be used to better interpret a run chart for improvement potential. There are several rules that can be applied to determine common versus special cause variation. Other more advanced rules exist to differentiate special from common cause variation (shifts, trends, and runs within the graph) that are beyond the scope of this chapter. Looking back at Figure 9.6, does any unit's data demonstrate an outlier or finding

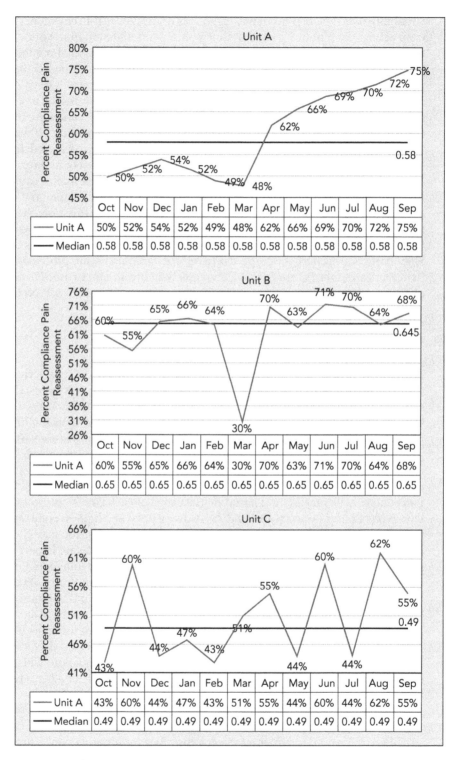

FIGURE 9.6 Run charts demonstrating pain reassessment compliance within 60 minutes of intravenous pain medication administration for three units.

different from the others? If you said Unit B, you would be correct. With a median of 65% compliance, the 30% seen in March is an outlier. In general, Unit B is relatively stable with most compliance scores hovering around the median line, except for March, which was a drastic drop from February (64%). Unit B should ask, what happened? Is there an explanation for this change? Also notice the improvement in April (70%). When the process is in control, which was the case for Unit B before March, and suddenly an outlier occurs, it may not need immediate attention. Perhaps Unit B was orienting new nurses who were not yet familiar with the pain policy. The outcome may have improved due to their completed orientation. Before mobilizing resources to improve an outlier representing special cause, first determine if there is explanation, if so, monitor the trend for the next few months to determine if that outlier was incidental or if there actually is a problem needing QI intervention. If one special cause data point cannot be explained that might place patients at risk, further QI interventions are needed.

How would you compare the units in Figure 9.6 regarding their compliance with pain reassessment? Unit A was below the median for the first 6 months then steadily improved over the last 6 months. What is not known is if the unit implemented an intervention in March with the following 6 months demonstrating positive improvement. If an intervention was implemented it should be sustained and celebrated. Also unknown is if the change from April (48%) to May (62%) was special cause variation. With the additional of subsequent data points, it appears that the process changed for the better and improved performance is being sustained. One challenge when interpreting a run chart for outliers or abnormal findings is that it is a guess. Unit B's process has been in control except for that one special cause finding in March. Unit C demonstrates lots of variability in outcomes. There is little consistency month by month. Although no special cause can be clearly defined, a QI intervention may be triggered to reduce or explain the variation.

When comparing units, knowing the goal or target that demonstrates success is necessary. If the goal is 90% compliance, no unit is meeting the goal. It may be helpful to include the goal on the run chart. Additionally, relative internal and external comparisons can provide benchmarking opportunities. Table 9.3 summarizes types of variation, analysis considerations, and potential QI actions. Prioritization is based on the volume and criticality of the outcomes and should include the consensus of QI

TABLE 9.3 VARIATION INTERPRETATIONS, ANALYSIS, AND QI ACTIONS

TYPE OF VARIATION	ANALYSIS	QI ACTIONS
Common cause variation (Process IN Control)	Is the process demonstrating acceptable variation/acceptable level of performance?	No QI actions is required
	Is the process in control but a wide-range or unacceptable variation exists?	QI actions may be required based on QI priorities
Special cause variation (Process OUT of Control)	Is the process statistically demonstrating a problem, a change that is not desirable?	Action is required
	Is the process is statistically demonstrating improvement based on QI efforts?	Continue to monitor to determine if efforts are sustained over time, if so, spread the lessons learned

experts and staff involved in the process. Although Unit C might like to reduce variation, other more critical problems may require attention first.

One advantage of using a run chart is ease in interpretation and it is commonly used by health care organizations. One disadvantage is that it is not as statistically sensitive as other tools with more specificity (Lloyd, 2010). There is another type of run chart, the Shewhart control chart described below, which adds a statistical advantage to the run chart that clearly detects outliers or astronomical findings eliminating the need for guessing. It takes time and practice to interpret run charts. For a closer look at interpreting a run chart, refer to Case Study 9.3.

CASE STUDY 9.3

Use the data from Figure 9.6. At a Unit C QI meeting, a nurse asks for assistance interpreting if the unit improved its pain reassessment compliance. The nurse notes that the first 3 months' results are October, 52%, November, 45%, and December, 50%, respectively (Figure 9.6, Unit C).

1. *How would you respond as to whether the pain reassessment compliance improved or not?*

The Shewhart Control Chart

The Shewhart control chart, often referred to as simply a control chart, is the same as the run chart but adds statistical control limits to the run chart using SD. As SD is used, the centerline is represented by the mean of the data set rather than the median that is seen on the run chart. The X- and Y-axis are set up the same on both charts, with the X-axis being the time points and the Y-axis being the variable or process under study. The control chart has the same purpose as the run chart, to distinguish common from special cause variation. Recall the discussion about SD and that "sigma" is another term used for SD. The control chart, created by software, will set SD control limits at 1, 2, and 3 SD above and below the mean of the data set. The advantage of the control chart is the addition of SD because there is no guessing if an outlier or abnormal data point is present, which will be demonstrated shortly. When analyzing a control chart, the **upper control limit** (UCL) is defined as the line 3 SD above the mean while the **lower control limit** (LCL) is the line 3 SD below the mean. A process that is considered to be in control or demonstrating common cause variability will have all data points between the UCL (+3 SD from the mean) and LCL (−3 SD from the mean). Together, the upper and LCLs represent Six Sigma. When a data point falls above or below the UCL or LCL, the process is said to have a statistically significant outcome (special cause variation, or abnormal finding).

Before examining the control chart, it is a good time to think about what we have already learned. Data can be displayed using a variety of formats, including histograms, Pareto charts, run charts, and control charts. Each format has a purpose and value within QI. Consider the Pareto chart in Figure 9.7. This data represents the annual contributing factors of incident reports of a large multisite organization. Medication errors are the leading cause of incidents over a 12-month period. That outcome could trigger a QI activity. However, we now know there are more sophisticated SPC methods available to better analyze these incident report data.

In Figure 9.8, aggregate medication errors are shown on a control chart using a time series design over 12 months. A range of outcomes, in this case from 8 to 37 medication errors, is depicted, which represents significant variation. In analyzing aggregate medication errors in Figure 9.8, what do you notice different in the control chart as opposed to a run chart? The major difference includes the addition of the UCL and LCL, which can be used to analyze the process range. As nearly 100% (specifically 99.8%) of

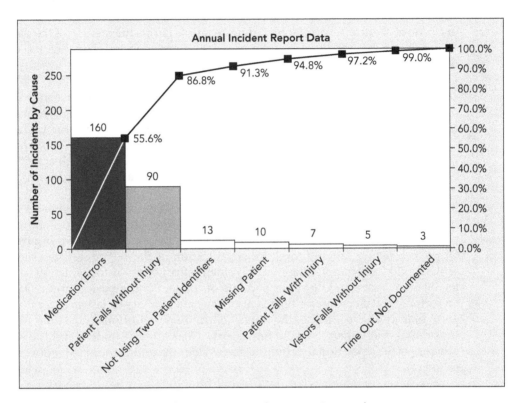

FIGURE 9.7 Incident report data over 12 months using a Pareto chart.

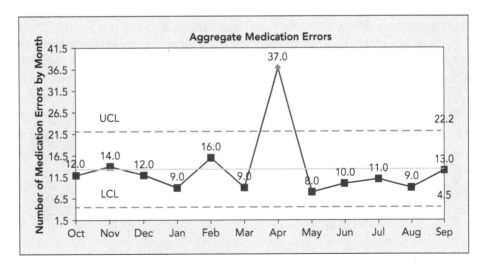

FIGURE 9.8 Aggregate incident report data over 12 months using a control chart.

outcomes are expected to fall within 3 SD from the mean, as seen in Figure 9.1, using 3 SD is generally acceptable when analyzing for special cause variation. In Figure 9.8, the UCL was established at 22.2 and the LCL at 4.5 automatically using specific software.

Evaluating the UCL and LCL is valuable because these limits specify the process range. In other words, 22 to nearly 5 medication errors could occur each month and be considered in control, or within Six Sigma of the mean. In this case, that alone might trigger a QI activity as 22 medication errors a month while being considered in control would be concerning. Also note in Figure 9.8 the centerline is the mean of the data points in a control chart, whereas the centerline on a run chart is the median of the data set.

There are several different types of control charts and interpretation rules. At this point, it is important to apply the same rule used with the run chart, identifying if an outlier or "astronomical" data point exists. With the control chart, your job is made easier as special cause is evident when a data point appears either above or below the control limits. Analysis and actions outlined in Table 9.3 also apply to the control chart. In Figure 9.8 (37 incidents in April) is nicely depicted above the UCL, there is no guessing required if the data point represents special cause variation. The control chart reduces interpretation errors and the risk of not implementing QI activities when necessary or implementing QI activities when not necessary, leading to inappropriate resource utilization.

Stratification is the process of breaking the data down into subsets to better interpret what is happening and where (Fowler Byers & Rosati, 2008). Suppose the patient safety officer is studying Figure 9.8 and prioritizes medication errors for a QI project. Before moving forward, stratification of the 160 aggregated medication errors could help target where improvement efforts should focus. To do so, the 160 medication errors could be stratified into outpatient and inpatient areas. Data could be further stratified among inpatient or outpatient units to better determine if one particular unit is leading to the abnormal finding. Additional questions should be considered: Were there truly so few errors? Does all staff understand the reporting process? Is the operational definition clear? Does the culture support reporting medication errors?

We have examined what data is and how data can be displayed for QI decision making and monitoring. Tools, such as those described in the SPC section, provide the QI team with the most efficient, systematic means of determining what health care process needs improvement or if a QI was sustained over time. Given the advantages of SPC, these methods should be applied to health care decision making whenever possible. Creating and analyzing data using run or control charts require time and practice. Collaborating with QI experts for assistance is recommended. The next step in the QI journey is to empower a team that utilizes outcomes for data-driven QIs.

Critical Thinking 9.2

Go to the Agency for Healthcare Research and Quality (AHRQ) website, http:// statesnapshots.ahrq.gov/snaps10/index.jsp. Select "state ranking for selected

(continued)

indicators." *Examine the state's overall performance, noting the definition of the indicator. Select another state and compare the two.*

1. How do you know the states are measuring the same thing the same way?
2. How would this information drive QI?

TEAM TOOLS

Interprofessional teams are often created to bring experts together to address problems and make improvements. Other QI tools, such as Gantt charts, parking lots, and flow maps help teams work through projects. Cause/effect or fishbone diagrams, Lean thinking, Six Sigma, Plan-Do-Study-Act (PDSA), health care failure mode effects analysis (HFMEA), and root cause analysis (RCA) are all QI tools used by teams and are discussed in Chapter 7.

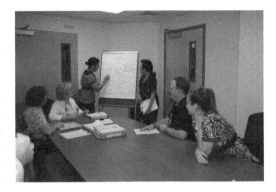

Quality improvement team.

Gantt Chart

A **Gantt chart** is a graph depicting the phases of a project over the project's time line and is used to keep the team on schedule (Table 9.4). All known project tasks are included in the Gantt chart, from beginning to end. As QI takes time and effort, line 16 nicely reminds us to celebrate and share success, something all teams should include.

Flow Map

QI is focused on improving the health care process; therefore, understanding each step within the process must be considered before interventions are identified. A **flow map**, or process flowchart, allows the QI team to diagram the actual sequence of a health care process from the beginning to the end. Clarifying a process reduces redundancy, unnecessary steps, and overly complex processes helping to identify a future improved process flow. Different steps or actions within a health care process are represented by specific symbols in a flow map, such as ovals to depict the beginning and end points, squares identify steps in the process, diamonds identify decision points, and arrows identify directional flow of the process. Figure 9.9 shows patient flow through an ED.

TABLE 9.4 THE GANTT CHART

Emergency Department Microsystem Redesign Project

ID	TASK NAME	START	FINISH	FEBRUARY 2010			MARCH 2010			APRIL 2010			MAY 2010			JUNE 2010			JULY 2010		
				1/24 1/31 2/7	2/14 2/21	2/28 3/7	3/14 3/21 3/28	4/4	4/11 4/18 4/25	5/2	5/9 5/16 5/23	5/30	6/6 6/13 6/20 6/27	7/4	7/11 7/18 7/25
1	Defined global aim of the project	1/29/2010	2/21/2010	▬▬▬▬											
2	Defined specific aim of the project	3/15/2010	3/24/2010				▬▬								
3	Created ED flow log	3/15/2010	3/19/2010				▬								
4	Team coaching regarding the tool	3/24/2010	3/24/2010				▮								
5	Data collection (Pre)	4/9/2010	4/29/2010					▬▬▬							
6	Study and evaluate ED tools	3/25/2010	4/8/2010					▬▬▬							
7	Satisfaction survey (Pre) for patients and ED Staff	4/26/2010	4/30/2010						▬						
8	Created share point access to data and satisfaction survey	4/26/2010	4/29/2010						▬						
9	Made changes to computerized triage template	5/7/2010	5/7/2010							▮					
10	Team coaching regarding the triage tool	5/7/2010	5/12/2010							▬					
11	Data collection (post)	5/8/2010	6/9/2010							▬▬▬▬				
12	Analyzed the data	6/10/2010	6/14/2010								▬			
13	Satisfaction survey (post) for patients and ED staff	6/23/2010	6/30/2010								▬		
14	Displayed the results to the team	7/7/2010	7/7/2010									▮
15	Report to management in PDSA format	7/1/2010	7/30/2010									▬▬▬▬
16	Celebrate and share success	7/14/2010	7/14/2010									▮

Courtesy of Providence VA Medical Center, Providence, RI.

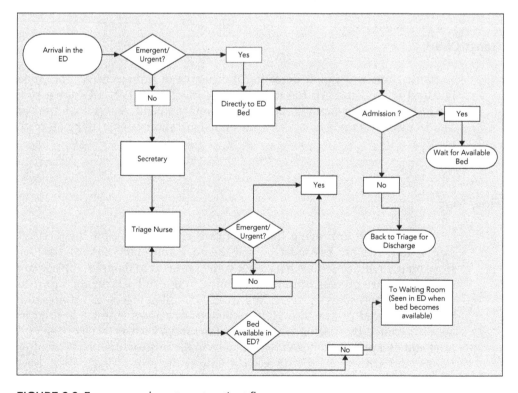

FIGURE 9.9 Emergency department patient flow map.

Courtesy of Providence VA Medical Center, Providence, RI.

REAL-WORLD INTERVIEW

I was asked to participate in Lean training. A group from our unit went to the training not knowing what Lean really referred to. None of us were sure what this Lean was or what it involved. Content was presented using lots of new terminology. We heard about PDSA but process mapping? Fishbone diagrams? As the program progressed, it became clear that the expectation of the participants was to complete a Lean project. Although nervous and wondering what did we commit to, we all were intrigued and believed we had lots of ways of making our unit more efficient.

We focused on brainstorming, process mapping, flow diagrams, and creating a PDSA. This was enlightening. Here we were flow mapping health care processes! What was most exciting was how we might use some of these tools on our unit. We were always so busy just responding to the many demands of patient care that we seldom took the time to discuss our unit and how we could make things better. We gained insight how to creatively make change. It was an amazing feeling!

After the training we were all energized and eager to continue our discussion on a project and to get others on the unit involved. We were successful in creating our first systems redesign project using Lean principles. We all shared similar frustrations with inefficiency in delivering patient care, particularly in our supply areas. Supplies were scattered instead of being grouped together. If a nasogastric tube needed to be inserted, it required travel to four different supply locations.

Our large clean supply area was changed due to construction. This gave us the impetus to improve the supply area layout for efficiency using Lean principles. We tagged unnecessary or duplicate supplies and eliminated them. We collaborated with other departments; had quality experts take pictures so we could compare the before and after changes; we worked with supply staff to consider how we might change the utility room layout, added photos of supplies, and logically arranged supplies together (e.g., oxygen administration supplies were all reorganized to the same bin area; patient care supplies, pajamas, toothbrushes, urinals, and any personal care items were all relocated in one spot, saving us time and frustration!)

What was amazing was our collaboration and success in working with other departments. We interacted with laundry, carpenters, infectious disease, pharmacy, central supply, quality experts, and housekeeping. Our group was on fire. We had actually implemented tools introduced to us in training. None of us ever collected data or worked through an improvement process from beginning to end. Yet we did it and had fun at the same time because we created a positive change for our unit. It has been exciting, overwhelming, and frustrating at times to be involved in such a project. I started off completely unprepared for such an activity. After all, I'm just a staff nurse, right? Never would I have imagined taking a lead role in the redesign project and now I can say I contributed to a successful change on my unit. What a journey!

Annette M Phillips, BSN, RN
Staff Nurse, Providence VA Medical Center
Providence, Rhode Island

KEY CONCEPTS

- QI is a continuous process used to prevent, recognize, and reduce harm. It includes the ongoing search for performance excellence.
- QI is defined using the QSEN definition, "Use data to monitor the outcomes of care processes and use improvement methods to design and test changes to continuously improve the quality and safety of health care systems."
- Quality initiatives are data driven and patient centered.
- Many sources of data exist, including internal, external, baseline, postintervention, incidence, prevalence, and aggregate.
- Data can be displayed using a variety of formats, including histograms, Pareto charts, scatter plot diagrams, and run and control charts).
- The science of QI, mainly SPC, is concerned with minimizing variability within health care processes.
- Teams, often interprofessional, bring expertise and innovation to improving outcomes.
- Teams can use a variety of tools (flow maps, parking lots, and Gantt charts) during the improvement process.

KEY TERMS

Aggregate data
Baseline data
Common cause variation
Data display
Descriptive statistics
External data
Flow map
Gantt chart
Histogram
Incidence measures
Information
Internal data
Interrater reliability
Lower control limit
Mean
Median
Mode

Objective data
Operational definition
Outliers
Pareto chart
Postintervention data
Prevalence measures
Quality improvement
Range
Run chart
Scatterplot diagram
Special cause variation
Standard deviation
Statistical process control
Stratification
Subjective data
Upper control limit
Variability

DISCUSSION OF OPENING SCENARIO

The ongoing collection and interpretation of patient data occurs relentlessly while practicing as a professional nurse. When interpreting data, it is necessary to know baseline findings for comparison to current findings. Based on the scenario, the only interpretation the day nurse can make is that the patient continues to have a fever and elevated white blood cell count. The day nurse did not receive a comprehensive hand-off. There is insufficient information to decide if the patient is responding to IV antibiotics or if his fever is improving or not. Without key data, analysis becomes subjective and potentially inaccurate. In this scenario, answering the physical therapist's basic question is difficult due to the poor handoff communication that occurred. Several important handoff questions may have been useful to better interpret the patient's data. What specifically was the night shift temperature? What are the trends or range in his temperature since admission? Was a sputum culture obtained to determine if the right antibiotic was prescribed? What lung sounds were heard on auscultation? When assessing data, trends are useful in identifying the range, or low and high values. If the patient had a maximum fever of 103 degrees on admission, a current fever of 101.1 degrees is an improvement despite being elevated. Thus, an elevated temperature and white blood cell count may actually be an improvement depending on baseline findings. Improvements depend on multiple factors, including if adequate time for treatment has passed, if the right antibiotic was prescribed, and if the patient's immune system is able to respond appropriately. In addition to improving communication and patient safety, handoffs are valuable opportunities to collect baseline data to assess the response to care and services. Always appreciate the patient's subjective responses as to how he or she feels despite normal or abnormal objective data findings. The patient's perceptions of improvement, his or her comfort and satisfaction with care and services impact the nursing plan of care. In this scenario, if the patient's perceptions were assessed, they were not shared during the handoff.

CRITICAL THINKING ANSWERS

Critical Thinking 9.1

1. Select the best operational definition for a fall and explain why you selected the option.

    The third option is the strongest operational definition because it includes visitors. Visitor falls need to be documented as an incident and aggregated along with patient falls. Root cause and elimination of contributing factors for patients and visitors may be necessary based on the results. Using a control chart will allow the unit practice council an opportunity to decide if common cause or special cause variation is evident in falls over time. The incident rate using the upper and lower control limits may suggest the need for improvement even if no special cause variation is evident. (In addition to not being a good operational definition, also note that in the first option, data reported annually is stated. Such a plan would be unacceptable as special cause may have occurred and the council would not be aware or have the opportunity to reduce fall incidence rates.)

Critical Thinking 9.2

1. How do you know the states are measuring the same thing the same way?

    It is impossible to tell if the states are measuring the same thing the same way. The standardized definition suggests that all organizations are measuring the same thing since the indicator is very specific, that is, breast cancer deaths per 100,000 female population. Other indicators are more general, that is, percentage of adult hemodialysis patients with adequate dialysis. In the hemodialysis definition, we do not know what "adequate dialysis" is, how it is quantified, how it is measured and how to report "adequate dialysis." This leaves room for hospitals to define the measure, which may or may not be the same for all hospitals.

2. How would this information drive QI?

Health care organizations can evaluate their outcomes of care data against other health care organizations. This may uncover a potential problem area that requires a QI project to improve the data.

CASE STUDY ANSWERS

Case Study 9.1

1. How would you write this plan and ensure both nurses are measuring their clinic no-shows consistently?

Begin by creating an operational definition of what a clinic no-show is defined as. In the operational definition, include a definition of the numerator and denominator. An example might look like this:

A clinic no-show includes all patients who call to cancel their appointment within 48 hours of the appointment date and time or who do not notify the clinic they are unable to make their appointment. (*Do not* count those who notify the clinic more than 48 hours of their scheduled appointment as the clinic can fill those appointments using a wait list.) The numerator is the number of no-shows and the denominator is the total number of clinic visits scheduled.

The two nurses might create a spreadsheet that looks like the following:

DATE	CLINIC A OR B	TOTAL SCHEDULED APPOINTMENTS	NUMBER OF NO SHOWS	PERCENTAGE OF NO SHOWS VS. TOTAL NUMBER OF APPOINTMENTS
May 1	Clinic A	26	2	7.7%
May 1	Clinic B	30	7	23.3%

Both nurses would pilot, or test, the usefulness of the spreadsheet to collect the needed information. They would agree to pilot for one complete week. Both nurses would gather at the closing of the clinic to compare their findings. They would determine if they were applying the operational definition consistently at each clinic. If unwanted, unexpected, or unplanned variations were discovered, clarification and revision of the operational definition, or further discussion/training with the reviewers might be necessary with continued IRR testing. If both nurses found no errors in their application of the operational definition, they have demonstrated IRR in the data collection process. In doing so, the team can be confident the data is accurate and represent the variable under improvement.

Case Study 9.2

1. Now that you have your outcomes, calculate the mean, median, mode, and range of these results.

Beginning with the mean, or average of your results, add all the number together and divide by that total number of observations. In the case above, there are nine data points (three each week by shift). When each data point is added together, the sum of those data is 18. Dividing observations (9) into data points (18), you can calculate the mean of the data (18/9 = 2). Based on your observations or results, over this 3-week time period of measurement, the average number of call-offs was 2. You can apply this same process and "drill-down" or look closer to assess if one shift has a higher average than another. *Drilling down* is a term used to help isolate where the problem may be. For example, even though the mean of this data is 2, there may be one shift that is an outlier, or much higher than the other two shifts causing the mean to be high. In the example above, looking at day shift, you can see the mean of those three data points is 8/3 = 2.67, which is higher than the mean of the entire set of data. The mean for night shift is 4/3 = 1.33, below the mean of the entire data set. Therefore, the improvement intervention may target day shift.

The median of a set of data is used to divide the data into two groups, low and high results. This is measured by listing the results from low to high. In the example above, the low to high results include 1–1-1–1-2–2-3–3-4, respectively. The median is the number directly in the middle of the set of data. In this case, it is at position five, resulting in the median value of 2. If for example you had an even number of data points, say we added another shift to our data above that had 2 calls-offs, our data would look like this: 1–1-1–1-2–2-2–3-3–4, respectively. The data median would be the average of the 3 middle points, points 4 through 6. Looking at our data, those points are 1–2-2 (5÷3 = 1.67).

The range of a set of data is a quick measure of variability or the spread of the data over time. Looking at the nine data points in the example, the range is simply the low (1) and high (4) value of your data set.

Case Study 9.3

1. How would you respond as to whether the pain reassessment compliance improved or not?

   There is no evidence of special cause if this data was added to the existing run chart with the median minimally changed (now 50%). The process of documenting pain reassessment within 60 minutes remains in control but variation within the process continues. You might suggest a QI action or not, depending if other outcomes are more concerning.

REVIEW QUESTIONS

Please see Appendix D for answers to Review Questions.

1. You are reviewing a control chart that depicts the number of falls over a 24-month period. You note a special cause variation occurred at month 6. Which characteristic below is indicative of a special cause variation?

   A. The 6th month data point is between the UCLs and LCLs.
   B. The 6th month data point is 2 SD below the mean.
   C. The 6th month data point is 1 SD above the mean.
   D. The 6th month data point is above the mean at 3 SDs.

2. At a staff meeting, your nurse manager reports patient satisfaction has declined on your unit. In analysis of the patient comments, 30% of the 100 discharged patients surveyed over the last month complained about the noise at night. You are asked to be a participant in an improvement team to increase patient satisfaction. Which of the following questions are most appropriate to ask your manager before the team begins their QI project? Select all that apply.

A. How many staff will be invited to participate in the team?
B. Is there evidence this finding is a special cause variation?
C. What time frame is permitted to complete the project?
D. Will there be overtime to attend meetings?
E. How will trends be measured?
F. How will participation affect my performance?

3. One of the key concepts of QI is how a need for change does actually become an improvement. Which of the following is not an appropriate option for launching a QI project?

A. High-priority findings from a proactive risk assessment such as the HFMEA recently completed on your mental health unit
B. Ongoing concerns identified in the medication usage review committee
C. A fellow staff nurse's poor performance that is negatively affecting patient care
D. Need for innovation to close the gap between your organization's restraint usage and that of the identified benchmark or best practice

4. Tardiness of evening shift staff has been a problem on your unit. This has led to excessive overtime to ensure that patient shift handoffs are conducted in a timely manner. Your manager invites you to monitor evening-shift tardiness for one week. There are eight evening nurses. You just completed data collection and are preparing a spread sheet to share with your manager. Using the findings in the table below, what is the mean time for tardiness and range of minutes that evening staff were tardy over this 7-day period?

TABLE: TARDINESS OF EVENING SHIFT

NURSE	SUNDAY	MONDAY	TUESDAY	WEDNESDAY	THURSDAY	FRIDAY	SATURDAY
A	OFF	OFF	OT	3 min	OT	OFF	OT
B	OT	12 min	5 min	OFF	13 min	11 min	OFF
C	OT	OFF	OT	5 min	OT	12 min	OFF
D	OT	OT	OFF	OT	OT	OT	OFF
E	OFF	3 min	OT	OT	3 min	OFF	5 min
F	OFF	OT	ILL	5 min	OFF	OT	15 min
G	OT	OFF	20 min	OT	OT	OT	OFF
H	OFF	OT	4 min	OFF	7 min	OT	OT

OT, on time. A, Mean = .75 minute, Range = 0–3; B, Mean = 8.2 minutes, Range = 0–13; C, Mean = 3.4 minutes, Range = 0–12; D, Mean = 0 minutes, Range = 0; E, Mean = 2.2 minutes, Range = 0–5; F, Mean = 5 minutes, Range = 0–15; G, Mean = 4 minutes, Range = 0–20; H, Mean = 2.2 minutes, Range = 0–7.

5. When considering data display options, which order of display, from least scientific to most scientific, exists when examining process variation?

   A. Range–run chart–control chart
   B. Run chart–Pareto chart–control chart
   C. Range–control chart–run chart
   D. Only a control chart allows for analysis of variability

6. The most distinguishing characteristic of a Pareto chart is that it

   A. Includes UCLs and LCLs
   B. Depicts 80% of the problem comes from 20% of the causes
   C. Displays data using a time series format
   D. Is used when determining if special cause variation exists
   E. Provides information about primary causes of a problem

7. Statistical process control is

   A. Assessed using a run or control chart
   B. Assessed only when data is presented in a control chart
   C. A sophisticated measurement using the data range as the centerline
   D. Easily assessed using a run chart (no, can make interpretation errors, many guesses)

8. Stratification of data refers to

   A. Averaging the number of data points
   B. Identifying the lowest and highest data point
   C. 3 SDs above or below the mean
   D. Segmenting the data from aggregate to more specific subsets

9. When a QI team wants to document a process from beginning to end, which of the following tools is most helpful?

   A. Flow map diagram
   B. Fishbone diagram
   C. Scatter plot diagram
   D. Pareto chart

10. Why is baseline data useful in QI activities?

    A. It is used to differentiate common from special cause variation.
    B. It is used as the operational definition.
    C. It is used to demonstrate a sustained improvement outcome.
    D. It is used to compare pre intervention to postintervention outcomes.

11. Of the options below, which is the most important requirement when creating an operational definition?

    A. Using the dictionary as a reference
    B. Creating a numerator/denominator for measurement purposes
    C. Listing the team member names
    D. Have the approval of the organization's director before defining the variable

REVIEW ACTIVITIES

Please see Appendix E for answers to Review Activities.

1. Robert Wood Johnson Foundation (RWJF), http://rwjf.org. Read about the RWJF mission and goal. Select Program areas—Explore Public Health and Quality/Equality areas. Appreciate the up-to-date news and headlines regarding these important topics. While exploring the Quality/Equality page, open the Aligning Forces for Quality (AF4Q) option. Consider how this program is working to reduce disparities in health care.

2. The Joint Commission (TJC), http://www.jointcomission.org. Select Sentinel Event Alert Issue—Explore the current alert. Consider the impact of this alert. Consider QI ideas that might eliminate this occurrence from happening? How would you approach preventing this incident in your organization?

3. Transforming Care at the Bedside (TCAB), http://www.ihi.org. Search TCAB on the Institute for Healthcare Improvements website. Select *Transforming Care at the Bedside How-to Guide: Engaging Front-Line Staff in Innovation and Quality Improvement.* Explore several options listed under Featured Content. While in this same section, select Case Studies and explore several interesting reports from the frontlines.

EXPLORING THE WEB

1. RWJF: http://rwjf.org
2. AHRQ; Data Sources: http://www.ahrq.gov/research/data/dataresources.html
3. The Healthcare Effectiveness Data and Information Set (HEDIS): http://www.ncqa.org/HEDISQualityMeasurement.aspx
4. Health-Related Datasets: http://www.hhs.gov/open/datasets

REFERENCES

Berwick, D. M. (1991). Controlling variation in health care: A consultation from Walter Shewhart. *Medical Care, 29*(12), 1212–1225.

Carey, R. G. (2003). *Improving healthcare with control charts.* Milwaukee, WI: ASQ Quality Press.

Cronenwett, L., Sherwood, G., Barnsteiner, J., Disch, J., Johnson, J., Mitchell, P., . . . Warren, J. (2007). Quality and safety education for nurses. *Nursing Outlook, 55*(3), 122–131.

Evans, J. R. (2008). *Quality and performance excellence: Management, organization, and strategy* (5th ed.). Mason, OH: Thompson South-Western.

Fowler Byers, J., & Rosati, R. J. (2008). Foundation, techniques, and tools. In L. R. Pelletier & C. L. Beaudin (Eds.), *Q solutions: Essential resources for the healthcare quality professional* (p. 66). Glenview, IL: National Association for Healthcare Quality.

Grube, J. A. (2008). Strategy and leadership. In L. R. Pelletier & C. L. Beaudin (Eds.), *Q solutions: Essential resources for the healthcare quality professional* (p. 79). Glenview, IL: National Association for Healthcare Quality.

Lloyd, R. C. (2010). Navigating in the turbulent sea of data: The quality measurement journey. *Clinics in Perinatology, 37,* 101–122.

Mohammed, M. A., Worthington, P., & Woodall, W. H. (2008). Plotting basic control charts: Tutorial notes for healthcare practitioners. *Quality and Safety in Healthcare, 17,* 137–145. doi:10.1136/qshc.2004.012047.

Nelson, E. C., Batalden, P. B., & Godfrey, M. M. (2007). The model for improvement: PDSA SDSA. In E. C. Nelson, P. B. Batalden, & M. M. Godfrey (Eds.), *Quality by design: A clinical microsystems approach* (pp. 271–283). San Francisco, CA: Jossey-Bass.

Pelletier, L. R., & Beaudin, C. L. (Eds.). (2008). *Q solutions: Essential resources for the healthcare quality professional* (2nd ed.). Glenview, IL: National Association for Healthcare Quality. Reprinted with permission.

SUGGESTED READING

Ashley, L., Dexter, R., Marshall, F., McKenzie, B., Ryan, M., & Armitage, G. (2011). Improving the safety of chemotherapy administration: An oncology nurse-led failure mode and effects analysis. *Oncology Nursing Forum, 38*(6), E436–E444.

Berwick, D. M. (2011). Preparing nurses for participation in and leadership of continual improvement. *Journal of Nursing Education, 50*(6), 322–327. doi:10.3928/01484834–20110519-05.

Berwick, D. M., Nolan, T. W., & Whittington, J. (2008). The triple aim: Care, health, and cost. *Health Affairs, 27*(3), 757–769.

Donaldson, M. S. (2008). An overview of to err is human: Re-emphasizing the message of patient safety. In R. G. Hughes (Ed.), *Patient safety and quality: An evidenced-based handbook for nurses* (pp. 1–9). Rockville, MD: Agency for Healthcare Research and Quality.

Duclos, A., & Voirin, N. (2010). The p-control chart: A tool for care improvement. *International Journal for Quality in Health Care, 22*(5), 402–407.

Goldmann, D. (2011). Ten tips for incorporating scientific quality improvement into everyday work. *British Medical Journal of Quality and Safety, 20*(Suppl 1), i69–i72. doi:10:1136/bmjqs.2010.046359

Kimsey, D. B. (2010). Lean methodology in health care. *American Journal of Perioperative Room Nurses, 92*(1), 53–60. doi:10.1016/j.aorn.2010.01.015

Oman, K. S., Flynn-Makic, M. B., Fink, R., Schraeder, N., Hulett, T., Keech, T., & Wald, H. (2011). Nurse-directed interventions to reduce catheter-associated urinary tract infections. *American Journal of Infection Control, 30,* 1–6.

Pocha, C. (2010). Lean six sigma in health care and the challenge of implementation of six sigma methodologies at a veterans affairs medical center. *Quality Management in Health Care, 19*(4), 312–318.

Shewhart, W. A., & Deming, W. E. (1939). *Statistical method from the viewpoint of quality control.* Washington, DC: Department of Agriculture.

Vest, J. R., & Gamm, L. D. (2009). A critical review of the research literature on six sigma, lean, and studer-group's hardwiring excellence in the United States: The need to demonstrate and communicate the effectiveness of transformation strategies in healthcare. *Implementation Science, 4*(35), 1–9.

vretveit, J. (2011). Understanding the conditions for improvement: Research to discover which context influences affect improvement success. *British Medical Journal of Quality and Safety, 20*(Suppl 1), i18–i23. doi:10:1136/bmjqs.2010.045955

10

INFORMATICS

Donna L. Silsbee and Francia I. Reed

In their daily practice, nurses are seeing the beginnings of a broad-based transformation of healthcare delivery. If they haven't already implemented an electronic health record (EHR), they're probably either in the midst of doing this or are planning for it. The time really is now for being a part of this transformation, helping it succeed, and making sure it reflects the priorities we've always counted on nursing to support. (Dr. Farzad Mostashari, National Coordinator for Health Information Technology [Mostashari interview as cited in Cipriani, 2011])

Upon completion of this chapter, the reader should be able to

1. Define health informatics
2. Discuss national initiatives that are taking place to implement electronic health records (EHRs)
3. Explain how hospital information systems supply data to the EHR
4. Discuss the Department of Veterans Affairs (VA) Veterans Health Information Systems and Technology Architecture (VISTA) system
5. Describe the role of other technologies within the hospital systems
7. Explain the role telehealth plays in the care of the homebound patient
8. Explain the advantages and disadvantages of clinical alerts in the EHR
9. Differentiate between the concepts of privacy, confidentiality, and security
10. Discuss the future of health informatics

*I*n *November 2007, actor Dennis Quaid and his wife Kimberly walked into Cedars-Sinai Medical Center to visit their newborn twins: Thomas Boone and Zoe Grace. To the Quaids' horror, they were immediately greeted by a nurse who informed them that the twins had been given an overdose of heparin (10,000 U/mL rather than 1,000 U/mL). Once the error was* *noticed, the children were treated with protamine sulfate and they apparently suffered no long-term effects of the incident. The Quaids' subsequently sued the drug company for using drug labels on the high- and the low-concentration heparin vials, which were very similar and could cause confusion. Although they did not sue the hospital, they did ask that the hospital review its policies and procedures (Rosen, 2008).*

- *Are any types of information systems used to help prevent medication errors like this?*
- *What is an alternative to using heparin to flush an IV?*
- *What types of policies and procedures may have not been followed to allow such an error to have occurred.*

H̲ealth informatics is one of the largest growing areas of specialty within health care. The growth is due in part to a national initiative to convert all health care records into electronic records within the next few years. The world of technological advances and information access is ever changing and health care is not immune from its effects. The result of merging health care and technology is known as the relatively new discipline of health informatics.

This chapter defines health informatics as well as discusses the various aspects of telecommunications, science, information, and the role health informatics has in helping providers to deliver safe and efficient health care. The impact of national initiatives is discussed relative to the implementation of EHRs. From that vantage point, the role of technologies in hospitals and other health care systems is illustrated, including the VISTA system. The description of technologies role includes explanation of how information systems within the hospital or health care organization supply data to the EHRs. In addition to inpatient examples of health informatics, the role telehealth plays in outpatient care is discussed. Specific technologies are introduced and discussed relative to advantages and disadvantages including clinical alerts within a patient's EHR. Federal law to protect identifiable information is detailed, providing differentiation between the concepts of privacy, confidentiality, and security. Lastly, the future of informatics is discussed.

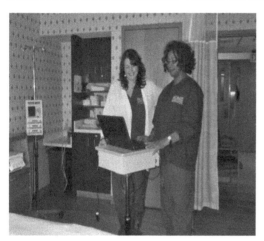

Nurses utilize a computer on wheels.

HEALTH INFORMATICS DEFINED

While informatics is simply the science of collecting, managing, and retrieving information, health informatics is "the interdisciplinary study of the design, development, adoption and application of IT-based innovations in healthcare services delivery, management and planning" (U.S. National Library of Medicine, 2012). Management of health records dominates the discussion of health informatics; however, computer technology offers a variety of ways to record and retrieve information to support the evidence-based needs and actions of the interprofessional team including

- Patient-decision support tools
- Laboratory and x-rays results, reporting and reviewing systems
- Quality improvement (QI) data collection/data summary systems
- Disease surveillance systems
- Electronic bed boards that monitor bed availability
- Simulation laboratories

The Health Care Information Management and Systems Society (HIMSS, 2011) defines an **electronic health record** (EHR) as a longitudinal electronic record of patient health information generated by one or more encounters in any care delivery setting. Included in this health information are patient demographics, progress notes, problems, medications, vital signs, past medical history, immunizations, laboratory data, and radiology reports. The EHR automates and streamlines the clinician's workflow. The EHR has the ability to generate a complete record of a clinical patient encounter, as well as supporting other care-related activities including evidence-based decision support, quality management, and outcomes reporting.

EHRs will form the basis of the National Health Information Network (NHIN), which is a plan to be able to exchange patient information electronically from one health care provider to another health care provider. NHIN will allow the health care provider to access previous information such as the patient's disease history, the list of medications, the known allergies, and the prior test results. The electronic exchange of patient information will eliminate delays that occur when paper records must be copied and sent to another provider. The NHIN will also help exchange patient information between health care providers and public health authorities. For example, submission of reports to government vaccination registries and the reporting of communicable diseases will be done from the EHR. The reports will be done at the same time care is provided (in real time) so agencies charged with protecting the health of the public will be able to act quickly. If a particular lot of a vaccine is recalled, health authorities will know which patients to contact. If a virulent strain of influenza occurs, health authorities can issue public health warnings and close some public places to prevent further spread of the disease. The electronic information exchange within NHIN must protect patient privacy and the content of the data. Health care providers have a legal and ethical duty to maintain the confidentiality of patient information. For patient safety, data cannot be altered in any way. For example, information regarding a medication must maintain the same name, dose, frequency, and route of administration as it is being transmitted to another provider. No one should be able to capture the data enroute and change it.

The Department of Health and Human Services predicts that the NHIN will enhance the quality of care by reducing health care errors (especially those related to medications), eliminating the need for duplicate testing thus subjecting the patient to less risk, and reducing delays that occur from lack of information. If the efficiency and effectiveness of care is improved, the costs of providing care should be reduced.

NATIONAL INITIATIVES TO IMPLEMENT HEALTH INFORMATICS

Although work in the informatics discipline started many decades ago, a landmark 1991 report by the Institute of Medicine (IOM) brought national attention to the topic of informatics. The report titled *The Computer-Based Patient Record: An Essential Technology for Health Care* stated it was time for the health care industry to catch up with other industries with regard to its use of information technology (Dick & Steen 1991; IOM, 1997). In 1991, almost all health care records were on paper. If a patient visited three different physician offices, there would be a paper health care record in each office. Similarly, if the patient was hospitalized, there would be yet another paper health care record at the hospital. The result was as follows:

- No one health care provider had a coordinated and complete view of the patient's health status; therefore, optimum care was more difficult to ensure.
- No one health care provider knew exactly what tests had been performed on the patient; thus, there was duplicate testing that wasted health care dollars, created an inconvenience for patients, and, in some cases, subjected patients to unnecessary risks.
- Paper health care records were mostly handwritten and frequently illegible; thus, important information about patients was not readable and mistakes in care resulted. In particular, physician orders for medications were sometimes incorrectly interpreted and/or sent to the pharmacy resulting in the wrong medications being given and/or incorrect doses being administered.
- Human intervention was required to predict when adverse drug reactions might occur due to contraindications and/or certain drug combinations. As the number of available medications grew, it became more difficult for humans to remember all the important aspects of each medication.
- Paper health care records were sometimes lost, resulting in no information being available about the patient. In the case of a health care emergency, the treatment team sometimes had to treat the patient symptomatically or just on the basis of findings at that time and without knowledge of the patient's past history, what medications the patient was on, or what chronic diseases the patient had.
- Patients who had not been seen before by a health care provider had no health care history on file with that provider. It was a manual process to try to obtain copies of records from other providers. There was a delay in receiving these records so there were also some delays in care.
- Documentation of the care given was a time-consuming process for all members of the health care team. Time spent documenting care left less time to actually care for the patient.

At the time of the 1991 IOM report mentioned above, the banking industry already used highly sophisticated electronic information systems for handling money and they were able to exchange information between banks with relative ease. Other industries such as the airlines also had initiated advanced electronic information systems that included the ability to make reservations and do flight scheduling. The airlines had access to information about all the passengers on each plane, the names of the staff members, and other important details about each flight. The 1991 IOM report urged health care organizations to look at the technology used by other industries and make investments in electronic information systems that would address some of the problems associated with paper records and to move to electronic patient records. With electronic patient records, information could be more easily exchanged in real time (i.e., as it is happening) among health care providers, with legible records, and documentation done at the point of care. Care could be streamlined somewhat through more efficient methods of data collection, and computer programs could be written to improve safety issues such as medication interactions.

Progress on implementing electronic patient records was slow following the 1991 IOM report in part because of concerns for patient privacy and the perceived lack of funding for information technology. In 1997, the IOM issued a revised version of the same report, which again called on the health care industry to make some forward progress on the use of information systems to support health care.

In 1999, the IOM published yet another landmark report that presented frightening statistics about the number of health care errors occurring. The report titled *To Err Is Human: Building a Safer Health Care System* looked at patient data collected in California, New York, and Utah. That data was used to derive an estimate of the number of health care errors occurring nationally. IOM stated that, "at least 44,000 and perhaps as many as 98,000 Americans die in hospitals each year as a result of medical errors." The health care system, itself, was identified as the cause of many errors. This meant the traditional way of doing work created situations where errors could occur (Kohn, Corrigan, & Donaldson, 2000, p. 26).

The IOM then started a series of landmark reports called the *Quality Chasm* series in which it identified ways the health care system could change to reduce the number of errors. The 2001 report titled *Crossing the Quality Chasm: A New Health System for the 21st Century* devoted an entire chapter to information technology (Committee on Quality of Health Care in America, 2001). Among the recommended changes for health care technology were

- Computerized provider order entry (CPOE) automated reminder systems to improve compliance with clinical practice guidelines
- Computer-assisted diagnosis
- Computer-assisted patient management
- Computer-assisted patient education
- Computerized clinical decision support systems (National Research Council, 2001, p. 164)

To effectively address this list of recommended changes, the computer system is used as a tool to alert the health care provider to problems with the patient; to remind the provider about clinical practice guidelines, allergies, or potential adverse effects of drug combinations; to help the provider arrive at an accurate diagnosis and an effective treatment plan; and to present educational information to patients either by an onsite computer or via the Internet.

Committee on Patient Safety and Health Information Technology

A 2011 IOM report titled *Health Information Technology and Patient Safety: Building Safer Systems for Better Care* identified a series of characteristics that computer software developers should use to make electronic information systems easier for the health care professional to use.

The suggestions made included the following characteristics:

- The data within the system is accurate, timely, reliable, and native.
- The system is easy to navigate and use as well as one that users want to interact with.
- The system, as well as data displays, is simple and intuitive to the user.
- The data displays are simple and, again, intuitive to the user.
- The evidence at the point of care be available to aid clinical decision making.

- The system works only to enhance workflow, automate mundane tasks, and stream-line work rather than increase physical or cognitive workload.
- The time required for upgrades is minimal and limited.
- The data is easily imported and exchanged between systems (Committee on Patient Safety and Health Information Technology, 2011, p. 62).

Native, Accurate, Reliable, and Timely Data

The Committee's work clearly focused on increasing the efficiency and efficacy of computer and electronic information systems to aid and augment the work of the clinician and health care professional. The Committee wanted to ensure the highest standards for protecting patient information. For example, in the first bullet above, "native data" is that information entered directly into the electronic computer system. Native data might include information about vital signs entered by the nursing staff; whereas imported data would include data coming from another electronic information system such as the electronic laboratory result information system. In most health care organizations, laboratory tests are done on a completely different electronic system specific to the laboratory within the health care organization, or they are done by a laboratory outside the organization. For the data to be considered "accurate and reliable," the data could not have been changed in any way. Within this requirement, assurance is needed that no one is able to hack into the computer system and/or alter the data.

The Committee also recognized the importance of "timely" data. Data is timely if it is available as soon as they are created. For example, laboratory test results are needed immediately for patients in critical-care units such as intensive care. Once a blood chemistry test such as the serum level of potassium is completed, the information must be relayed to the health care provider immediately, especially if it is abnormal. For example, if the potassium level in a patient is low, IV administration of potassium would probably be necessary (low potassium levels may cause the patient's heart to beat irregularly). Quality care depends on having the results as soon as possible so interventions can be taken as the patient's condition warrants. A laboratory result sent 2 weeks after the blood chemistry was drawn will be of little use in caring for the intensive care patient.

Easy to Use

An electronic record system must be easy to learn and easy to use so health care providers will want to use it as part of patient care activities. Health care providers will not want to work with electronic systems that are difficult to learn and that don't make sense to them. The way information is entered and used in the electronic system should match the way the provider works. For example, a provider might have a standard set of questions to ask a patient with diabetes. The electronic record system should have the same set of questions in the same order so the provider can easily add the patient's answers as they are given. In some cases, a checklist of probable answers can be listed in the electronic patient record so all the provider has to do is check off the applicable answer. Ideally, providers should be able to customize the electronic record system to match the way they do their work.

Intuitive Displays

The Committee suggested that the computer system utilize "simple and intuitive" data displays referring to what is usually on a computer screen and/or on a personal data assistant (PDA) or a smartphone. Intuitive data displays are those that present the information in the form the user needs it. For example, a nurse might want to see the blood pressure readings displayed in a table, whereas a physician might prefer that same information be displayed on a graph. If either the physician or the nurse wants to change the display format, it should be easy to toggle or change between the table and the graph. The master electronic information system will need to know what device the user has, so that the information will be properly displayed on their device. Some information such as graphs can easily be read on a personal computer (PC) screen but may not be easily adapted to small displays such as on a smartphone.

Navigation

Another characteristic the Committee suggested was that EHRs be easy to "navigate." Navigation refers to the way the computer user moves from one part of the electronic patient record to the next part. For example, if a nurse wants to look first at patient assessment data and then look at the care plan data, it should be easy to make that move in the patient's electronic record. This is usually done through a navigation bar that may be on the side of the screen or across the top of the screen.

Evidence at the Point of Care

Availability of "evidence at the point of care" was yet another characteristic suggested by the Committee. Evidence at the point of care refers to the availability of scientific evidence at the bedside or in the exam room to aid the provider. The availability of this evidence to aid with decision making is crucial to providing quality care. For example, the provider may be confronted with an unusual clinical situation and may want to consult the existing professional literature on that topic. The provider should be able to access the literature or "evidence" from the same computer or workstation they are using to enter data into the patient's EHR. In another instance, a wound care nurse who is treating a Stage IV decubitus ulcer may want to see the latest articles available in full text from the National Library of Medicine. The nurse should be able to access those articles at the patient's bedside without having to go to the organization's library. This process is known as knowledge utilization, a method of bringing evidence to the bedside. Informatics is uniquely positioned to provide this knowledge utilization feature.

Enhance Workflow

Electronic information systems transform data into information that is meaningful for the user. A simple example of the electronic transformation of data into information is the list of deposits and withdrawals made to a bank account. The transactions of deposits and withdrawals are the data. When those transactions result in an addition and/or subtraction of the money in the account, the data is processed electronically and information results. The information is the balance in the bank account. The balance information guides the owner of the bank account in managing finances. Likewise in health care, when information is combined with experience and understanding, it becomes knowledge that can be used to make informed decisions (LaTour & Maki, 2010). Knowledge becomes wisdom when it is "applied in a practical way or translated into actions" (McGonigle & Mastrian, 2012, p. 63). While Kenney and Androwich (2012) state that a nurse is applying knowledge in a practical way when a patient care plan is developed (p. 124).

Limit Inefficiencies

Electronic information systems should introduce efficiencies in the way work is done so no new physical demands will be placed on the nurse. For example, a nurse should not have to travel to a separate computer or be required to be in a library to access scientific literature. Likewise, it is important not to make work anymore mentally demanding than it already is. Rather than create a delay in patient care, new electronic technologies should enhance patient care efficiently for all involved. Information in health care is expanding exponentially and although health care providers are highly educated, no one provider can be expected to know everything. Point-of-care technology, for example, provides reliable information to fill the knowledge gap of providers at the time they need it most—while they are interacting with the patient.

All electronic information systems will need some downtime for routine hardware and software updates and/or maintenance. The computer will not be available during those times.

However, this downtime should be for a short duration of time and the nursing and health care staff needs to know when this downtime will occur. Planned downtime is usually in the middle of the night when the least number of users will be affected. As health care is delivered round the clock, any necessary downtime should be for a relatively short duration. Health care facilities try to prevent excessive downtime by having backup generators for power failures and by running parallel computer systems so if one computer system goes down, another computer system immediately kicks into action. Disaster planning requires that provisions be made for unusual situations such as hurricanes, power outages, and other large-scale problems. Accreditation standards also require health care facilities to determine how they will provide essential services under extreme conditions. "Provisions" and "essential services" must include protecting data within electronic health systems from unauthorized access or getting lost due to systems failure.

Exchange of Information

Since patients are often treated across many different health care organizations, it should be quick and easy to obtain information from another organization. The coordination of the access and exchange of patient information occurs through the establishment of health information exchanges (HIEs) on both a regional and national level. HIEs usually operate on a regional level such as by cities or counties since most health information is shared between local health care providers. HIEs are not-for-profit organizations formed by a variety of vested health care professionals from health care organizations, institutions, and practices. At the regional level, these HIEs are referred to as regional health information organizations (RHIOs). When health information is shared over a longer distance, it is shared between HIEs. Thus, information about a patient in Syracuse, New York, can be shared with providers in Los Angeles, California. The RHIOs or network of HIEs forms the basis of the NHIN discussed earlier in this chapter. Patients have a choice to sign an authorization to have their information shared or can opt out of the HIE if they do not want their information shared (Bass, 2011).

Health Informatics Legislation

The reports of the IOM inform Congress about important legislation needed to bring about change in health informatics. As a result, several important laws have been passed to advance the health informatics agenda. These laws include:

- Health Insurance Portability and Accountability Act (HIPAA, 1996), which contains important provisions for privacy and security of health information (Pub. L. 104–191, Aug. 21, 1996, 110 Stat. 1936).
- Health Information Technology for Economic and Clinical Health Act (HITECH Act; Pub. Law 111–5, div. A, title XIII, div. B, title IV, February 17, 2009, 123 Stat. 226, 467 [42 U.S.C. 300jj et seq.; 17901 et seq.]), which was part of the American Recovery and Reinvestment Act of 2009 (ARRA; Pub. L. 111–5). The HITECH Act provided billions of dollars of federal money in the form of grants to advance widespread use of health information technology.
- The Patient Protection and Affordable Care Act (PPACA) of 2010 (Public Law 111–148), often called the Affordable Care Act (ACA). The PPACA provides ongoing funding for health information technology (Health Services Research Administration, 2012).

EHR

The vision for the EHR is that it will be composed of input from many different health care facilities and/or individual health care practitioners. The EHR is to be a longitudinal record that will show the patient's health record across his or her lifespan. In other words, it will be a birth-to-death record. Some EHR proponents would even say it is a before-birth-to-after-death record. That is because there is some prenatal information in the birth record and there may be an autopsy report in a death record.

EHRs are not yet fully available for all patients. The EHR will be a decentralized record because it will not all be housed in one location. Instead, data will be pulled from multiple other computer systems and networks as the need arises. For the most part, this will not be visible to the user. To the EHR user, it will appear as just one record on the computer.

Clinical Decision Support System

As the name implies, a **clinical decision support sysytem** (CDSS) is an integrated database of clinical and scientific information to aid health care professionals in providing care. The CDSS is designed to look at a set of data and then lead the user through a decision-making process. This may be done by asking the user a set of questions that narrow possible choices to one choice that is the most effective. A CDSS might be used to arrive at a correct diagnosis or it might be used to determine the most effective treatment plan for the patient. For example, a doctor might be treating a patient who is a recovering drug addict with postoperative pain. Utilizing the CDSS on the hospital's health information system, the provider is able to enter assessment data and confounding factors such as opiate addiction to decide the best alternative medication to prescribe.

Standards for Interoperability

Interoperability is an agreed-upon standard of communication between hardware and software companies that allows for the effective exchange of patient information between various health information systems. For example, different hospitals use different electronic medical record (EMR) vendors; however, with interoperability standards in place, these various EMRs are able to exchange patient information seamlessly and accurately. The telephone system is an excellent example of interoperability. Regardless of the type of phone used or the service vendor selected, anyone is able to communicate via phone. That is because all the phone makers and all the service providers adhere to a common set of standards. The same level of interoperability is needed for the computer exchange of health information.

Many computer standards are currently available to facilitate communication between different health information systems and even more standards are under development. Policies, procedures, and development of standards for health information systems is coordinated by the American National Standards Institute (ANSI; http://ansi.org) and its Healthcare Information Technology Standards Panel (HITSP; http://www.hitsp.org). Standards development groups include representatives from government, the health care industry, and health informatics system vendors.

NHIN

A federal certification program is now in place to make sure vendors develop EHR products that meet interoperability and formatting standards. ANSI sets the standards, however; the federal government provides the certification that the health information system meets meaningful use provisions. Meaningful use is applying certified EHR technology to

- Improve quality, safety, efficiency, and reduce health disparities
- Engage patients and family
- Improve care coordination, and population and public health
- Maintain privacy and security of patient health information

Ultimately, it is hoped that the meaningful use compliance will result in

- Better clinical outcomes
- Improved population health outcomes
- Increased transparency and efficiency
- Empowered individuals
- More robust research data on health systems (HealthIT.gov, n.d., p. 1)

For an EHR product to be certified, the vendor must submit the product for a technical evaluation by an expert panel from a certifying organization recognized by the federal government. Medicare and Medicaid are currently offering enhanced payments to health care providers who adopt certified EHRs. These financial incentives are being used to speed EHR adoption so the vision of a NHIN can become a reality. As discussed earlier, the NHIN would be a structure that would allow for secure sharing of confidential health care information among health care providers across the country.

REAL-WORLD INTERVIEW

Cardiac surgery patient data is used nationally to provide a measure of comparison for individual physician's or hospital's performance. In addition, physicians and hospitals can use the raw patient data to identify trends and quality gaps that may require changes to current processes or practice to improve the quality of patient care. Trends in inappropriate intervention or surgeries as well as adverse event rates, allow hospitals to closely monitor individual and departmental practice in support of patient safety. Data collected on medication administration and device utilization (such as pacemakers) provide information to track device and medication safety.

Denise Famolaro, RN
Cardiac Care Data Coordinator, Bassett Medical Center
Cooperstown, New York

Centers for Medicare and Medicaid Services (CMS) Incentive Programs

As previously mentioned, the **HITECH** Act is a federal law that provides money to health care providers, institutions, and organizations to encourage the use of EHRs. However, the federal government also wanted to make sure its money was wisely spent. It will only give providers enhanced payments if they use certified EHRs. In addition, the provider must show the EHR is being used in a meaningful way. To assist providers in determining if their use of the EHR met the federal expectation, CMS of the U.S. Department of Health and Human Services developed criteria showing meaningful use; these criteria are being added to each year for the next several years. Examples of some of the first meaningful use criteria were that the EHR must be able to

- Implement drug–drug and drug-allergy checks
- Generate and transmit permissible prescriptions electronically to pharmacies in a facility and to retail pharmacies. This is called e-prescribing. Whenever the letter "e" precedes a word it means "electronic."
- Maintain an active medication allergy list (CMS, 2011)

The CMS financial incentives to providers and health care organizations for meaningful use continue through 2016. However, if by 2015 a health care provider has not shown meaningful use of a certified EHR, there will be financial penalties in the form of less reimbursement from these payers. This is an extremely strong catalyst to move the country to EHRs within a relatively short period of time.

REAL-WORLD INTERVIEW

I work with multiple clinical systems. My duties involve setting up new computer systems, building computer files, testing computer systems, training computer users, getting the computer system ready to go live, supporting computer users, helping them troubleshoot problems, making changes in the workflow, selecting, and designing computer systems. I teach other clinicians about what to look at when selecting a new computer system. There is so much work to do that we now have six nurses doing these duties in our computer department. We are also active in the vendor's user groups to help the vendor improve the products. Our involvement with the vendor is important because we are able to keep informed of state and federal regulations. We were just certified for meaningful use of our EHR systems by Medicare. Meaningful use means our hospital qualifies for increased reimbursement on all our Medicare patients. The increased meaningful use funding is the federal government's way of helping us implement the computer systems. Certification for meaningful use of our EHR systems means our computer systems meet the federal government's criteria for what an EHR should be able to do.

Joan Farmer, RN
Clinical Analyst, Network Data Systems
Utica, New York

VISTA

The VA took an early lead in 2008 in developing an EHR that can be accessed from any its facilities across the country. When the clinician logs in to VISTA, a summary screen is shown that can be reviewed to prepare for the patient visit. The summary screen contains a list of the patient's active problems, known allergies, current medications, laboratory results, vital signs, and visit history. VISTA includes a real time order checking system that issues a clinical alert if the order might be dangerous to the patient. VISTA also notifies clinicians any time a significant change occurs in the patient. Every VISTA computer screen notifies the clinician of the patient's status with regard to advance directives, warnings, adverse drug reactions, and important notes. The clinical reminder system assists the clinician in remembering when to perform tests to track the patient's progress and when to recommend preventive health care, such as influenza vaccines.

The VISTA system is also unique in using its web-based patient portal called MyHealtheVet. The MyHealtheVet patient portal allows the patient to access some personal health information directly and it allows the patient to enter some data for reporting on chronic conditions, such as diabetes, in a secure eVault accessible only to the patient and the health care providers he or she receives care from. Patients can track their own progress on controlling blood sugars and cholesterol as well as manage their prescription refills and renewals online. My HealtheVet makes the patient a partner in the care process and improves communication between the patient and the clinician.

VISTA also generates patient acuity and QI reports. Patient acuity reports identify the severity of the patient's condition and the appropriate number and type of nursing staff needed on each patient care unit to ensure optimum patient care. In addition, as a health information system, VISTA collects and analyzes patient information, such as length of patient stay, which allows VA hospitals to generate QI reports and plans. VISTA is a good model of a health information system that could be implemented throughout the country to exchange information on all patients. MyHealtheVet, as well as the patient portal VISTA, could be used for patients in other hospital systems or even private practices. The VA is currently working with the U.S. Department of Defense (DOD) to develop new EHR technology that can be used by both the VA and the DOD (Miles, 2011). This will be especially useful as the DOD health information system has patients spread around the world.

TECHNOLOGIES AND INFORMATION SYSTEMS IN HOSPITALS

A hospital has many information systems that feed into the EHR and that support health care safety and quality. Among the information systems of most interest to nursing staff are admission/discharge/transfer (ADT) and patient registration systems; **computerized provider order entry** (CPOE); **bar-code medication administration** (BCMA); and **radio-frequency identification** (RFID).

The ADT and patient registration systems are used to collect demographic data about patients being admitted to the hospital or being registered as an outpatient. ADT systems are used for inpatients. Patient registration systems are used for outpatients. Demographic data contain facts that identify a patient as a unique individual. They include name, address, phone numbers, date of birth, sex, race, ethnicity, religion, and insurance information. In addition, ADT and patient registration systems collect dates and times health care services were provided. If a patient is transferred from one inpatient unit to another, that will also be tracked by the ADT system. Data accuracy in these systems is extremely important to make sure appropriate care is given to the correct patient.

Medical identity theft is an increasing problem within the U.S. health care system. **Medical identity theft** is a crime that occurs when a patient poses as a different person to receive free medical care. The imposter often knows the health insurance numbers for the other person. Medical identity theft is dangerous because if care is provided to one person based on another person's medical history, adverse outcomes may occur. This is a dangerous situation for both the patient and for the imposter.

CPOE

Another component of hospital's health information systems is the CPOE. The CPOE is a software component of an EMR that allows the clinician to enter patient care orders directly into the computer system, thus eliminating any illegibility problems that can potentially occur with handwritten orders. Patient orders can be entered from any location so there is no longer a need for verbal orders or telephone orders. In addition, the CPOE will issue alerts about various aspects of the patient's condition. For example, the CPOE might alert the clinician to a low heart rate currently being experienced by a patient. The CPOE will also check orders against the hospital formulary to determine if a medication is stocked by the hospital pharmacy and then it will check known allergies, medication–medication interactions, and appropriate dosages of medication. Delays in care are avoided because orders for lab tests are immediately transmitted to the lab, medication orders are immediately transmitted to the pharmacy, and blood transfusion orders are immediately transmitted to the blood bank.

CASE STUDY 10.1

The nursing staff at your hospital is upset because CPOE was implemented 3 months ago. However, only about half of the health care providers are using the new system. The rest of the health care providers continue to handwrite orders as well as only give verbal and/or telephone orders. This creates confusion for the nursing staff because they have to remember which providers are using the new system. For providers not using the new CPOE system, the nurses must read the handwritten orders and make sure they are properly executed. In addition, the nurses feel that they have a greater liability when they receive verbal or telephone orders and the physician has not yet signed them.

1. *What should the nurses do in this situation?*
2. *What could have prevented this problem?*

BCMA

BCMA is a system that receives orders from the CPOE system, which prints bar-coded labels that contain the patient's identification number (usually the patient's health care record number). BCMAs may also print the specifics of the medication order (i.e., name of the medication and dose). The patient identification bar-code label is then attached to the medication sent from the pharmacy to the nursing unit. Before the nurse administers the medication, the bar code on the patient's wrist bracelet is scanned and the bar code on the medication packet is scanned. The computer system will check to make sure that the packet contains the right medication for the patient and that the medication is being given according to the clinician's order; that is, the right time and frequency, right dose, and the right route of administration (McGonigle & Mastrian, 2012, p. 386). Poon et al. (2010) studied an academic medical center and found BCMA systems reduced the number of potential adverse drug events by more than half.

RFID

RFID is technology used in health care involving the use of a small computer chip worn on the patient's body like a bracelet or necklace. The RFID device transmits radio waves that can be picked up by sensors located throughout a health care facility. A common application of RFID is with Alzheimer patients in a nursing home setting. RFID technology used in the patients' wrist bracelets can be used to sound an alarm when patients try to leave the unit or when an external door is opened. The computer chip used in RFID can also store much more information than a bar code so RFID provides the ability to have even more detail about the patient in a medication administration system. This additional information comes at a higher cost than associated with bar-code technology.

A relatively new technology is the use of RFID chips in surgical sponges to determine if any sponges are left in the patient at the end of the surgical procedure. This RFID technology ensures the patient will not have to return to surgery to remove a missed sponge (Steelman, 2011). It also protects the health care facility from liability and unnecessary costs. In 2008, the CMS determined it would no longer pay for higher costs of hospitalization associated with events such as objects left in an operative wound.

Technology in Direct Patient Care

Electrophysiological monitoring technology collects vital signs and other related data such as heart rhythms about the patient and immediately sends them to the EHR to give the clinician faster access to the data. The EHR can also issue clinical alerts to the clinician. The alerts might be present when the clinician signs on to the EHR or the EHR might send an electronic page, an e-mail message, or a phone call to the clinician. The EHR systems eliminate the transcription errors that occur when vital signs data is handwritten and then later documented in the record.

Smart Health Care Devices

The miniaturization of computer chips allows their use in a number of health care devices. These devices are called smart devices because they are able to monitor certain parameters about a patient and transmit that information to the health care provider. In some cases, the smart devices are programmed to take corrective action when problems occur. An implantable cardioverter defibrillator (ICD) is one example. If the patient experiences ventricular tachycardia or ventricular fibrillation, the smart device will immediately evaluate the situation and deliver an electric impulse to the heart. If the heart rhythm does not convert to an acceptable level, the smart device will deliver another, stronger impulse (National Heart, Lung, and Blood Institute, 2012). These smart devices save lives because they can identify and/or treat abnormal conditions much faster than the health care provider can. Other devices with smart technology include cardiac pacemakers, infusion pumps, and implantable insulin pumps. In each case, a computer processor is an essential component of the smart device. The use of smart devices will continue to expand with the advent of nanotechnology. According to the National Nanotechnology Initiative (2012), a nanometer is one billionth the size of a meter. It describes nanotechnology as the science involved with understanding, manipulating, and manufacturing materials of this small size. This will make it possible to have extremely small computer processors for smart devices.

TELEHEALTH

Telehealth is "a telecommunications system that links health care organizations and patients from diverse geographic locations and transmits text and images for (medical) consultation and treatment" (LaTour & Maki, 2010). Telehealth uses some type of computer devise at both the sending end and the receiving end of the communication. Cameras and microphones may also be used to send pictures and sound. This innovative technology allows a patient's home to serve as an extension of the health care facility (Dewsburys, 2012) in that it removes time and distance barriers in the provision of health care services. The typical telehealth scenario has nurses interacting with patients over telephone systems. The patients are usually in their homes and they may have home monitoring equipment connected to their phone lines. This monitoring equipment is used to gather data on the patient such as blood pressure, pulse oximetry, blood glucose, and weight. Originally, only telephones with landlines were used but now it is possible to use mobile devices such as cellular phones, satellite phones, phones connected over television cable systems, and the Internet (Dewsburys, 2012). Telehealth devices prompt the patient at a certain time of the day to obtain the various readings. For example, the patient may attach a blood pressure cuff to his or her arm, press a button, and then wait while the cuff inflates. The monitoring device records the blood pressure and transmits it over phone lines to the nurse who usually works for a home care agency. A pulse oximeter is attached to the patient's finger and, again, the data is transmitted to the nurse. For patients with conditions such as congestive heart failure, it is important to check the patient's weight to determine if he or she is retaining fluid. Thus, a scale may also be attached to the monitoring device. Patient data may be transmitted through cables attached to the home monitoring station or the data may be transmitted wirelessly to the station.

On the receiving end, a nurse uses a telehealth computer workstation to monitor the data coming in from the patient. The telehealth computer software will provide alerts if any information falls outside the parameters set for that patient. The nurse will usually phone the patient after the data arrives to discuss how the patient is feeling and to see if there are any problems that need to be addressed. If the nurse is unable to reach the patient, the nurse may contact family members and/or call 911 to check on the patient. The home health agency may also send a nurse to the patient's home.

Bowels (2010) cites one of the many benefits in telehealth use is among patients with chronic diseases. The prompt attention to the patient's health care status helps to decrease their risk of exacerbation of the disease. Telehealth can improve patient outcomes and can be delivered at a lower cost than home health care. Along with reducing the burden on patients to travel to receive health care, Aguida (2012) notes other benefits of telehealth. These include increased patient independence, increased collaboration with other community organizations and increased opportunities for nurses to provide education to patients and families. An innovative example of telehealth can be seen with the Medicare and Medicaid Program of All-Inclusive Care for the Elderly (PACE). PACE takes patients who are medically certified as needing nursing home care and keeps them in their homes as much as possible by providing them with home-based services such as telehealth monitoring, and community-based services.

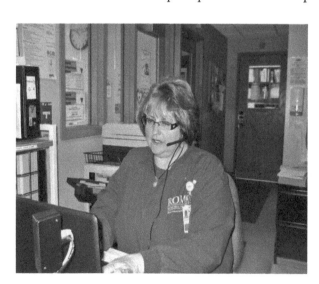

Nurse at a typical telehealth workstation.

EVIDENCE FROM THE LITERATURE

Citation

Dansky, K. H., Vasey, J., & Bowles, K. (2008). Impact of telehealth on clinical outcomes in patients with heart failure. *Clinical Nursing Research, 17*(3), 182–199.

Discussion

The purpose of this study was to determine the effects of telehomecare on hospitalization, ED use, mortality, and symptoms related to sodium and fluid intake, medication use, and physical activity.

The authors studied 284 patients with heart failure and noted the effects of telehomecare on health services utilization and mortality and changes in self-reported symptoms. They found that after 60 days of telehealth services, the telehomecare patients had statistically significant, lower rates of rehospitalization, and ED use. Differences were statistically significant at 60 days but not 120 days. The technology enables frequent monitoring of clinical indices and permits the home health care nurse to detect changes in cardiac status and intervene when necessary.

Implications for Practice

The trend toward the increased use of technology has created a need for nurses to learn additional methods of delivering nursing care. Nurses need to become educated on the benefits and responsibilities of providing care using telehealth. This method of health care provision will require different skills in patient assessment, patient education, and equipment utilization.

CASE STUDY 10.2

A newly hired nurse is assigned to work at the telehealth workstation. The nurse is monitoring the data coming in from home-based patients, checking to see if there are any situations that require nurse intervention, and taking action as appropriate. One patient with type 2 diabetes reports fasting blood glucose of 52. Another patient who has congestive heart failure and normally reports in on a daily basis does not transmit any data.

1. *What is the best course of action for the nurse to take regarding the patient with diabetes?*
2. *How should the nurse proceed regarding the lack of information obtained from the patient with congestive heart failure?*

REAL-WORLD INTERVIEW

Telehealth patient monitoring supplements regular home health visits with daily, state-of-the-art monitoring that allows patients to stay in their own homes. Information about the patient can be sent electronically to the physician and to the home health nurse via the telehealth monitor. Telehealth is an integrated and collaborative approach used by health care providers. Through enhanced patient assessment, self-management, and patient education by the telehealth nurse appropriate treatment can be initiated more quickly when problems are identified. This can potentially avert an ED visit or hospitalization. It is a good way to monitor a patient who has comorbid conditions (more than one illness occurring at the same time) such as congestive heart failure and diabetes, lives alone or in a remote location.

Dorothy Hailston, RN
Disease Management and Telehealth Coordinator, Visiting Nurse Association
Utica, New York

TO ALERT OR NOT TO ALERT

Although automatic EHR alerts within hospitals can be very helpful, care should be taken in the electronic system design and implementation to make sure the physicians and the nursing staff are not receiving too many alerts. Otherwise, there is a tendency for staff to start to ignore the alerts (Hoonakker, Wetterneck, Carayon, Cartmill, & Walker, 2011). Staff may try to turn the alerts off and they can become increasingly annoyed with the system. The actual users of the electronic system should determine which alerts will be the most beneficial to them. For example, in a cardiac intensive care unit (ICU) the interprofessional team may determine cardiac parameters they want alarms for such as heart rates decreasing or increasing by 10%. The presence or absence of an alert does not relieve the nurse or the providers of the duty to provide quality care. Alerts are only tools. The responsibility to deliver quality care remains with the health care professional rather than the device.

EVIDENCE FROM THE LITERATURE

Citation

Hoonakker, P., Wetterneck, T. B., Carayon, P., Cartmill, R., & Walker, J. M. (2011). Drug alerts override from a human factors perspective. In S. Albolino, S. Bagnara, T. Bellandi, J. Llanez, G. Rosal-Lopez, & R. Tartaglia (Eds.), *Health care systems ergonomics and patient safety*. London, UK: Taylor & Francis Group. Retrieved from http://cqpi.engr.wisc.edu/system/files/Hoonakkeretal_2011_CPOE.pdf-date

(continued)

Discussion

This study looked at health care provider reactions to drug alerts in four ICUs using EHRs. Data was collected on two different occasions and represented the views of attending physicians, physicians in various stages of training, and nurse practitioners. The first data collection involved 56 subjects and the second data collection involved 57 subjects. Subjects were asked how often they overrode drug alerts using a scale of 1 to 7 where 1 was *never* and 7 was *always*. The first data collection showed that 90% of the respondents chose to override drug alerts. Similar results were obtained in the second data collection. The results show that the drug alerts are often not helpful and that the actual users of the system should determine the type of alerts programmed in the EHR. Ideally, an alert should represent a real hazard to the patient that can be avoided if a meaningful and appropriate alert is issued such as with when a patient's heart rhythm indicates a decline in cardiac status.

Implications for Practice

Nurses as well as other interprofessional members of the health care team should be directly involved with information technologists in creating systems that are user friendly and promote patient safety. They should then monitor meaningful and appropriate system alerts and investigate any potential for adverse outcomes to the patient.

Critical Thinking 10.1

The nurse is reviewing orders and completing the medication reconciliation in the EHR on a patient just admitted to the medical–surgical floor. Medication reconciliation is a process for double checking medications, where the nurse verifies that the details of the medications written on the provider's orders match those recorded in the medication administration record used by the nurse. During the reconciliation process, several system alerts go off.

1. Does the use of EHRs guarantee error-free patient care?
2. What types of nursing behavior regarding the use of EHRs might contribute to jeopardizing patient safety?
3. What are the dangers of excessive system alerts in computer charting systems? How can the nurse guard against the potential effect?

PRIVACY AND CONFIDENTIALITY

Information privacy is the patient's right to limit the amount of personal health care information accessible to and known by others. Within this right of patients, providers are mandated to maintain confidentiality. Confidentiality is the duty the provider has to hold patient information private. Although the patient's right to information privacy is not stated in the U.S. Constitution, various court cases such as *Griswold v. Connecticut* (1965) interpret sections of the Bill of Rights (the first 10 amendments to the Constitution) as giving the patient this right. In particular, the fourth amendment to the Constitution, which protects against unreasonable search and seizure of papers and effects, is thought to provide information privacy. Attention to privacy is extremely important because if patients think their privacy will not be protected, they will be reluctant to share information needed to provide quality care. The **HIPAA** of 1996 is a federal law requiring health care providers to use several privacy protections for patients and their records. HIPAA protects an individual's identifiable health information that is in oral, written, and/or electronic form. HIPAA also requires that each health care facility have a designated privacy officer. An excellent online resource for staff training on privacy is available from the National Institutes of Health (NIH). Users can take the course on the website http://irtsectraining.nih.gov/publicUser0.aspx and receive a certificate of completion.

CASE STUDY 10.3

A patient complains to the nurse about the amount of personal data collected in the admissions office. The patient states that too much data is collected and he is concerned about the protection of his privacy.

1. *What should the nurse explain to the patient about the amount of personal data collected?*
2. *What should the nurse explain to the patient about how his data is protected?*

SECURITY

Security is the set of protections placed on a computer system to prohibit unauthorized access and to prevent any loss or distortion of the data. HIPAA also requires that security measures be in place in an organization and that there is a designated security officer. The NIH training website (http://irtsectraining.nih.gov/publicUser0.aspx) also offers a course to the public on the topic of computer security.

Critical Thinking 10.2

A nurse is using the EHR to document the findings from her patient assessment. She has entered approximately half of the information when suddenly the computer screen freezes, with the patient's information in full view on the screen.

1. What is the nurse's most appropriate response to a frozen computer screen?
2. What are the governing principles in documenting care during computer down-time?
3. Who would be the most appropriate resource for the nurse to contact within the facility?

FUTURE OF INFORMATICS

Nursing curricula at both the undergraduate and graduate level are changing to include more knowledge of informatics. This is due in large part to the work of the Technology Informatics Guiding Educational Reform (**TIGER**) which is a national plan

> to enable practicing nurses and nursing students to fully engage in the unfolding digital electronic era in healthcare. The purpose of the initiative is to identify information/knowledge management best practices and effective technology capabilities for nurses. TIGER's goal is to create and disseminate action plans that can be duplicated within nursing and other multidisciplinary healthcare training and workplace settings…and is focused on using informatics tools, principles, theories and practices to enable nurses to make healthcare safer, more effective, efficient, patient-centered, timely and equitable. (TIGER, 2012, para. 1)

Today's nurse must be prepared to embrace rapidly changing technology. Technology in all forms, including informatics, is the future of health care which when used properly can effectively help to ensure patient safety and quality of care nurses.

Critical Thinking 10.3

It has been a very busy shift and the nurse is a bit overwhelmed with five assigned patients. It is 6 hours into the shift and the nurse has only charted initial assessments. She must remain in a room to monitor an IV medication but believes she can also begin charting, even if just for the patient whose room she is in. The challenge is the patient's family is also in the room.

1. What principles should the nurse consider in completing bedside charting in the presence of the patient's family?

KEY CONCEPTS

1. EHRs are replacing paper records, as a result of a federal initiative.
2. EHRs (if properly implemented) improve the quality of care and reduce health care costs.
3. EHR is the preferred term that is replacing the term EMR.
4. The VA VISTA EHR system is a model of a future NHIN.
5. Several different information systems in a hospital feed data to the EHR.
6. Telehealth keeps patients in their homes, improves patient outcomes, reduces the number of hospital days used, and reduces health care costs.

7. Nurses should participate in the development of computer system alerts to make sure they are useful and not an annoyance. Nurses retain responsibility for the care they provide, regardless of the presence or the absence of an alert.
8. The HIPAA and its rules on privacy and security apply to EHRs. Nurses have a duty to protect patient privacy.
9. Nursing curricula must change to incorporate the study of new technologies.
10. Lifelong learning is essential for practicing nurses to keep up with technology.

KEY TERMS

Bar-code medication administration

Clinical decision support system

Computerized provider order entry

Electronic health record

HIPAA

HITECH

Medical identity theft

Radio frequency identification

Telehealth

TIGER

DISCUSSION OF OPENING SCENARIO

1. Are any types of information systems used to help prevent medication errors like this?

CPOE systems, BCMA systems, and also automated medication dispensing units are linked to the medication administration system. The medications are stored by bulk in drawers or bins, and as the nurse selects a medication to be administered, only the bin or drawer for the selected drug will open.

2. What is an alternative to using heparin to flush an IV?

This hospital switched to a saline solution. The standard procedure is to use saline flush for all IV locks, and as a flush before and after medication is administered via the IV.

3. What types of policies and procedures may have not been followed to allow such an error to have occurred?

In this case, the error was the result of a chain of events where two different pharmacy technicians failed to check the strength of the drug that was delivered to the pediatrics unit and where the nurse also failed to check the drug before administering it to the twins. Actually, in addition to the violating one of the 5 Rs (right dose), the policy of double checking in pediatrics was likely violated as well. In pediatrics, all medications must be double checked by another nurse, prior to administration. Each nurse is supposed to independently check the math, and come to an agreement, then each check the label, and then each check the syringe, all prior to administration.

CRITICAL THINKING ANSWERS

Critical Thinking 10.1

1. Does the use of EHRs guarantee error-free patient care?

No. Although studies have shown a reduction in errors with the introduction of the EHR, it is not foolproof and errors may still occur. Nurses still need to remain vigilant, check for potential errors, and safeguard the patient from possible mistakes in the health care environment.

2. What types of nursing behavior regarding the use of EHRs might contribute to jeopardizing patient safety?

Some of these may include:

- Ignoring or suppressing system alerts may lead to possible mistakes in patient care
- Failing to check the patient's identity using at least two reliable methods
- Failing to navigate to additional screens within the EHR may lead to late and/or omitted medications or treatment
- Developing bad habits of attempting to circumvent the system safeguards
- Failing to check the 5 Rs of patient care
- Failing to provide complete documentation due to time constraints or inefficient systems

3. What are the dangers of excessive system alerts in computer charting systems? How can the nurse guard against this potential effect?

A danger of excessive alerts promotes the habit of nurses ignoring them, or attempting to suppress them. A more effective approach would be to work with the informaticist in your facility to adjust the number of systems alerts, to prevent overload on the user, but remain effective in promoting patient safety.

Critical Thinking 10.2

1. What is the nurse's most appropriate response to a frozen computer screen?

Although computer systems are efficient tools, they are not perfect. Problems can and will occur from time to time. Facilities are responsible for educated and training users on appropriate responses to system failures. Each user should become familiar with how to contact his or her IT help desk, super user, or informaticist in cases of emergencies. One option may be to restart the device. It is important for the user to know the implications of restarting a device, and to double check the completeness of the record. It is the responsibility of the nurse to protect patient information and safeguard the file against inadvertent viewing by unauthorized persons. Nurses should also have a voice in the system design, to promote ease of use at the point of care.

2. What are the governing principles in documenting care during computer down time?

Ideally nurses should document care, as soon as possible after it is provided. Point of care access systems, portable computers make it possible for the nurse to document care before leaving the patient bedside. Computer downtime will interfere with the nurse's ability to complete timely documentation. Local policies should identify the documentation procedure to be followed in the event computer down times last longer than expected. Usually facilities will have an alternate method of documentation, such as pen and paper records, that may be added to the database when the system comes back online.

3. Who would be the most appropriate resource for the nurse to contact within the facility?

Several resources exist including colleagues and administrators associated with the department the nurse is affiliated with. However, the most appropriate resource to contact for definitive help would be the IT Help Desk of the facilty.

Critical Thinking 10.3

1. What principles should the nurse consider in completing bedside charting in the presence of the patient's family?

   The nurse should always keep in mind the need to promote and provide patient privacy and maintain his or her confidentiality, regardless of the mechanism of documentation. Although the ideal situation might be to chart at the bedside, there may be times when it will not be appropriate to have the computer screen display the patient's personal information where it may be viewed by visitors. It may be necessary to delay charting in the interest of promoting patient privacy. An alternative approach may be to take the computer to an area with controlled access, or to chart at the nurses' station. It is important for the nurse not to become lax in considering when and where charting is completed.

CASE STUDY ANSWERS

Case Study 10.1

1. What should the nurses do in this situation?

   The nurses should work through the appropriate chains of command to report this issue to nursing administration and to the nurse informaticist (if there is one). The director of nursing and the nurse informaticist can bring this issue to the attention of the medical staff organization and can work with the physicians to resolve it.

2. What could have prevented this problem?

   The nurses should have been involved with the implementation plan for the CPOE before it was implemented so their concerns would have been addressed in the initial planning phase.

Case Study 10.2

1. What is the best course of action for the nurse to take regarding the patient with diabetes?

   The nurse should call the patient to see how the patient is feeling. The nurse should determine if the patient ate after taking the low blood glucose reading and if the reading increased after eating. If the patient did not eat, the nurse can advise the patient on the best foods to increase the blood glucose level. If the patient ate appropriate food and the reading is still low, the nurse should take further action, which might involve: asking the patient about the presence of symptoms indicating hypoglycemia, asking the patient about when and how she took her diabetic medication, asking the patient to repeat the test and report the results, asking a home health nurse to make a visit to the patient that day, calling the primary care physician, and calling 911. The nurse should continue to monitor the situation until the patient's condition improves. If the situation is continuing at the end of the nurse's shift, the nurse should report the situation to the next shift of nurses who will be working with the telehealth patients.

   If there is no answer at the patient's home, the nurse should contact a family member or friend who is close by and who can check on the patient. The nurse should ask that person to report back on the patient's condition. If the contact person cannot be reached or if the contact person cannot get into the patient's home, the nurse should call 911 and provide all the information needed by the first responder. The nurse should also call 911 and/or give the contact person appropriate treatment information if the contact person finds the patient in an apparent medical emergency

2. How should the nurse proceed regarding the lack of information obtained from the patient with congestive heart failure?

The nurse should attempt to contact the patient by phone. If the patient answers, the nurse can ask questions to determine why the transmission was not received. It may be an equipment malfunction or the patient may have forgotten. The nurse should problem solve with the patient to get the necessary data for the day. If the patient is ill, the nurse should ask questions to determine the nature and severity of the illness. As in the previous answer above, the nurse should continue to monitor the patient until the situation is resolved. If needed, the nurse can call the emergency contact for the patient and/or call 911.

Case Study 10.3

1. What should the nurse explain to the patient about the amount of personal data collected?

The nurse should explain to the patient that it is very important to collect enough information to verify the patient's identity. Treatment must be given to the correct person. The nurse should also explain medical identity theft.

2. What should the nurse explain to the patient about how his data is protected?

The nurse should explain the HIPAA requirements for protecting the privacy and security of patient information.

REVIEW QUESTIONS

Please see Appendix D for answers to Review Questions.

1. The nurse is caring for a patient and preparing to administer scheduled medications. Which of the following represents a benefit of using informatics technology with regard to medication administration?

   A. Automated medication systems alleviate the need for cross-checking allergies.
   B. Using automated medication systems prevents medication errors.
   C. Automated medication systems provide decision-making aids that alert the nurse to potential problems.
   D. Automated medication administration systems prevent the nurse from administering the wrong medication.

2. The nurse uses the EMR to review key components of the patient's health. What most directly impacts the nurse's ability to effectively utilize the EMR?

   A. The functional design of the EMR system as described by the manufacturer
   B. The national guidelines for every nurse using an EMR system
   C. The state and federal initiatives mandating the use of EMR systems
   D. Local policies, training, and institutional guidelines on the EMR

3. The facility is using a newly implemented EMR for patient care. The nurses have expressed some frustrations with the high volume of system alerts that are generated

throughout the day. Which of the following demonstrates the most appropriate response to excessive alerts by the nurse?

A. Turn alerts off so they do not slow down the data processing capability.
B. Report excessive alerts to the software designer.
C. Collaborate with the nurse informaticist in the institution to make necessary adjustments.
D. Just ignore the alerts and they will eventually go away.

4. The nurse wants to decrease the rate of medication errors for patients and advocates for use of a CPOE system. Which of the following best indicates the benefit of CPOE systems?

A. Eliminates the need for the nurse to decipher illegible handwriting
B. Assists the nurse in receiving verbal orders from the providers
C. Eliminates the need for the nurse to chart
D. Takes the guesswork out of knowing when to call the provider

5. A patient presents to the ambulatory surgery clinic for scheduled rhinoplasty. During the admission interview, the patient notes a history of an allergic reaction to an antibiotic medication 3 years prior. The patient states that she does not know the name of the drug. Which of the following actions is best for the nurse to take?

A. Call the surgeon and share that the patient's allergy history remains incomplete.
B. Ask the patient to describe what the pills looked like.
C. Consult the patient's EHR.
D. Chart that the patient has an allergy to antibiotics.

6. A nurse on the cardiac unit overhears the licensed practical nurse (LPN) explain to a coworker how to check the status of patients in the labor and delivery unit even though the computer system should not provide this access. Where does the responsibility for system security reside to guard against this type of access?

A. With the nurse who will maintain patient privacy and avoid HIPAA violations
B. With the nurse informaticist who will make certain the EMR maintains confidentiality
C. With the federal government who will make sure no laws are violated
D. With the designated security officer who will make sure the entire system is secure

7. One feature of some EMR is decision-making pop ups. For example, the nurse will be alerted to the patient's medication allergies when administering medications. Which of the following best describes the potential work place benefit for the nurse?

A. It is time saving and eliminates the need to ask the patient about allergies.
B. It is safer and provides a double check opportunity for the nurse to remember to ask the patient.
C. It helps with communication. It eliminates cross-checking with pharmacy.
D. It is cost-effective and reduces the time the nurse spends in transcribing medications.

8. The nurse is preparing a patient for discharge. Which of the following represents the nurse's most effective application of the information technology at the bedside?

A. Accessing current research materials in preparation to answer the patient's questions upon discharge

B. Using the computer to print a list of websites that may be of interest to the patient

C. Posting the patient's questions to a social media website and compiling the response for the patient

D. Referring the patient to his health care provider so the provider can answer the patient's questions

9. The nurse is monitoring the telehealth computer and notices that the patient's pulse oximetry reading drops below 90%, which is the predetermined action criteria for this patient. Which of the following depicts the most appropriate next step the nurse should take?

A. Call the patient's family and alert them to administer oxygen immediately.

B. Call 911 to send emergency responders to the home.

C. Call the patient and assess how the patient is feeling and what is currently happening.

D. Call the primary care provider to obtain treatment orders.

10. Nurses need to increase awareness of the implementation of technology and informatics in patient care. Which of the following best represents a collaborative effort to ensure best practices in nursing informatics?

A. HIPAA

B. TIGER

C. VISTA

D. EHR

REVIEW ACTIVITIES

Please see Appendix E for answers to Review Activities.

A. Match the Following Terms to Their Most Appropriate Definition

1. Navigation	a. Availability of patient information as it is occurring
2. Real time	b. Computer data chip that sends information directly to the computer via transmitted waves
3. Computerized Provider Order Entry	c. Information technology that removes time and distance barriers
4. Radio-Frequency Identifier	d. Describes the way a computer user can move from one part of the patient's electronic record to another
5. Telehealth	e. System for providers to directly input instructions into computer systems

B. Fill in the Blank

In addition to HIPAA, the _____ act provides guidelines that govern access to patient health information with the use of technology.

The need for a nurse to receive verbal orders is eliminated by the provider's use of a _____.

The _____ _____ (two words) is the name of a series of reports that has stimulated increased efforts in utilization of informatics in health care.

_____ took an early lead in utilizing an effective EHR.

C. Short Answer

- Discuss some of the issues noted in the IOM report regarding the dangers or pitfalls of paper charting.
- Discuss the intended use of point of care decision prompts.
- Identify and explain three advantages of using the EHR.
- Differentiate between confidentiality and security.
- Explore some of the features and benefits of VISTA.

EXPLORING THE WEB

1. Visit the HealthIT Buzz Blog at http://www.healthit.gov/buzz-blog. This blog is run by the Office of the National Coordinator (ONC) of Health Information Technology. It contains blogs on the latest topics in health informatics. Follow the links to read three blogs. Be prepared to participate in a class discussion on these topics.
2. Visit the ONC's YouTube channel on http://www.youtube.com/user/HHSONC. Watch five videos about patients and their experiences with health information technology. Most videos are only 2 to 3 minutes long.
3. Prepare a list of five benefits that patients might experience as a result of the implementation of this health information technology. Draft a one-page, double-sided, trifold brochure that could be given to patients to educate them on the topic. Title the brochure "Health IT and You." Insert photos or graphics as you think appropriate.

REFERENCES

American Recovery and Reinvestment Act of 2009 (ARRA) (Pub. L. 111–5). Anguita, M. (2012). Opportunities for nurse-led telehealth and telecare. *Nurse Prescribing, 10*(1), 6–8.

Bass, D. (2011). Opting for opt out: How one HIE manages patient consent. *Journal of AHIMA, 8*(5), 34–36.

Bowels, K. H. (2010). Achieving meaningful use with information technology: Telehealth research. *Online Journal of Nursing Informatics, 14*(3).

Centers for Medicare and Medicaid Services (CMS). (2011). *Eligible professional meaningful use table of contents core and menu set objectives.* Retrieved from https://www.cms.gov/EHRIncentivePrograms/Downloads/EP-MU-TOC.pdf

Cipriani, P. (2011). Transforming care through health information technology: A conversation with Dr. Farzad Mostashari, national coordinator for health information technology. *American Nurse Today, 6*(11), 10.

Committee on Quality of Health Care in America. (2001). *Crossing the quality chasm: A new health system for the 21st century.* Washington, DC: National Academy Press. Retrieved from http://books.nap.edu/openbook.php?record_id=10027&page=R1

Dansky, K. H., Vasey, J., & Bowles, K. (2008). Impact of telehealth on clinical outcomes in patients with heart failure. *Clinical Nursing Research, 17*(3), 182–199.

Dewsburys, G. (2012). Telehealth: The hospital in your home. *British Journal of Healthcare Assistants, 6*(7), 338–340.

Dick, R. S., & Steen, E. B. (Eds.). (1991). *The computer-based patient record.* Washington, DC: National Academies Press.

Griswold v. Connecticut, 381 U.S. 479, (1965).

Healthcare Information Management and Systems Society (HIMSS). (2011). *Electronic health record*. Retrieved from http://www.himss.org/ASP/topics_ehr.asp

HealthIT.gov. (n.d.). *EHR incentives and certifications*. Retrieved from http://www.healthit.gov/providers-professionals/meaningful-use-definition-objectives

Health Information Technology for Economic and Clinical Health Act (HITECH Act) (Pub. L. 111 5, div. A, title XIII, div. B, title IV, February 17, 2009, 123 Stat. 226, 467 [42 U.S.C. 300jj et seq.; 17901 et seq.]).

Health Insurance Portability and Accountability Act (HIPAA). (1996). (Pub. L. 104–191).

Hoonakker, P., Wetterneck, T. B., Carayon, P., Cartmill, R., & Walker, J. M. (2011). Drug alerts override from a human factors perspective. In S. Albolino, S. Bagnara, T. Bellandi, J. Llanez, G. Rosal-Lopez, & R. Tartaglia (Eds.), *Healthcare systems ergonomics and patient safety* (pp. 367–371). London, UK: Taylor & Francis Group. Retrieved from http://cqpi.engr.wisc.edu/system/files/Hoonakkeretal_2011_CPOE.pdf-date

Institute of Medicine (IOM). (1997). *The computer based patient record: An essential technology for health care*. Retrieved from http://iom.edu/Reports/1997/The-Computer-Based-Patient-Record-An-Essential-Technology-for-Health-Care-Revised-Edition.aspx

Kenney, J. A., & Androwich, I. (2012). *Nursing informatics roles, competencies, and skills*. In D. McGonigle & K. G. Mastrian (Eds.). *Nursing informatics and the foundation of knowledge* (2nd ed., pp. 121–145). Burlington, MA: Jones & Bartlett Learning.

Kohn, L., Corrigan, T., & Donaldson, M. (Eds.). (2000). *To err is human: Building a safer health system*. Washington, DC: National Academies Press. Retrieved from http://www.nap.edu/catalog.php?record_id=9728

LaTour, K. M., & Maki, S. M. (Eds.). (2010). *Health information management concepts, principles and practice* (3rd ed.). Chicago, IL: American Health Information Management Association.

McGonigle, D., & Mastrian, K. G. (2012). Introduction to cognitive science and cognitive informatics. In D. McGonigle & K. G. Mastrian (Eds.), *Nursing informatics and the foundation of knowledge* (2nd ed., pp. 121–145). Burlington, MA: Jones & Bartlett Learning.

Miles, D. (2011). *Gates, Shinseki agree to joint electronic records*. Armed Forces Press Service. Retrieved from http://www.defense.gov/news/newsarticle.aspx?id=63435

National Heart, Lung, and Blood Institute. (2012). *What is an implantable cardioverter defibrillator?* Retrieved from http://www.nhlbi.nih.gov/health/health-topics/topics/icd

National Nanotechnology Initiative. (2012). *What it is and how it works*. Retrieved from http://www.nano.gov/nanotech-101/what

National Research Council. (2001). *Appendix A: Report of the technical panel on the state of quality to the quality of health care in America committee. Crossing the quality chasm: A new health system for the 21st century*. Washington, DC: The National Academies Press. Retrieved from http://www.nap.edu/openbook.php?record_id=10027&page=225

National Research Council. (2012). *Health IT and Patient Safety: Building Safer Systems for Better Committee on Patient Care*. Washington, DC: The National Academies Press.

Patient Protection and Affordable Care Act (PPACA) of 2010 (Public Law 111–148).

Poon, E. G., Keohane, C. A., Yoon, C. S., Ditmore, M., Bane, A., Levtzion-Korach, O., . . . Gandhi, T. K. (2010). Effect of bar-code technology on the safety of medication administration. *The New England Journal of Medicine, 362*(18), 1698–1707. doi:10.1056/NEJMsa0907115

Rosen, I. (Producer). (2008, March 16, 2008; updated August 22, 2008). *60 minutes* [Television Broadcast]. New York, NY: CBS News.

Steelman, V. M. (2011). Sensitivity of detection of radiofrequency surgical sponges: A prospective cross-over study. *The American Journal of Surgery, 201*(2), 233–237.

Technology Informatics Guiding Educational Reform (TIGER). (2012). Retrieved from http://www.tigersummit.com/About.Us.html

TIGER. (2012). *The TIGER collaborative teams—Stage II activities*. Retrieved from http://www.tigersummit.com/9_Collaboratives.html

U.S. National Library of Medicine. (2012). *National information center on health services research and health care technology (NICHSR): Definition of health informatics*. Retrieved from http://www.nlm.nih.gov/hsrinfo/informatics.html

SUGGESTED READING

Akridge, J. (2010). Carts roll with the flow of healthcare challenges. *Healthcare Purchasing News, 34*(8), 52–62.

Bar-code/eMAR combo reduces errors. (2010). *Healthcare Benchmarks & Quality Improvement, 17*(9), 100–102.

Bedouch, P., Allenet, B., Grass, A., Labarère, J., Brudieu, E., Bosson, J., & Calop, J. (2009). Drug-related problems in medical wards with a computerized physician order entry system. *Journal of Clinical Pharmacy & Therapeutics, 34*(2), 187–195. doi:10.1111/j.1365–2710.2008.00990.x

Braccia, D. (2008). Web connect; Online resources will help you use informatics in your nursing practice. *ONS Connect, 23*(7), 16.

Chaffee, B., & Zimmerman, C. (2010). Developing and implementing clinical decision support for use in a computerized prescriber-order-entry system. *American Journal of Health-System Pharmacy, 67*(5), 391–400. doi:10.2146/ajhp090153

Flood, L., Gasiewicz, N., & Delpier, T. (2010). Integrating information literacy across a BSN curriculum. *Journal of Nursing Education, 49*(2), 101–104. doi:10.3928/01484834–20091023-01

Green, S., & Thomas, J. (2008). Interdisciplinary collaboration and the electronic medical record. *Pediatric Nursing, 34*(3), 225.

Headlines from the NLN. (2008). Informatics in the nursing curriculum: A national survey of nursing informatics requirements in nursing curricula. *Nursing Education Perspectives, 29*(5), 312–317.

McIntire, S., & Clark, T. (2009). Essential steps in super user education for ambulatory clinic nurses. *Urologic Nursing, 29*(5), 337–343.

Murphy, J. (2011). Nursing informatics: Engaging patients and families in eHealth. *Nursing Economics, 29*(6), 339–341.

Patient Protection and Affordable Care Act (PPACA) of 2010 (Public Law 111–148).

Russo, M. (2008). eMAR and mobile computing: Why nursing homes need to get wired now. *Nursing Homes: Long Term Care Management, 57*(1), 32.

Schleyer, R., & Beaudry, S. (2009). Data to wisdom: Informatics in telephone triage nursing practice. *AAACN Viewpoint, 31*(5), 1.

BASIC LITERATURE SEARCH STRATEGIES

J. Scott Thomson, Ashley Currier, and Mary Gillaspy

Beginning researchers might be tempted to start developing a research study without a thorough literature search, assuming that the answer to their problem does not exist. At the opposite extreme, they might copy a research study without any literature search because they have heard that research study replication is valuable. In the world of science, the literature review provides the foundation for every study, guides every aspect of study development, and must therefore never be omitted. (Schmelzer, 2008)

Upon completion of this chapter, the reader should be able to

1. Review basic literature search strategies
2. Discuss how to search electronic databases for health care literature using key words and subject headings
3. Discuss the use of Boolean commands in electronic databases
4. Discuss the importance of developing broad literature searches
5. Discuss the patient/population, intervention, comparison, outcome (PICO) model for searching the literature
6. Discuss electronic databases
7. Discuss point-of-care information tools, for example, electronic databases and practice guidelines, used for basic literature searches
8. Identify critical appraisal guides used for literature evaluation
9. Identify Internet guides available to evaluate websites
10. Discuss resources for lifelong learning

You are spending time on a surgical inpatient unit as one of your clinical rotation assignments. You observe that peripheral IV catheters are left in patients for 3 days prior to being changed. In a previous clinical rotation at a different organization, you recall that the policy for changing peripheral IV catheters was to change them every 4 days. You ask your preceptor about this as part of your efforts to better understand which organization has the safer practice. The preceptor appreciates your question and reports wondering the same thing. The preceptor comments that patients often dread having their IVs restarted on the third day when most of them are going home the next day. You and your preceptor decide to speak with your nurse manager about wanting to look into the recommended frequency for peripheral IV catheter changes. You review the literature and find that many studies report no increase in infection rates, infiltration risk, and so on, if an IV is changed every 96 hours instead of every 72 hours. You and your preceptor summarize key points from the literature, determine the expected cost savings from fewer IV replacements, and highlight the potential impact on patient satisfaction. You present your findings to the nursing practice committee. As a result, nursing practice is modified to reflect the best evidence for a safe experience for patients requiring peripheral IV catheters.

- *What opportunities are there in nursing to facilitate dissemination of information?*
- *What other nursing actions should you take when adopting new practice changes like this?*

Basic literature search strategies are used by health care practitioners to search the literature for research and evidence that will improve patient care and fill knowledge

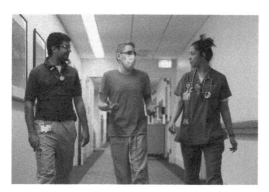

Two nurses walking with a patient.

gaps. High-quality literature searches are needed to ensure that the most up-to-date research and information are being used to shape patient care. A literature search is "a systematic and explicit approach to the identification, retrieval, and bibliographic management of independent studies (usually drawn from published sources) for the purpose of locating information on a topic, synthesizing conclusions, identifying areas for future study, and developing guidelines for clinical practice" (Auston, Cahn, & Selden, 1998).

Nursing research is a process of inquiry that is systematic, adheres to rigorous guidelines, and, at the most significant level, produces unbiased answers to questions of nursing practice (Houser, 2008). Nurses and health care delivery institutions consistently use research to shape practice and ensure that the care they deliver is at the forefront in terms of safety and quality. Thus, patients can be reassured that the care rendered to them is of the highest quality, is patient centered, and is tailored to fit their unique needs.

This chapter discusses basic literature search strategies as they relate to nursing. It discusses how to search electronic databases for health care literature using key words and subject headings. The use of Boolean commands in electronic databases and the importance of developing broad literature searches are explored. The PICO model and electronic databases for searching the literature are discussed. Point-of-care information tools, for example, electronic databases and practice guidelines, and critical appraisal guides used for literature evaluation are explored. Finally, the chapter identifies Internet guides available to evaluate health information websites and identify resources for lifelong learning.

BASIC LITERATURE SEARCH STRATEGIES

As mentioned earlier, basic literature search strategies are used by health care practitioners to search the literature for research and evidence that will improve patient care. The first and most important resource in searching the literature for peer-reviewed evidence is your institution's librarians. Speak to your librarian and ask him or her to tell you about your library's key journals and electronic databases for nursing. If your institution does not have a library or reference librarians, you may still have access to library services through a university or health care system affiliation with your school of nursing. Public libraries are also a viable option for stand-alone health care institutions that lack library resources. Health care questions are common at public libraries. Many public librarians are well versed in health care electronic databases and how to search them. They can help the nurse or patients identify peer-reviewed literature and become proficient at searching electronic databases.

Need for Administrative and Computer Support

Administrative and computer support for literature searches is a resource that is increasingly necessary for working nursing professionals. Administrative support can take the form of making computers and library resources available or it can take the form of providing for time away from patient care to examine the literature. Administrative support can also provide funding for paid time away from the unit, mentorship, statistician support, or money to conduct studies. Often, scholarships through charitable boards or endowments are offered to those who aim to investigate and improve health care practice. Some of these scholarships and supports are offered for broad research interests, such as best practices, while others are offered to support certain patient populations, that is, patients with cancer, neonates, and so on. An important recommendation for novice nursing researchers is to seek a mentor who has the ability to coach you through the research process and assist you in securing any needed funds, resources, or other necessary support.

Many health care organizations have a specific department or committee responsible for the advancement of nursing practice through evidence-based practice (EBP) and research. This department or committee is often a great place to begin when seeking to use literature to improve your nursing practice. Note also that these committees or departments will often have funds allocated to support nurses interested in conducting research.

Other necessary supports for searching the literature are access to a computer with Internet connectivity and access to electronic databases. Some electronic databases discussed in this chapter are free (e.g., PubMed at http://www.ncbi.nlm.nih.gov/pubmed). Other electronic databases will only be available to you if you have access to them through an institution that subscribes to the electronic database. Most searching of the literature takes place using Internet-based electronic databases. It is therefore necessary to learn a few literature search concepts to successful conduct a literature search on an electronic database.

Literature Search Tutorials

It is helpful to review how to use electronic databases through tutorials at the website of the database, if available. For example, when you visit the PubMed electronic database site, http://www.ncbi.nlm.nih.gov/pubmed, click on the "PubMed Quick Start Guide." Note the tutorials, Frequently Asked Questions (FAQ), PubMed Quick Start Tips, How Do I Search PubMed, and Medical Subject Headings (MeSH) terms discussed there. These tutorials will improve your ability to use the electronic database.

Searching Like a Librarian

Librarians and other experienced literature searchers approach the literature search process differently than novice or inexperienced literature searchers. Before librarians begin a literature search, they usually think about the subject in which they are interested and brainstorm possible search terms for a topic. Note the example in Table 11.1 of searching the literature. The PubMed literature database is used in this example.

LITERATURE SEARCHING WITH KEY WORDS OR SUBJECT HEADINGS

Literature searching can be done with key words or with subject headings. A **key word** is a self-identified literature search term that uses your own personal natural language to search the literature. It is often necessary to conduct your literature search with key words. The electronic database looks for matches to the key word or words entered. Key word searching allows the literature searcher to enter any key words or groups of key words for the electronic database to search. The electronic database then looks for matches to the key word or key words entered; it does not evaluate the usefulness or relevancy of the search term to the focus of your literature search (Sherwill-Navarro, 2010). Searching with key words frequently identifies more literature citations than searching with subject headings; however, there is a greater possibility that there will be more nonuseful, nonrelevant literature citations returned with the key words literature search.

Using Subject Headings to Search the Literature

In a literature search, a **subject heading** is a word picked to represent a concept that is then used consistently for data organization and retrieval. Subject headings are part of a larger system of a controlled electronic database vocabulary, that is, a database vocabulary through which a single term is used consistently to represent a concept. The National Library of Medicine (NLM) MeSH–controlled vocabulary of biomedical terms is used to describe the subject of each journal article in Medline. MeSH contains approximately 26,000 subject headings and is updated annually to reflect changes in medical terminology. MeSH subject headings are arranged hierarchically by subject categories with more specific subject headings arranged beneath broader subject headings. PubMed allows you to view this subject heading hierarchy and select subject headings for searching in the MeSH Database. An outline of the

TABLE 11.1 SEARCHING THE LITERATURE

QUESTION: IS AN INSULIN PUMP A GOOD CHOICE FOR A PATIENT WITH TYPE 2 DIABETES WHO IS HAVING PROBLEMS KEEPING HER BLOOD GLUCOSE UNDER CONTROL?

1. Start by brainstorming possible search terms for this topic, for example,
   - Insulin pump
   - Uncontrolled blood glucose
   - Type 2 diabetes
2. Identify possible literature databases for your literature search. Databases frequently chosen for nursing related literature searching include:
   - CINAHL, http://www.ebscohost.com/public/the-cinahl-database
   - PubMed, http://www.ncbi.nlm.nih.gov/pubmed
   - Ovid Medline, http://www.ovid.com/webapp/wcs/stores/servlet/ProductDisplay?sto reId=13051&catalogId=13151&partNumber=Prod-901
3. Go to the website of the literature database. For example, PubMed, http://www.ncbi. nlm.nih.gov/pubmed
   - Then, on PubMed, click the "Advanced Search" link at the top of your literature database website page and type your first literature search term, identified above in step 1. For example, type 'Insulin pump' in the "PubMed Advanced Search Builder" on the PubMed website.

Note that when a literature search for the term "insulin pump" was done on June 27, 2013, in PubMed, 2,605 search results were returned for this literature search.

4. Limit your literature search further, as needed, by choosing filters from the left column of the PubMed search results page, for example, choose:
   - Review articles, and,
   - "5 years" from "publication dates."

Note that when the above search limits were applied to the above literature search, 93 articles were returned. This is a much more manageable and, hopefully, relevant set of articles to review than the 2,605 articles returned from the above search of "insulin pump."

Note that you can also filter your search results further by making use of the "Related Searches" feature on the right. For example, on the date that we completed the above "insulin pump" search, "Related Searches" included "insulin pump, type 2." When we clicked on "insulin pump, type 2," 32 articles were returned. Depending on your needs (a thorough literature search compared to a small focused literature search), this process can help to quickly narrow your literature search results down to a highly relevant and usable set set of literature.

NLM subject heading classification is available at http://www.nlm.nih.gov/class// OutlineofNLMClassificationSchedule.html.

Anyone who has used the Yellow Pages has searched a database that employs controlled vocabulary subject headings. When looking for a place to buy a new car, you might begin in the "c" section of the Yellow Pages for car dealers. There may be a "see" reference that says to also "see automobile dealers." The term "automobile dealers" is the subject heading for the concept of a business that sells new cars. When you turn to that automobile dealers section, the entries will be automobile dealers and nothing else. Using subject headings makes searching more efficient and precise because it groups similar information together (Sherwill-Navarro, 2010). Because of this, it is important to understand how to search the literature using subject headings.

Literature searching in an electronic database with subject headings that are straightforward and clear usually identifies relevant literature easily while literature searches that are less clear will likely need to be searched with key words as well. For example, a definite, clear health care disease subject heading topic such as "type 2 diabetes" lends itself well to being searched using subject headings. A literature search on less clear, broader terms such as "family involvement in patient care," however, might be best searched initially with key words; for example, family involvement, since family involvement can mean several things and isn't easily described with a definite, clear subject heading like the health care topic of "type 2 diabetes." Remember that key word searches frequently identify more literature citations than searching with subject headings; however, there is a greater possibility that there will be more nonrelevant literature citations that are not helpful to your search (Anders & Evans, 2010).

Key Word Searches

Different electronic databases use slightly different techniques for key word searches, but in PubMed, for example, you would accomplish a key word literature search by entering each of your key words in the PubMed search bar. After each key word literature search, you can then click on "Advanced." Then, on the "Results" screen, scroll down to "History" and click "Add" to combine your search results together. For example, a search today on PubMed for type 2 diabetes retrieved 91,156 articles; then, a search for weight loss surgery retrieved 24,797 articles. When the author then clicked on "Advanced" on the "Results" screen and scrolled down to "History," and clicked on "Add" to combine these two search topics together, that is, combine type 2 diabetes, and weight loss surgery, the combined search of these two topics retrieved 1,080 articles.

Subject Heading Searches

Click on the MeSH Database link found under "More Resources" on the front page of PubMed. This is a good place to check your search terms to see if they will work well with your literature search. Type your search terms, for example, heart attack, into the search bar and click "Search." Note the results. If the database has matched the search term that you have chosen with a subject heading, for example, myocardial infarction, then your search will probably work well with that subject heading. Note that the term, family involvement, does not give you any relevant search results in the subject headings listing.

Creators of electronic literature databases will usually employ a controlled subject heading vocabulary. They will index articles with a single controlled subject heading whenever possible, regardless of what terminology is used by the author of a journal article or other example from the literature. Because of this, a user wishing to search for articles on weight loss surgery, for example, in an electronic literature database using a controlled subject heading vocabulary will not need to search for "weight loss surgery," "weight loss surgeries," "gastric bypass," "jejunoileal bypass," "roux-en-Y surgery," and so on. Instead, the user can identify the subject heading used by the electronic database, for example, "bariatric surgery," and know that all relevant literature search results will be returned. There are a few subject headings related to weight loss surgery in the Medline database, but the best choice if one wanted a broad term is probably the subject heading, "bariatric surgery." The user can often select that subject heading, ignore all the other terms, and be reasonably sure that all relevant articles will be retrieved.

REAL-WORLD INTERVIEW

As a medical librarian in a hospital health learning center, I help nurses and other health care professionals access the resources they need to conduct literature reviews and explore topics for new evidence-based research. Our learning center team also empowers patients and members of the community by helping them find accurate, reliable sources of health information. Patients can use this information to better understand their treatment and care.

Nurses often seek assistance after they've developed a potential research topic and conducted an initial search of databases such as Medline or the Cumulative Index to Nursing and Allied Health Literature (CINAHL) but are having trouble identifying enough relevant articles for a literature review. I work with these nurses to demonstrate how they can refine their search results through the use of limits and controlled vocabularies like MeSH.

If you don't know where to begin a search or just aren't finding what you need, consult with a librarian who can help you troubleshoot your search strategy. Seeking guidance early in the search process can save you time you might otherwise spend sorting through a large number of irrelevant citations. When nurses understand how to effectively search the literature, they can apply that knowledge to develop best practices for their organization and improve patient safety and satisfaction.

Nora St. Peter, MSIS
Manager, Alberto Culver Health Learning Center
Northwestern Memorial Hospital
Chicago, Illinois

Critical Thinking 11.1

Go to the PubMed website, http://www.ncbi.nlm.nih.gov/pubmed, click on "PubMed Quick Start Guide." Review the many tips there for getting started with your literature searches.

1. What did you find?
2. How will this information help you with your clinical practice?

Searching Separate Key Words or Subject Headings in a Literature Search

Some of the electronic databases discussed later in this chapter allow the user to combine key words or subject heading search terms during an initial literature search on one search line, for example, weight loss surgery *and* type 2 diabetes. However, when working with an electronic database that allows this function, it is generally much

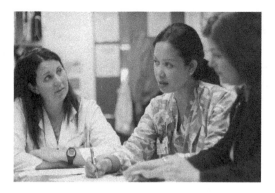

Health care team meeting.

better to conduct a literature search for each main search term separately and then combine the terms after the initial search results are retrieved for each. This allows for much greater flexibility in literature search design and eliminates the need to start over completely if your initial efforts do not produce the desired results. For example, when searching for evidence on the effectiveness of weight loss surgery as a treatment for type 2 diabetes compared to traditional treatment, your best literature search results will be achieved by first searching for weight loss surgery, getting a set of results, searching again for type 2 diabetes, and then combining the literature search results of both search sets. In many electronic databases, searching for several topics at one time will introduce too many variables into the literature search and will not produce optimum results.

In PubMed, for example, you can control when your literature search terms are added to the search. To do this, click the "Advanced" link found on the PubMed front page and type your first search term into the "Builder" search bar. Click the "Add to History" button, and you will begin to build your literature search. When you are ready to add another search term to your literature search strategy, use the "Add" link and click the "Search" button. Click the "Advanced" link again to go back to your list of saved literature search terms. Techniques like these are particularly important with literature searches that involve many terms. If you conduct your initial literature search with all terms and do not obtain satisfactory results, it will be difficult to determine why. However, if you make use of literature search builder tools like the "Add to History" search feature of PubMed, for example, and add your search terms to your literature search individually, it will be easy to identify the terms that are negatively affecting your literature search results.

Critical Thinking 11.2

Identify an area of nursing that interests you. Using your web browser, for example, http://www.google.com, search for a professional nursing organization that represents the clinical practice area that you have chosen, for example, Emergency Nurses' Association, Association of periOperative Registered Nurses, and so on. Visit the professional organization's web page. Can you find any content on literature and research?

1. What are some common topics currently being investigated by the professional organization in the clinical practice area that you have chosen?

Critical Thinking 11.3

Go to www.ahrq.gov/clinic/epcix.htm. This is the EBP content maintained by the Agency for Healthcare Research and Quality (AHRQ). Go to "Completed Reports" and select a clinical category that is related to your area of practice. Click on an abstract for a research study that interests you and read it.

1. What was the objective?
2. What were the results?
3. What were the conclusions from the research?
4. What are potential implications of this research for your practice?

USE OF BOOLEAN COMMANDS IN ELECTRONIC DATABASES

Almost all electronic databases make use of Boolean logic to define relationships between relevant terms in literature searches. **Boolean commands** are terms such as **AND, OR,** or **NOT** that are used to either expand or limit your literature search results when searching the literature in most electronic databases. For example, a literature search in an electronic database using the phrases, weight loss surgery **AND** type 2 diabetes is making use of the Boolean command, **AND.**

The specific attributes of the **AND** and **OR** Boolean commands are frequently confused. Note that the **AND** Boolean command means that all terms linked by the **AND** Boolean command must be present in the title or the abstract of the literature to be included in the search results. For example, if conducting a literature search for myocardial infarction **AND** aspirin, both terms must be present in the title or abstract in order for the evidence to be retrieved in a literature search.

When the **OR** Boolean command is used to connect a list of terms, literature search results will be returned if either term is present in the title or abstract, for example, aspirin **OR** ibuprofen. Only literature search results with the terms aspirin or ibuprofen in the title or abstract will be returned. The **NOT** Boolean command will eliminate the term that follows the **NOT** Boolean command from your literature search results, for example, aspirin **OR** ibuprofen **NOT** acetaminophen. Only literature search results with the terms aspirin **OR** ibuprofen, but **NOT** acetaminophen in the title or abstract will be returned.

DEVELOPING BROAD LITERATURE SEARCHES

When searching electronic databases for literature, especially when using databases that employ a controlled vocabulary like subject headings, it is often best to start your search more broadly and see what initial results are returned before searching for every term of your search. It is also often helpful to get an initial sense of how much published literature exists on your chosen topic before you begin narrowing results (Price, 2009). If you were working with a search question that had four terms, for example, it is often best to search initially for the two most important terms and see how many relevant search results you get. For example, if you are interested in finding evidence to indicate whether or not weight loss surgery is a more effective treatment option for type 2 diabetes compared to traditional treatments specifically with normal-weight or nonobese patients, it would be best to initially search an electronic database for the terms "weight loss surgery" and "type 2 diabetes." If a large enough data set is returned, then add the additional term of ideal or normal body weight. If the literature is abundant, add the additional term of traditional treatments. If the first two search terms return a small set of literature, adding more terms, and thus limiting your search further, will likely not be helpful.

When searching with subject headings, it is often beneficial to pick a broad subject heading, since more specific subtopics will automatically be included in the literature search in most cases. For example, in the Medline electronic database, a literature search using the subject heading "bariatric surgery" will also automatically include the subject heading "gastric bypass," a specific type of bariatric surgery. Many electronic databases make this hierarchy of subject headings clearly visible while searching, although the location of this hierarchy will vary from database to database. As mentioned earlier, in PubMed, the hierarchy of subject headings will be visible when using the MeSH Database. Type your literature search term into the search bar and click "Search." Look at the subject heading literature search results on the left side of the screen. Click any subject heading to view the complete record for it, including where it falls in the hierarchy of related subject headings.

Use of Literature Search Limit Commands

When using electronic databases, be sure to look for literature search limit commands. **Literature search limit commands** will edit your literature search results to only include results that meet your limiting criteria, for example, articles published in the last 5 years. In most databases, "search limits are added later and are not included in the initial search" (Sherwill-Navarro, 2010). Every database will have slightly different literature search limit commands, but examples of common search limit commands, found on www.pubmed.gov, include the following:

- Limit search results to English language publications. Note that larger electronic databases often index foreign language material.
- Limit search results by the date of publication, for example, current year, past 5 years, and so on.
- Limit search results to meta-analysis or practice guideline articles.

Even the most basic of literature search limits can lower the number of retrieved literature search results considerably. It is often best to start with basic literature search limits, for example, limit to "English language" and limit by publication date. You can add other more specific literature search limits, for example, meta-analysis articles only, as needed.

THE PICO MODEL

Developing a question for your literature search can be helped by using the PICO model (pronounced peak-o). PICO can be a very effective way to systematically approach the identification and retrieval of independent nursing and health care published studies (Table 11.2).

A PICO question for a literature search can be, "Does treatment of patients with type 2 diabetes with weight loss surgery provide better outcomes compared to traditional

TABLE 11.2 PICO

(P) Patient/Population of interest	Answers the question, "who?"	Example: patients with type 2 diabetes
(I) Intervention of interest	Answers the question, "what?"	Example: weight loss surgery
(C) Comparison	Used in evaluation of the intervention of interest	Example: compared to traditional management with pharmaceuticals, diet, and exercise
(O) Outcome	Used to describe desired outcome pertaining to what is being evaluated	Example: provide better outcomes?

Developed with information from Stillwell, Fineout-Overholt, Melnyk, and Williamson (2010).

patient management with pharmaceuticals, diet, and exercise?" The PICO model can be very helpful in insuring that your literature search question remains organized and that you address all aspects of it.

Use of PICO to Search for Evidence in PubMed

The PICO question, "Does treatment of patients with type 2 diabetes with weight loss surgery provide better outcomes compared to traditional management with pharmaceuticals, diet, and exercise?," when searched in PubMed using MeSH subject headings would be structured as follows:

If you click the "MeSH Database" link found under "More Resources," on the front page of http://www.PubMed.gov, and enter the search term "weight loss surgery" into the search bar, you will see that the MeSH Database will match this term with the subject heading "bariatric surgery." You can then use the "Add to Search Builder" button to add the subject heading "bariatric surgery" to your list of search commands. Repeat the same steps and you will see that the search term "type 2 diabetes" matches up best with the subject heading "diabetes mellitus, type 2."

PubMed's Search Builder is a small window that is visible on the right-hand side of the MeSH Database page once a search term has been entered in the search bar at the top. This window is where the MeSH Database builds your search using a format it can understand. You will see commands appear in the Search Builder box that do not look familiar, but don't worry about this at first. Once you have gained some experience, the Search Builder box can be edited by hand if desired.

When PICO search terms are entered into the search bar on the MeSH Database page and the search button is clicked, possible matches to MeSH Database subject headings will be displayed on the left side of the screen in a list. Each possible match can be clicked to learn more information about it, such as the exact definition of the term, what other subject headings are related to the term, and any entry terms, which are key words or synonyms that the MeSH Database considers to be covered by the subject heading. For example, entry terms for "diabetes mellitus, type 2," include "diabetes mellitus, ketosis-resistant" and "diabetes mellitus, maturity-onset."

Critical Thinking 11.4

Note the examples of asking different types of PICO questions at http://libguides.ohsu.edu/ content.php?pid=249886&sid=2079612. Put this clinical question in the PICO format.

1. What is the impact of exercise on patients with type 2 diabetes?

Subheadings

When you click on a subject heading to learn more about it, one important piece of information that will be displayed in the complete record for the subject heading is a list of the subheadings for that subject heading. Subheadings are subtopics that can be used to increase relevancy for your literature search. For example, the subject heading "diabetes mellitus, type 2" has the subheading "prevention and control." If the "prevention and control" subheading is selected, all search results that do not discuss the prevention and control of type 2 diabetes will be eliminated from the search result set.

Once a subject heading has been selected and relevant subheadings have also been selected, they can be added to the search builder box with the desired Boolean operator AND, OR, or NOT using the links provided on the MeSH database screen. When a new term is added to the search builder box, subject headings that were previously added to the search builder box on the screen will remain until the literature search is executed.

Checking for Usefulness or Relevancy

Once literature search results have been returned, the resulting literature set can be evaluated for usefulness or relevancy. Is the literature what you are looking for useful and relevant to your search? The literature search can be limited further using some of the common search limit commands, for example, date of publication, language, and so on.

If the relevancy of your search results is not high enough, there are several things that can be done, as follows:

- Check the subject headings used in the literature search. Are they too broad for what you are seeking? Too specific? Not relevant enough? It may be necessary to select additional subheadings or to search for other subject headings. For example, "glucose metabolism disorders" and "diabetes mellitus, lipoatrophic" are both subject headings that are related to "diabetes mellitus, type 2," with "glucose metabolism disorders" being a broader subject heading than "diabetes mellitus, type 2," and "diabetes mellitus, lipoatrophic" being a more specific subject heading. "Drug therapy," "diet therapy," and "genetics," are all subheadings that can be used with the subject heading "diabetes mellitus, type 2."
- If certain individual search results are relevant to your literature search, but the overall data set is not highly relevant, examine the complete article record for each relevant individual search result for additional help. Most databases that make use of subject headings will show which subject headings were used to index the article in the complete article record. The complete record is usually accessed by clicking the title of the desired article in the set of search results. Seeing how one highly relevant article is indexed usually provides clues for refining a literature search. This technique is often called "pearl growing." **Pearl growing** is a technique for refining

Critical Thinking 11.5

You're a nurse on an adult patient unit, frequently working with patients who are receiving dialysis. You'd like to determine which mechanism is best for patients to receive dialysis treatment.

1. Where would you start looking for this information?
2. What might be the terms from your PICO question that you will use to search a database?
3. How will you plan to use the information that you find?

a literature search through examining the complete record of one highly relevant article to see which subject headings have been attached to it, thus finding clues for how to search the literature for other relevant articles.

- Remember that while searching with subject headings is preferable whenever possible, some topics are better searched with key words. As with the example above of family member involvement in patient care, "family involvement" does not match with a subject heading. Therefore, initial key word searching of this topic to identify relevant articles can be beneficial.

REAL-WORLD INTERVIEW

One of the most challenging but essential parts of literature searching is making sure you use the right resources and techniques to find the best evidence, such as practice guidelines and research articles, to inform your clinical decisions. I once aided a medical student who struggled with treating a patient's uncontrolled diabetes. He wondered if there was any literature indicating that the medication, Janumet, a combination medication of the diabetes medications metformin and sitagliptin, would better control the blood glucose levels than metformin used alone. The student used www.google.com, but he was bombarded by too many unrelated resources and materials of questionable validity. I guided him to the biomedical database Medline via PubMed (http://www.PubMed.gov). He began to discover literature through searching that answered his PICO question, that is, would a patient with uncontrolled diabetes (patient/population of interest) taking Janumet (issue of interest) instead of metformin alone (comparison) have better blood glucose levels (outcome)? With this PICO question, he could move forward with his literature search process. This is an example of how using a specialized resource such as Medline or CINAHL, instead of simply searching the Internet, can help you get to the evidence you need more efficiently so that patients can be helped. If unsure of how to use these resources or where to find them, do not hesitate to ask your hospital librarian.

Charlotte M. Beyer, MSIS, AHIP
Instruction and Reference Librarian, Learning Resource Center
Rosalind Franklin University of Medicine and Science
North Chicago, Illinois

ELECTRONIC DATABASES

There are two main types of electronic databases; bibliographic databases and full-text databases. **Bibliographic databases**, such as Medline, provide a basic record, or citation, for an article and often provide an abstract or brief summary of the article; they do not necessarily contain the complete text of the article itself (Rosenberg & Donald, 1995). Whether or not you will be able to access the full text of an item found in a bibliographic database depends on which publications your parent institution subscribes to. Bibliographic databases are very important for EBP because they allow the user to search a wide range of relevant literature without limiting the results only to articles that the user would be able to access in full text.

Full-text databases provide the complete text of an article as well as the article citation. When using a full-text database, search results will still be presented in a list with basic information about each article, but unlike a bibliographic database, the user should be able to access the complete text of every search result when using a full-text database.

The type of database that is best to use depends on the needs of the user. Involvement in a large-scale research study would necessitate searching multiple bibliographic databases because it would be necessary to see all research relevant to the topic to create a good study design, to ensure that the idea in question has not already been studied, and to ensure that there are no major safety concerns. A student in need of a few recent articles for a school paper might only require a full-text database.

REAL-WORLD INTERVIEW

In today's fast-paced and outcomes-driven health care environment, nurses play an increasingly critical role in delivering safe and effective care to patients. This role requires nurses to become experts in finding and using the best evidence available. They need to be able to access the literature, understand how to evaluate the evidence, and develop policies, procedures, and processes that put the evidence into practice. Further, in those instances where solid evidence is not readily available, nurses need to add to the nursing profession's body of evidence through research, quality improvement, and EBP projects. While this is a tall order, nurses are more than up to the task. What they need is appropriate education, support, and mentoring to ensure their success. With the right resources, nurses at all levels can and do become champions of EBP and use their newfound knowledge to benefit the patients they serve.

Jill K. Rogers, PhD, RN, NEA-BC
Director of Professional Practice and Development,
Northwestern Memorial Hospital
Chicago, Illinois

EVIDENCE FROM THE LITERATURE

Citation

Scher, M. S., Ludington-Hoe, S., Kaffashi, F., Johnson, M. W., Holditch-Davis, D., & Loparo, K. A. (2009). Neurophysiologic assessment of brain maturation after an 8-week trial of skin-to-skin-contact on preterm infants. *Clinical Neurophysiology, 120*(10), 1812–1818.

Discussion

EBP involves either testing a new idea against existing practice or extending a proven EBP into real-world use. Published research studies in the literature are the evidence used to inform EBP. This study of the care of preterm infants is a good example of how searching the literature can shape and inform patient care.

Beginning in the 1970s, nurses in neonatal intensive care units (NICUs) began experimenting with what is sometimes called "kangaroo care." Kangaroo care is a technique practiced on newborn, usually preterm, infants wherein the infant is held skin-to-skin with an adult. The NICU nurses explored whether there would be a positive difference in fragile preterm infants' conditions if there was skin-to-skin contact between parents and preterm infants.

Initial studies demonstrated improved social development (Kramer, Chamorro, Green, & Kundston, 1975), food intake, and weight gain (White & Labarba, 1976; Rausch, 1981) in neonates, all of which lead to decreased length of stay, resulting in significant cost savings for both families and institutions (Field, et al., 1986). By 2002, research studies indicated that positive cognitive, perceptual, and motor development in the infant and parental behaviors were attributed to kangaroo care (Feldman, Eidelman, Sirota, & Weller, 2002). Trials continue today to test variations of physiologic and developmental milestones (Scher, et al., 2009) and have even extended the use of kangaroo care to help manage pain in these very fragile patients (Cong, Ludington-Hoe, McCain, & Fu, 2009; Johnston et al., 2008; Xiaomei Cong, Ludington-Hoe, & Walsh, 2011). Forty years of developing, testing, and extending the evidence of the beneficial effects of kangaroo care is part of the success that today emerges from NICU settings.

Implications for Practice

Investigating new and improved ways to care for different patient populations is what continues to elevate the standards of care. As evidenced from the example above, this can start with a simple question and lead to years of research, knowledge generation, and best practice dissemination. This culture of inquiry is important to the profession of nursing as it encourages bedside practitioners to consistently question the efficacy of their current practice; this inquiry can often lead to improvements in care that improve outcomes for patients.

CASE STUDY 11.1

You have been caring for overweight patients with type 2 diabetes. You note the following: Type 2 diabetes is a widespread disease, and traditional treatments often fail to provide adequate control (Nathan, et al., 2009). Treatment failure can lead to the use of drugs that cause weight gain, exacerbating the problem (Dixon, le Roux, Rubino, & Zimmet, 2012). You have heard other discussions in the news and are wondering if treatment of patients with type 2 diabetes with weight loss surgery provides better outcomes than traditional management of type 2 diabetes with pharmaceuticals, diet, and exercise. Conduct a literature search to find evidence to help answer this question.

1. *What did you find?*
2. *How will you proceed to share these results?*

Electronic Databases for Searching the Literature

There are many electronic databases that are available for searching the literature.

This is not intended to be an exhaustive list; rather, it is a snapshot of some of the electronic databases that can be used to search the literature. A few of these electronic databases are free, although most require subscriptions. Due to cost, access to these electronic databases is provided by large organizations such as universities and hospitals. It is necessary to have an affiliation with these organizations to have access. Access is usually provided through a resource website, such as a university library web page, and an institutional login will be required for access. The cost of these products will vary greatly for the institutions that subscribe to them. Cost is based on factors such as number of students (for a university) or beds (for a hospital) and the nature of the institution (community college, medical school, etc.). Personal subscriptions to these types of electronic databases are not practical or even possible in most cases. Students may not have access to all of these electronic databases, but hopefully a few electronic databases will be accessible to students and maybe even familiar.

Medline via PubMed and Ovid Medline and Other Vendors

Medline is the U.S. National Library of Medicine's (NLM's) bibliographic electronic journal database, indexing thousands of journal publications in the fields of medicine, nursing, dentistry, veterinary medicine, the health care system, and the preclinical sciences (Thomson, 2011). Medline can be accessed both through a free interface, www. PubMed.gov, and through subscription-based products such as Ovid Medline, http:// www.ovid.com/site/catalog/DataBase/901.jsp. Medline provides a complete citation for each article within the electronic journal database. An abstract is also provided in most cases. Medline is by far the largest bibliographic database in the medical, nursing, and scientific fields and is an essential starting point when conducting a literature search. PubMed, http://www.PubMed.gov, is the free search engine for Medline.

PubMed searches Medline using both key words and subject headings. PubMed has many other features in addition to searching Medline. These features include a database of journals included in Medline, and single and batch citation matchers, tools that can help identify articles when you have incomplete references.

PubMed's default search bar for Medline is at the top of the web page when you go to http://www.PubMed.gov. This search bar will perform a key word search. If the "MeSH Database" link on the front page of http://www.PubMed.gov is clicked, the user will be directed to a different search bar where the electronic database will attempt to match up the key words of your literature search terms, for example, match the key words from your PICO search, to a subject heading.

Ovid Medline, www.ovid.com/site/catalog/DataBase/901.jsp, is a subscription-based interface for searching Medline. Unlike PubMed, which has separate search areas for searching with key words and searching with subject headings, Ovid Medline has a feature called "map term to subject heading." This feature gives the user the opportunity to match his or her natural language, that is, the key words from a PICO search, with relevant subject headings as they search. Ovid Medline searches can be saved, and searches can be re-executed in other Ovid-owned products, such as Embase, without leaving the search screen or retyping search commands. As with PubMed, it is possible to apply subheadings for each subject heading used. Table 11.3 provides basic information about other electronic databases for literature searching. As mentioned earlier, this is not a complete list of electronic databases for literature but the following tables combined with the Medline database will provide a solid foundation of resources for the beginning literature searcher.

TABLE 11.3 ELECTRONIC DATABASES FOR LITERATURE SEARCHES

Cumulative Index to Nursing and Allied Health Literature (CINAHL), http://www.ebscohost.com/cinahl, is a bibliographic database that indexes the contents of nursing and allied health publications, including journals, dissertations, and other materials. While Medline indexes content from a wide variety of medical, nursing, and scientific fields, CINAHL is much more nursing-focused, making it essential for any research related to nursing.	Medline, http://www.nlm.nih.gov/bsd/pmresources.html The United States National Library of Medicine's (NLM) database of journal articles related to biomedicine. The NLM is a component of the National Institutes of Health, http://www.ncbi.nlm.nih.gov/pubmed
The Cochrane Collaboration, http://www.cochrane.org, is responsible for the Cochrane Library, a full-text database of systematic reviews on a wide variety of clinical topics designed especially to help practitioners make health care decisions. Thousands of clinicians, researchers, providers, and consumers across the world have been adding to this body of evidence-based reviews since 1993.	The National Center for Biotechnology Information resource of biomedical literature from Medline, life science journals, and online books, http://www.ncbi.nlm.nih.gov

(continued)

TABLE 11.3 ELECTRONIC DATABASES FOR LITERATURE SEARCHES *(continued)*

Joanna Briggs Institute (JBI) began in 1996, http://www.joannabriggs.edu.au, is similar to the Cochrane Collaboration. Through the JBI database, the Institute provides systematic reviews, Best Practice Information Sheets, Evidence Summaries, and Evidence-Based Recommended Practices. The original focus of JBI was nursing; this emphasis remains, but in recent years JBI has expanded to include evidence-based tools for medical and allied health researchers, clinicians, academics, quality managers, and consumers.

EMBASE, http://www.elsevier.com/online-tools/embase, is a bibliographic database indexing peer-reviewed literature in the biomedical and pharmaceutical sciences. For the most comprehensive coverage of a biomedical topic, and especially for literature on drugs or medical devices, EMBASE is essential. It contains more than 1,800 journal titles not indexed by Medline, Google, and Google Scholar.

PsycINFO, http://www.apa.org/pubs/databases/psycinfo/index.aspx?, is a bibliographic database of peer-reviewed literature in the fields of mental health and the behavioral sciences. Historical records are available here, dating from 1597, with comprehensive coverage from the 1880s. References for books, book chapters, and dissertations are included along with literature from journals.

Google, http://www.google.com and Google Scholar, http://scholar.google.com, are Internet search engines. Google is a general Internet search engine, while Google Scholar is specifically geared toward finding scholarly literature. One should never feel bad about using these resources to find evidence; these sophisticated systems can provide quick information. However, it is very important to avoid situations where these Internet search engines are the ONLY tools used in the search for evidence.

SELECTED PATIENT CARE INFORMATION TOOLS

Many patient care information tools are accessed online. Some are accessed at the bedside point of care to provide immediate information for patient diagnosis, treatment, and procedure. Patient care information tools are divided into two main types, that is, electronic databases (Table 11.4) and practice guidelines and other EBP tools (Table 11.5). Both tools are similar in that they are designed to provide objective, evidence-based information to assist health care practitioners in clinical decision making. Many electronic databases are only available by subscription. They often contain enhanced content, such as pictures, videos, and patient education materials.

CRITICAL APPRAISAL GUIDES

Once literature has been retrieved from electronic databases, a critical appraisal guide is an excellent tool to evaluate the literature and to determine how applicable the literature is to the situation to which it will be applied. A **critical appraisal guide to the literature** is essentially a checklist containing questions to ask about key aspects of a study (Fineout-Overholt, Melnyk, Stillwell, & Williamson, 2010). A critical appraisal guide is designed to help clinicians appraise literature and determine if the information really can be considered evidence upon which to base a change in practice. There are many such critical appraisal guides available. A 2004 study counted 121 published critical appraisal guides (Katrak, Bialocerkowski, Massy-Westropp, Kumar, & Grimmer, 2004). Table 11.6 provides selected critical appraisal questions that should be asked when evaluating literature.

TABLE 11.4 SELECTED ELECTRONIC DATABASES

Mosby's Nursing Consult, http://www.nursingconsult.com/nursing/index, and Lippincott's Nursing Advisor http://www.lwwnursingsolutions.com/content/lippincotts-nursing-advisor, are point-of-care tools developed specifically for nursing. Both tools include drug information, patient education handouts, and evidence-based care guidelines and care plans. Both can be tailored as needed to reflect local practice.

UpToDate, http://www.uptodate.com, is designed primarily for health care practitioners. It is a valuable point-of-care tool containing frequently updated information on hundreds of conditions and treatments. Patient education materials are also available.

Essential Evidence Plus, http://www.essentialevidenceplus.com, is a point-of-care database that utilizes a unique evaluation criteria called POEMS, Patient-Oriented Evidence that Matters, to determine if the content is worthy of addition to the database.

TABLE 11.5 SELECTED PRACTICE GUIDELINES AND EBP TOOLS

Agency for Healthcare Research and Quality, National Guidelines Clearinghouse http://www.guideline.gov	National Institute for Health and Clinical Excellence (NICE) http://www.nice.org/uk
Guidelines International Network http://www.g-i-n.net	Registered Nurses' Association of Ontario http://www.rnao.org
The Critical Appraisal Skills Programme http://www.casp-uk.net	Clinical Evidence http://clinicalevidence.bmj.com/ceweb/index.jsp
Evidence-based Nursing http://ebn.bmj.com	Evidence-Based Mental Health http://ebmh.bmj.com
Registered Nurses' Association of Ontario www.rnao.org	Joanna Briggs Institute http://www.joannabriggs.edu.au
Sarah Cole Hirsh Institute http://fpb.case.edu/Centers/Hirsh/index.shtm	Center for Evidence-Based Medicine at the University of Oxford http://www.cebm.net
Knowledge Translation Clearinghouse http://ktclearinghouse.ca	Sigma Theta Tau International http://www.nursinglibrary.org/vhl
Academic Center for Evidence-Based Nursing (ACE) http://www.acestar.uthscsa.edu	McGill University Health Centre http://muhc-ebn.mcgill.ca
National Institute for Health and Clinical Excellence (NICE) http://www.nice.org.uk	Oncology Nursing Society (ONS) www.ons.org

TABLE 11.6 SELECTED CRITICAL APPRAISAL QUESTIONS

- Why was the study conducted?
- How many subjects were involved in the study?
- Are the instruments used for data collection valid and reliable?
- How were the data analyzed?
- Did anything unexpected happen during the study?
- Do the results fit with previous research in the area?
- What does this research mean for clinical practice?

Compiled with information from Melnyk and Fineout-Overholt (2010).

INTERNET GUIDES FOR EVALUATING WEBSITES

There are many guides available on the Internet to help users evaluate the quality and trustworthiness of websites providing health care information (Table 11.7).

Each of these Internet guides for evaluating websites has different information to offer, but here are some of main points to consider that are common to all:

- *Sponsorship*: Is it apparent who wrote and posted the information? Is it clear which persons or organization is responsible for the content? Quality Internet-based sources should make this clear. Remember that websites that end in .org are usually organizations; websites that end in .edu are educational institutions; and websites that end in .gov are U.S. government websites. Websites ending in .com usually denote commercial or for-profit organizations.
- *Currency*: Is the information on the website updated regularly? Are dates given for the last update of individual sections/articles/guides?
- *Bias*: Is the information presented as a fact or as an opinion? Do you feel that the information is trying to influence your opinion on a subject or sell you a product? Be wary of information that is presented with a bias.
- *Audience*: Is it clear whom the information is for? Is it for health care professionals? Patients? Others?

LIFELONG LEARNING

Many electronic databases have a feature that allows you to save literature searches that are either automatically run at specific intervals or allow you to run them manually when you choose to do so. This literature search feature can help you maintain your lifelong learning. PubMed from the NLM has a feature called "My NCBI." My

TABLE 11.7 INTERNET GUIDES FOR EVALUATING WEBSITES

Health on the Net Foundation. HONCode	Available at http://www.hon.ch/HONcode/ Pro/Conduct.html
Quality Guidelines from MedlinePlus	Available at http://www.nlm.nih.gov/ medlineplus/criteria.html
Evaluating Online Sources of Health Information from the National Cancer Institute	Available at http://www.cancer.gov/ cancertopics/factsheet/Information/internet
How to Evaluate Health Information on the Internet: Questions and Answers from the National Institutes of Health Office of Dietary Supplements	Available at http://ods.od.nih.gov/Health_ Information/How_To_Evaluate_Health_ Information_on_the_Internet_Questions_ and_Answers.aspx
How to Evaluate Health Information on the Internet from the U.S. Food and Drug Administration	Available at http://www.fda.gov/ Drugs/ResourcesForYou/Consumers/ BuyingUsingMedicineSafely/ BuyingMedicinesOvertheInternet/ ucm202863.htm
A User's Guide to Finding and Evaluating Health Information on the Web from the Medical Library Association	Available at http://www.mlanet.org/resources/ userguide.html

NCBI has two major functions. It allows you to save complex search strategies with limits. The searches can be automatically run on a schedule that you determine and e-mailed to you, or you can run the search when you choose. Using My NCBI requires free and simple registration. Your search strategies are saved on the NLM servers and not your computer, so they can be accessed from any computer with Internet access. My NCBI also allows you to save collections of literature citations. These features can be very useful. CINAHL and PsychInfo via the EBSCO platform and OVID Medline also allows you to create an account and save literature searches that can be accessed and rerun when you wish. There are several other databases on the EBSCO platform that utilize this feature. Utilizing this can save you time and make it easy to stay current on topics of interest with a minimum of time and effort (Sherwill-Navarro, 2010).

Nurse Linx

Nurse Linx is a service for nurses that monitors the major journals for each profession and sends a daily e-mail with summaries of approximately five current articles. To sign up for Nurse Linx, go to http://www.mdlinx.com and select "nursing" from the list of specialties on the left sidebar (Sherwill-Navarro, 2010).

Other E-mail Services

The American Nurses Association (ANA) has developed ANA SmartBrief, available at https://www.smartbrief.com/ana. This service shares news items that may be of interest to nurses. Medscape, available at http://www.medscape.com/nurses, offers nursing news and review articles, and so on. (Sherwill-Navarro, 2010).

Continuing Education Websites

There are also several helpful continuing education websites for nurses to examine. They include:

- www.nurseceu.com
- www.nursingceu.com
- nursingworld.org/MainMenuCategories/CertificationandAccreditation/Continuing-Professional-Development
- www.nursingcenter.com/lnc/ceconnection

KEY CONCEPTS

1. Research and literature serve a distinct purpose, that is, to generate new knowledge that fills a gap.
2. Developing a good research question is necessary to ensure a clear, purposeful research direction.

3. Basic literature search strategies are used to search electronic literature databases for health care literature using key words and subject headings.
4. While searching with controlled vocabulary subject headings is preferable whenever possible, some literature search topics are better searched with key words in one's own natural language.
5. Using Boolean commands and developing broad literature searches can help identify important content when conducting literature searches in electronic literature databases.
6. It is often better to first approach a literature search broadly and then narrow the search after the initial literature search results are returned to you.
7. Once literature has been retrieved from relevant electronic literature databases, the evidence must be evaluated to determine how relevant and applicable it is to the situation to which it will be applied.
8. The PICO model for searching the literature helps identify important evidence for review.
9. There are several electronic literature databases for searching the literature.
10. Point-of-care information tools, for example, electronic literature databases and practice guidelines, can be used for basic literature searches.
11. Critical appraisal guides are useful in literature evaluation.
12. There are many guides available on the Internet to help users evaluate the quality and trustworthiness of websites providing health care information.
13. Lifelong learning is facilitated with the use of resources on the Internet.

KEY TERMS

Bibliographic databases	Key word
Boolean commands	Literature search limit commands
Critical appraisal guide to the literature	Pearl growing
Full-text databases	Subject heading

DISCUSSION OF OPENING SCENARIO

1. What opportunities are there in the nursing profession to facilitate dissemination of information?

Perhaps one of the best mechanisms to disseminate information locally is through your organization's shared leadership structures and committees. Shared leadership structures and committees are effective when there is a systematic approach to membership that includes representatives from all key areas. Ensuring a diverse and representative membership will make certain discussion filters up and down from all relevant areas and reaches all necessary interprofessional practitioners who are impacted. In addition, external dissemination of information is equally important. Venues such as conferences and webinars for professional organizations and professional journals provide great platforms to access and share evidence-based work! The nursing profession will only continue to flourish when people contribute to growing the body of knowledge by facilitating dissemination of evidence-based information.

2. What other nursing actions should you take when adopting new practice changes like this?

Adopting new successful practice changes begins at the step of inquiry! Ensuring necessary key stakeholders are involved from the inception of an idea ensures that all relevant facets of a problem or concern are discussed and addressed. Synthesizing the literature for useful and applicable practice improvements should always be a step taken early on—no need to "reinvent the wheel" if a best practice already exists. Lastly, a step often overlooked in the change process is taking action to ensure there is a sustainable control plan in place to ensure that new practice changes stick. Making the safest and best practice into the easiest thing to do, for example, by using standardized bundles and guidelines, is also a tactic that can be helpful in setting up practice changes for long-term success.

CRITICAL THINKING ANSWERS

Critical Thinking 11.1

1. What did you find?

You can find much information that will help you with literature searches, for example, how to search by author, journal name, specific citation, and so on.

2. How will this information help you with your clinical practice?

This information will help your with your clinical practice as it will allow you to search the literature for up-to-date literature to improve your practice in an on-going fashion.

Critical Thinking 11.2

1. What are some common topics currently being investigated by the professional organization in the clinical practice area that you have chosen?

Here's an example of content on literature and research at one site. The website of the National Association of Neonatal Nurses (www.nann.org) has a section called Resources for Clinical and Professional Practice (http://www.nannp.org/Content/resources-for-clinical-and-professional-practice.html). This site discusses many topics and has links to use to several current practice guidelines.

Critical Thinking 11.3

1. What was the objective?

When you access www.ahrq.gov/clinic/epcix.htm and click on the section for lung conditions, you would be linked to a report titled "Exercise-Induced Bronchoconstriction and Asthma" (Dryden et al., 2010). Objectives for the study are listed.

2. What were the results?

The objective of the study is to compare alternative index tests with a standardized exercise challenge test in patients with exercise-induced bronchoconstriction or exercise-induced asthma (EIB/EIA), determine the effectiveness of four pharmaceutical and one nonpharmaceutical treatment versus placebo to reduce symptoms in EIB/EIA patients, and to determine if daily treatment with beta-agonists causes patients with EIB/EIA to develop a diminishing response to the drug.

3. What were the conclusions from the research?

The research tells us that there is no clear evidence that any of the alternative index tests are more effective than the standardized exercise challenge test; that the examined pharmaceutical and nonpharmaceutical treatments measured were significantly better than placebo; and that the effectiveness of beta-agonists does decrease with daily use.

4. What are potential implications of this research for your practice?

The potential implications from this research are that the literature indicates that no change in standard practice is warranted at this time.

Critical Thinking 11.4

1. What is the impact of exercise on patients with type 2 diabetes?

Your PICO question would be set up like this:

P—patients with type 2 diabetes
I—impact of exercise in patients with type 2 diabetes
C—no exercise in patients with type 2 diabetes
O—impact of exercise on morbidity and mortality in type 2 diabetes

Critical Thinking 11.5

1. Where would you start looking for this information?

The CINAHL and Medline would both be good databases to consult for literature to use as evidence for possible practice change.

2. What might be the terms from your PICO question that you will use to search a database?

Your PICO question probably includes terms such as "kidney dialysis," "best practice," "adults," and "compared to standard care." The terms "kidney dialysis " and "best practice" would be very good terms to use to start your literature search.

3. How will you plan to use the information that you find?

Examine the information you find and look for common themes in the research. Are there consistent trends? Are the populations studied similar to your population of patients? Is there enough consistent evidence to support a possible practice change? If change is indicated, you can start by discussing your findings with the interprofessional team and your nurse manager.

CASE STUDY ANSWERS

Case Study 11.1

1. What did you find?

When you conduct your literature search, you may find support for a change in practice for these patients. Before such a change in practice can be safely recommended, it is necessary to proceed by discussing this with the interprofessional team caring for patients with type 2 diabetes.

2. How will you proceed to share these results?

Start by talking with your nurse manager and share the results of your literature search and make plans together for the next step.

REVIEW QUESTIONS

Please see Appendix D for answers to Review Questions.

1. Which of the following best describes the purpose of Boolean commands in electronic database searching?

A. Define relationships between relevant search terms
B. Tell the database to provide only high-quality results
C. Are necessary to start the search
D. Are not used when searching most electronic databases

2. While caring for Mr. Blake and Mr. Otto, two patients with similar surgical procedures, you notice that Mr. Blake's pain level has been more consistently controlled than Mr. Otto's pain level. Both patients are receiving the same type and dose of medication with the same frequency. In addition to this pain management regimen, Mr. Blake has walked two laps around the hall each hour while Mr. Otto has remained in bed. Based on this, you would like to change practice and incorporate an ambulation protocol into the care of these two patients. What would your first action be to achieve this?

A. Meet with physicians to have them add this to the postoperative order set any time pain medication is ordered.
B. Tell your patients about your recommendation and encourage integration of ambulation into their postoperative care.
C. Perform a literature search to see if there is evidence to validate the efficacy of more frequent ambulation of patients to control pain.
D. Arrange for a pilot study on your unit that compares a control group (pain medication) to an experimental group (pain medication and ambulation).

3. You are a nurse who works on an orthopedic surgical floor primarily caring for patients who are post–artificial knee replacement. In your experience, you have noticed that patients who perform a stand-pivot-sit on the day of surgery, with ambulation on postoperative Day 1, appear to be more prepared functionally for discharge. You note that these patients have achieved more milestones quicker in physical therapy and often report less pain. You wish to see if any published literature exists to back up this observation. Which of the following statements is the most helpful to your search?

A. It is only necessary to search for literature with an Internet search engine, since most major Internet search engines cover everything available on the web.
B. Not all published research can be found with an Internet search engine.
C. In order to find the greatest amount of literature, it is necessary to consult at least one, and ideally more than one, specialized literature databases like PubMed or CINAHL.
D. If you find a few studies that support your theory, that is probably enough to justify practice change.

4. Lisa, a novice nurse-researcher, seeks to better understand the potential implications of a different wound dressing technique on postsurgical healing. Lisa's research mentor is assisting her in developing a PICO question. Which question best demonstrates the PICO framework?

   A. For postprocedural patients, does dressing the flap with a moist bandage, rather than a dry bandage decrease healing time?
   B. For patients who have undergone a flap procedure following a single mastectomy, does dressing the flap with a moist bandage, rather than a dry bandage decrease healing time?
   C. Does dressing a surgical site with a moist bandage, rather than a dry bandage decrease healing time?
   D. For patients who have undergone a flap procedure following a single mastectomy, does dressing the flap with a moist bandage decrease healing time?

5. The nurses on five south wish to design a research study to test the most effective model for assigning patients to the nursing staff for care. They are wondering if a model that bases assignments on patient location might be more effective than models that base assignments on patient acuity. A member of the team suggests performing a literature search to see if any previous research has been done on the topic before designing the study. Why is this important?

   A. Searching the literature could help provide methods for study design, help avoid duplicating previous research, and help identify patient assignment models to study.
   B. A literature search can help protect against legal liability in the event of an accident, even if no further action is taken.
   C. A literature search will eliminate the need to make choices, since a convenient patient assignment model can be picked.
   D. A literature search would not be important in this scenario.

6. You are a nurse on a general medical–surgical floor and are interested in improving the outcomes of your patients who have a tracheostomy. Your first step should be which of the following?

   A. Review your hospital's current policy and practice for how best to care for tracheostomy patients.
   B. Review available literature for best practices.
   C. Solicit the thoughts and opinions of experts around you.
   D. Implement a best practice highlighted in a medical–surgical nursing journal.

7. You are conducting a literature review and you plan to search for literature on your topic in both Medline and CINAHL. For best search results, it is important to remember which of the following?

   A. The search interface will not be as easy to use as an Internet search engine.
   B. In most cases, the best search results will be returned if you search using the database's system of controlled vocabulary subject headings, instead of simply using key words.
   C. Using the Internet for your literature search is often just as good as searching an electronic database.
   D. You should use whichever database you find easier to use, since your search results will be better if you are comfortable with the interface.

8. You are searching for evidence in an electronic database and you notice that it makes use of a system of controlled vocabulary. Because of this, it is usually best to do which of the following?

    A. Combine all search terms on to the same search command line, as one would with an Internet search engine.
    B. Disregard the system of controlled vocabulary and search using your natural language of key words.
    C. When the database allows it, break your search question down into separate subject headings and search for each subject heading separately before combining search results.
    D. Search using many subject headings at once to maximize results.

9. Members of a nursing unit are planning to search the literature, but their PICO question is very broad and involves many concepts. Searches of this type are best approached in which of the following ways?

    A. All concepts should be included in initial searches to maximize results.
    B. It is often best to initially search for only the core concepts of a question and then add the more specific criteria as needed after initial results are retrieved.
    C. Search only for the core concepts of your question and disregard anything that isn't absolutely essential.
    D. Search for the specific criteria first to maximize unique results.

10. You are working with a principal investigator on a study to improve how frequently used nursing supplies and equipment are ordered and stored through your organization. You have been asked to conduct a literature search to look for journal articles discussing best practices. What kind of database will best serve your needs?

    A. A bibliographic database
    B. A full-text database
    C. The Internet
    D. A list of relevant print journals

REVIEW ACTIVITIES

Please see Appendix E for answers to Review Activities.

1. Some literature searches work best with subject headings. For example, finding evidence to support the use of aspirin with patients who have had a heart attack. In most databases, myocardial infarction is the subject heading for heart attack. Searching for myocardial infarction and aspirin will produce high-quality, relevant results and produce them more quickly than searching for heart attack, cardiac arrest, and so on. Other literature searches work best using one or more key words. For example, finding literature to measure if getting the family members of patients in ICUs involved in the patient's care has a positive impact on outcomes is a broad search topic that would probably work best when searched with key words. Note that the concept of family involvement does not connect easily to a single MeSH subject heading. Try searching for literature on myocardial infarction and aspirin and then try search for family involvement of patients in the ICU in Medline to see what results you retrieve. What did you find?

2. Go back to the example of using aspirin with patients with myocardial infarction. Try searching this topic using PubMed (http://www.PubMed.gov). Type myocardial infarction AND aspirin into the search bar at the top of your computer screen. See how many results you get. Assess the usefulness and relevancy of those results. Then, click the MeSH Database link found on the front page of the website under More Resources and redo the search. This time, instead of typing both terms together with AND, type one term at a time, that is, type in myocardial infarction, search for it, select the best match from the results on the left side of the screen, click the link on the screen to add a term to the search builder, repeat the process with the term, aspirin, and then click the Search PubMed button to run the search. Assess the quality of relevant results returned with this search. What did you find?

3. You are working with the nurse manager. She is looking for research on the ideal patient-to-staff ratio for night shift charge nurses who practice in NICUs. In this situation, it is probably best to look for evidence on patient-to-staff ratio AND NICU. Once you see the number, quality, and relevancy of search results returned, you can then decide whether or not to add the additional criteria of charge nurses and night shifts. Try this in CINAHL or PubMed and see what results you retrieve. What did you find?

EXPLORING THE WEB

1. Review the three PubMed tutorials How It Works, Building Blocks, and Search Tools, at the "Building the Search" PubMed Tutorial section. http://www.nlm.nih.gov/bsd/disted/pubmedtutorial/020_010.html

2. Review the Literature Search Methods for the Development of Clinical Practice Guidelines from the NLM, http://www.nlm.nih.gov/nichsr/litsrch.html

3. Review the Searching CINAHL Tutorials from the University of Illinois at Chicago University Library, http://researchguides.uic.edu/content.php?pid=31366&sid=243338

4. Review the User's Guide to Finding and Evaluating Health Information on the Web from the Medical Library Association, http://www.mlanet.org/resources/userguide.html

REFERENCES

Anders, M. E., & Evans, D. P. (2010). Comparison of PubMed and Google scholar literature searches. *Respiratory Care, 55*(5), 578–583.

Auston, I., Cahn, M. A., & Selden, C. R. (1998, May 20). *Literature search methods for the development of clinical practice guidelines*. Retrieved from http://www.nlm.nih.gov/nichsr/litsrch.html

Cong, X., Ludington-Hoe, S. M., McCain, G., & Fu, P. (2009). Kangaroo care modifies preterm infant heart rate variability in response to heel stick pain: A pilot study. *Early Human Development, 85*(9), 561–567.

Dixon, J. B., le Roux, C. W., Rubino, F., & Zimmet, P. (2012). Bariatric surgery for type 2 diabetes. *Lancet, 379*(9833), 2300–2311.

Dryden, D. M., Spooner, C. H., Stickland, M. K., Vandermeer, B., Tjosvold, L., Bialy, L.,...Rowe, B. H. (2010, January). *Exercise-induced bronchoconstriction and asthma*. Retrieved from http://www.ncbi.nlm.nih.gov/books/NBK44508

Feldman, R., Eidelman, A. I., Sirota, L., & Weller, A. (2002). Comparison of skin-to-skin (kangaroo) and traditional care: parenting outcomes and preterm infant development. *Pediatrics, 110*(1 pt. 1), 16–26.

Field, T. M., Schanberg, S. M., Scafidi, C. R., Bauer, C. R., Vega-Lahr, N., Garcia, R.,... Kuhn, C. M. (1986) Tactile/kinesthetic stimulation effects on preterm neonates. *Pediatrics, 77*(5), 654–658.

Fineout-Overholt, E., Melnyk, B. M., Stillwell, S. B., & Williamson, K. M. (2010). Evidence-based practice, step by step: Critical appraisal of the evidence: Part I. *American Journal of Nursing, 110*(7), 47–52.

Houser, J. (2008). *Nursing research: Reading, using and creating evidence*. Retrieved from http://www.nursing.jbpub.com/book/houser/index.cfm

Johnston, C. C., Filion, F., Campbell-Yeo, M., Goulet, C., Bell, L., McNaughton, K.,... Walker, C. (2008). Kangaroo mother care diminishes pain from heel lance in very preterm neonates: A crossover trial. *BMC Pediatrics, 8*(13). Retrieved from http://www.ncbi.nlm.nih.gov/pmc/articles/PMC2383886

Katrak, P., Bialocerkowski, A. E., Massy-Westropp, N., Kumar, S., & Grimmer, K. A. (2004). A systematic review of the content of critical appraisal tools. *BMC Medical Research Methodology 4*, 22. doi:10.1186/1471–2288-4–22.

Kramer, M., Chamorro, I., Green, D., & Kundston, F. (1975). Extra tactile stimulation of the premature infant. *Nursing Research, 24*(5), 324–334.

Melnyk, B., & Fineout-Overholt, E. (2010). *Evidence-based practice in nursing & healthcare* (3rd ed.). Philadelphia, PA: Lippincott Williams and Wilkins.

Nathan, D. M., Buse, J. B., Davidson, M. B., Ferrannini, E., Holman, R. R., Sherwin, R., Zinman, B; American Diabetes Association; European Association for Study of Diabetes et al. (2009). Medical management of hyperglycaemia in type 2 diabetes mellitus: A consensus algorithm for the initiation and adjustment of therapy: a consensus statement from the American Diabetes Association and the European Association for the Study of Diabetes. *Diabetologia, 52*(1), 17–30.

Price, B. (2009). Guidance on conducting a literature search and reviewing mixed literature. *Nursing Standard, 23*(24), 43–50.

Rausch, P. B. (1981). Effects of tactile and kinesthetic stimulation on premature infants. *JOGN Nursing, Journal of Obstetric, Gynecologic, and Neonatal Nursing, 10*(1), 34–37.

Rosenberg, W., & Donald, A. (1995). Evidence-based practice: an approach to clinical problem solving. *British Medical Journal, 310*(6987), 1122–1126.

Scher, M. S., Ludington-Hoe, S., Kaffashi, F., Johnson M. W., Holditch-Davis, D., & Loparo, K. A. (2009). Neurophysiologic assessment of brain maturation after an 8-week trial of skin-to-skin contact on preterm infants. *Clinical Neurophysiology, 120*(10), 1812–1818.

Schmelzer, M. (2008). The importance of the literature search. *Gastroenterology Nursing, 31*(2), 151–153.

Sherwill-Navarro, P. (2010). Information and life-long learning. In K. A. Polifko (Eds.), *The practice environment of nursing*. Clifton Park, NY: Delmar Cengage Learning.

Stillwell, S. B., Fineout-Overholt, E., Melnyk, B. M., & Williamson, K. M. (2010). Evidence-based practice, step by step: asking the clinical question: A key step in evidence-based practice. *American Journal of Nursing, 110*(3), 58–61.

Thomson, S. (2011). Real world interview. In P. Kelly (Eds.), *Nursing leadership and management* (3rd ed., p. 125). Clifton Park, NY: Delmar Cengage Learning.

White, J. L., & Labarba, R. C. (1976). The effect of tactile and kinesthetic stimulation on neonatal development in the premature infant. *Developmental Psychobiology, 9*(6), 569–577.

Xiaomei Cong, Ludington-Hoe, S. M., & Walsh, S. (2011). Randomized crossover trial of kangaroo care to reduce biobehavioral pain responses in preterm infants: A pilot study. *Biological Research for Nursing, 13*(2), 204–216.

SUGGESTED READING

Brusco, J. M. (2010). Effectively conducting an advanced literature search. *AORN Journal, 92*(3), 264–271.

Ehrlich-Jones, L., O'Dwyer, L., Stevens, K., & Deutsch, A. (2008). Searching the literature for evidence. *Rehabilitation Nursing, 33*(4), 163–169.

Falagas, M. E., Pitsouni, E. L., Malietzia, G. A., & Pappas, G. (2008). Comparison of PubMed, Scopus, Web of Science, and Google Scholar: Strengths and weaknesses. *FASEB Journal, 22*(2), 338–342.

Fineout-Overholt, E., Melnyk, B. M., Stillwell, S. B., & Williamson, K. M. (2010a). Evidence-based practice, step by step: Critical appraisal of the evidence: Part I. *American Journal of Nursing, 110*(7), 47–52.

Fineout-Overholt, E., Melnyk, B. M., Stillwell, S. B., & Williamson, K. M. (2010b). Evidence-based practice, step by step: Critical appraisal of the evidence: Part II. Digging deeper—Examining the "keeper" studies. *American Journal of Nursing, 110*(9), 41–48.

Fineout-Overholt, E., Melnyk, B. M., Stillwell, S. B., & Williamson, K. M. (2010c). Evidence-based practice, step by step: Critical appraisal of the evidence: Part III. Digging deeper—Examining the "keeper" studies. *American Journal of Nursing, 110*(11), 43–51.

Finfgeld-Connett, D., & Johnson, E. D. (2013). Literature search strategies for conducting knowledge-building and theory-generating qualitative systematic reviews. *Journal of Advanced Nursing, 69*(1), 194–204.

Joseph, T., Saipradeep, V. G., Raghavan, G. S., Srinivasan, R., Rao, A., Kotte, S., & Sivadasan, N. (2012). TPX: Biomedical literature search made easy. *Bioinformation, 8*(12), 578–580.

Nourbakhsh, E., Nugent, R., Wang, H. Cevik, C., & Nugent, K. (2012). Medical literature searches: a comparison of PubMed and Google scholar. *Health Information and Libraries Journal, 29*(3), 214–222.

O'Malley, D. L. (2008). A survey of scholarly literature databases for clinical laboratory science. *Clinical Laboratory Science, 21*(1), 49–57.

Smith, M. L., & Shurtz, S. (2012). Search and ye shall find: practical literature review techniques for health educators. *Health Promotion Practice, 13*(5), 666–669.

Stillwell, S. B., Fineout-Overholt, E., Melnyk, B. M., & Williamson, K. M. (2010). Evidence-based practice, step by step: searching for the evidence. *American Journal of Nursing, 110*(5), 41–47.

Young, S., & Duffull, S. B. (2011). A learning-based approach for performing an in-depth literature search using MEDLINE. *Journal of Clinical Pharmacy and Therapeutics, 36*(4), 504–512.

Younger, P. (2010). Using Google scholar to conduct a literature search. *Nursing Standard, 24*(45), 40–46, 48.

12

EVIDENCE-BASED PRACTICE

Kathleen Fischer Sellers and Karen L. McCrea

At first people refuse to believe that a strange new thing can be done, then they begin to hope it can be done, then they see it can be done—*then it is done and all the world wonders why it was not done centuries ago.* (Frances Hodgson Burnett, 1911, *The Secret Garden*)

Upon completion of this chapter, the reader should be able to

1. Define evidence-based practice (EBP)
2. Identify relevant sources of research information
3. Describe appropriate methods for the evaluation of information
4. Discuss various models for implementing EBP
5. Utilize Titler's Iowa Model of Quality Care to explore the implementation process of EBP
6. Discuss Rogers's Diffusion of Innovation framework as a method to expedite the adoption of evidence

---

*A*t the quarterly nursing practice committee meeting, the research facilitator asks what issues you as a clinician have been concerned about. You think of the recent increase in urinary tract infections (UTI) that you have observed on the surgical unit. You know that per the Centers for Medicare and Medicaid Services (CMS) that there will be no reimbursement for any hospital-acquired UTIs. You wonder if the current standard of practice regarding care of patients with indwelling catheters is based on best practices. You wonder what the evidence is to support these practices.

- *How would you find out?*
- *What would you do if there was a difference between your organization's practice and the evidence?*

Nurses, other health care professionals, and health care institutions are constantly striving to improve patient safety and health outcomes. This goal requires the cultivation, implementation, and maintenance of evidence-based best practice. Best practices are continually changing and evolving as new evidence and research becomes available. This chapter defines and describes what EBP is. It also discusses methods and resources available to evaluate current research information. Several models for implementing EBPs are discussed. Titler's Iowa Model of Quality Care is utilized to explore the implementation process of EBP. Finally, the chapter explores methods to expedite the adoption of evidence into practice through Rogers's Diffusion of Innovation framework.

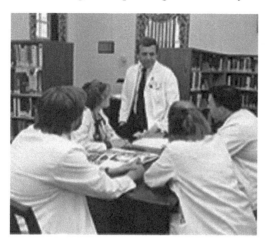

Interprofessional EBP task force defining the issue.

DEFINING EBP

Nurses and other health care providers (HCPs) employ EBP to promote the well-being and safety of patients. **EBP** is the delivery of optimal health care through the integration of best current evidence, clinical expertise, and patient/family values (Quality and Safety Education for Nurses [QSEN], 2012; Figure 12.1).

Much of this chapter is dedicated to the EBP concept of best current evidence. This process involves locating and analyzing high-quality, relevant scientific information. Today's practicing nurse must be able to determine how evidence can be incorporated into the particular setting of interest. This may mean a hospital-wide policy change or change on a much smaller scale.

Several common misperceptions regarding EBP exist. Misperceptions include ideas that EBP relies solely on current evidence and should be manifested by every patient receiving identical care, or that EBP ignores patient preferences and values (Dicenso, Guyatt, & Ciliska, 2005). These perceptions are not true! In addition to current evidence, it is important to recognize that clinical expertise and patient/family values are equally important in the provision of evidence-based, optimal care. Each component of the EBP model should be explored and integrated into practice by nurses and other HCPs.

In 1984, Benner published a landmark book in which she disseminated the idea that nurses constantly evolve in their practice along a continuum from novice to expert. This evolution occurs with the acquisition of advanced skills, experience, and understanding of patients, families, and their unique needs as well as additional education (Benner, 1984). Benner further stated that regardless of how much education a nurse possessed, the nurse could never become an expert without actual clinical experience.

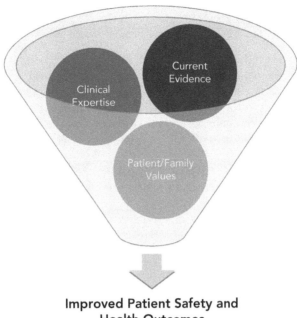

**Improved Patient Safety and
Health Outcomes**

FIGURE 12.1 The components of current evidence, clinical expertise, and patient/family values are funneled through a shared decision-making process and the result is improved patient safety and health outcomes.

In practical terms, what this implies is that based on knowledge and experience, each nurse brings unique perceptions and strengths to the health care arena. It is indisputable that every nurse must possess the skills and knowledge to be a safe provider of care. However, each nurse, through personal and clinical experiences, will be able to apply unique information and care as they promote patient safety and well-being.

For example, a physically debilitated patient requires assistance transferring from the chair to the bed. The patient has been using a gait belt to assist with this procedure. Two nurses with differing experience and background can approach the care of this patient differently while at the same time ensuring the safety and well-being of the patient. A novice nurse, with limited practical experience and knowledge related to the patient, decides to ask the physical therapist to assist her, and to ask the physical therapist to show her the proper techniques needed for the safe transfer of the patient to the bed. A more experienced nurse, familiar with proper body mechanics, gait belt transfers, and the patient's physical ability, opts to assist the patient to bed by herself. Both nurses achieved the same goal of safely transferring the patient to bed; however, they approached the issue differently based on personal experience and knowledge. This example demonstrates how individual nurses' varying clinical expertise can impact how care is delivered. To ensure optimal patient outcomes and patient safety, all nurses need to be constantly aware of their strengths and limitations as they plan and implement care.

CASE STUDY 12.1

As a nurse on the medical–surgical floor, you are caring for an Amish patient with end-stage renal disease (ESRD). The patient's attending physician has been talking about the need to start hemodialysis. The patient is asking you many questions related to this treatment recommendation. After listening to your explanations, which you give based on evidence from the research literature, the patient states that he would prefer to go home, and if he dies, then it is God's will.

1. *Is it appropriate to tell the patient that he needs to do what the physician ordered because dialysis can extend life expectancy?*
2. *Why or why not?*
3. *What would be the most appropriate action to take?*

Incorporating Research Into Clinical Practice

Caring is the essence of nursing according to Madeleine Leininger, a nurse theorist (Leininger & McFarland, 2006). Leininger does not stand alone in championing caring, as many other nurse theorists espouse theories that incorporate the concepts of caring as well as patient advocacy. Nurses actualize these caring concepts every day, which helps set nursing apart as the most trusted profession in the United States for the past 11 years (Gallup, Inc., 2010). Nurses have long placed themselves in the role of patient advocate by taking time to explain issues and educate patients and by speaking up for patients and their rights when the patient is unwilling or unable to verbalize concerns. At the core of patient advocacy is the elemental knowledge that each patient is an individual with unique feelings, beliefs, and thoughts. This patient individuality takes into account individuals' life experiences, cultural backgrounds, ethnic backgrounds, socioeconomic issues, and support structure. Since every patient has unique needs and challenges, there is no possibility that one plan of care can be utilized to optimize patient safety and outcomes for all patients. Incorporating EBP into patient care requires the nurse to utilize optimal data obtained through science and research and then work collaboratively with patients, families, community resources, and other HCPs to create a plan of care that is acceptable to the patient, maximizes patient health, and provides care safely.

For example, two patients with identical past health care histories are diagnosed with Stage IV lung cancer. Data identifies the optimal treatment to maximize their life expectancies but also indicates that mortality for this condition is very high. After learning all of the facts related to the disease, treatment, and prognosis, each patient chooses a different treatment course. The first patient states that he has led a good life, is very spiritual, and wishes to die peacefully at home with his family at his side. The second patient states that he has life goals that are unachieved and that he is also very spiritual and his family's support will assist him as he does whatever is necessary to beat the cancer. The nurse opts in both instances to help the patients achieve their desired plan of care. This scenario indicates that although research and scientific data is important in the decision-making process and EBP, personal beliefs and values also play a key role.

Critical Thinking 12.1

You work on a medical–surgical unit delivering care to patients. You want to be sure your care delivery is based on evidence and is state of the art.

1. How will you, as a new nurse, begin to promote EBP?
2. What contributions can you make to EBP?
3. How can nurses help to overcome potential resistance to EBP?

Best Practice

Evidence related to best clinical practice is continuously growing, changing, and evolving. Unfortunately, nurses and other HCPs often follow outdated policies, procedures, and treatment modalities (Melnyk, Fineout-Overholt, Stillwell, & Williamson, 2009). Balas (2001) indicates it takes an average of 17 years for clinical research to be fully integrated into everyday practice. It is imperative that all HCPs minimize the time from discovery to application of new research. This will lead to improved patient safety and outcomes. In efforts to improve patient safety and outcomes, the Institute of Medicine (IOM) is promoting the goal that 90% of all health decisions be evidence based by the year 2020 (Olsen, Aisner, & McGinnis, 2007). Melnyk and colleagues (2009) suggest that health care settings that promote curiosity regarding clinical decision making are optimally situated to discover and incorporate EBP, thereby improving patient outcomes.

As described earlier, the implementation of EBP incorporates three factors: patient/family values, clinical expertise, and the integration of best current evidence. There are some basic, essential requirements that must be available to assist the inquiring nurse or other health care professional. A computer with Internet connection is a primary necessity. The Internet provides access to vast amounts of data with amazing speed. The bygone days of spending hours, and days, in library stacks with dusty journals has, thankfully, evolved into the ability to locate data with relative ease.

CASE STUDY 12.2

As a nurse in the operating room, you are asked to change the method used to position patients during surgical procedures. You have been educated and trained in the new procedure that is being implemented as an evidence-based change. After several days of using the new positioning technique, you have noticed several patients with increased areas of skin erythema on key pressure points.

1. *Since this change is evidence based, will you just keep utilizing the new method despite concerns?*
2. *Why or why not?*
3. *What would be the most appropriate action to take?*

RELEVANT SOURCES OF RESEARCH INFORMATION

Although the time required to locate evidence-based literature has significantly lessened with the advent of the computer and Internet, it is important to note that seeking information still is a process that takes time and concentration. Therefore, to promote inquiry and EBP, there needs to be institutional, managerial, and library support for the acquisition of knowledge. A nurse manager needs to be willing to provide time and support for nurses to explore evidence related to an important issue. This typically includes releasing nurses from patient care duties to provide time for exploration of data. This is discussed more in Chapter 11.

While utilizing the Internet, the nurse or other HCP seeking information, requires access to online electronic databases as they seek the most current data. Table 12.1 provides information on a variety of available databases that can assist the nurse who is seeking relevant research for a topic of interest.

Another essential element for locating high-quality research based on evidence is a librarian. A librarian with a background in locating information related to health care issues is invaluable. Universities and large health care institutions typically have a librarian on staff that can provide valuable advice and information on how to best locate the specific information that is being sought. Often librarians are available for either personal consultations or tutorial sessions.

REAL-WORLD INTERVIEW

Utilizing evidence-based measures as part of the interprofessional team is crucial to establishing adequate substantiation for necessary changes to policies and procedures. As a nurse administrator, I utilize evidence from the literature when a clinical question comes up; if the department needs more background for an issue being addressed; and, when developing and implementing policies and procedures. When asking nurses, ancillary staff and/or other members of the health care team to change how things are done, questions regarding the value and merit are appropriate and often asked. Having sound rationale based on what the literature shows provides a strong foundation for explanation. It also helps provide credibility for the suggested change to team members who resist change or tend to be skeptical about changing from the way "things have always been done."

Most importantly, providing documentation of the evidence within or at the end the actual policy or procedure creates a standard the members of the team can count on. The registered nurse (RN) is accountable for any and all interventions provided to a patient; thus, having documentation of the literature supporting a policy provides an element of safety and professional comfort. Including documentation of the source and the strength of the evidence also creates an expectation that all policies, procedures, and change will include credible substantiation.

As a nurse administrator, I count on the evidence to guide how I lead my staff as well as, plan for change on a larger scale with my colleagues from other areas of the institution. I consider it my responsibility and obligation to consult and utilize appropriate evidence to guide how I lead and manage; as well as

(continued)

believe it sets an example for others to follow. At my institution, we are fortunate to have access to credible databases of literature anytime, which I encourage my staff, as well as interprofessional team members, to utilize.

Karen Callahan
Nurse Administrator
Oneida, New York

CASE STUDY 12.3

Your head nurse has asked you to investigate what the best EBPs are related to the prevention of pressure sores. The unit protocol for pressure sore prevention was last updated 5 years ago. You implement a search of the literature but are unable to locate any articles relevant to your topic of interest.

1. *What factor has most likely hampered your ability to locate relevant information?*
2. *What is your next step?*
3. *Who can assist you with this?*

EVALUATING THE EVIDENCE

When searching for the best evidence that is available, the nurse needs to review the quality of research evidence. Since the purpose of implementing evidence-based care is to improve patient safety and high-quality outcomes, a nurse or other HCP needs to be certain that enough rigor exists in located research to provide confidence the evidence is indeed factual and accurate. Rigor refers to the quality of the evidence and infers a high degree of thoroughness and merit or strength. It would be detrimental to patient safety and high-quality outcomes to base changes in patient care on poor quality, erroneous research.

Levels of Evidence

Existing evidence is classified into levels of evidence based on the rigor and strength. As such, **levels of evidence** is a ranking of evidence based on the strength and reliability of a study's findings. Evidence that is considered to be the strongest is referred to as Level I evidence and includes systematic reviews, meta-analyses of randomized, controlled trials and practice guidelines. Level II evidence generally consists of randomized controlled trials. Level III evidence is generated from well-controlled trials not utilizing randomization. Examples of Level IV evidence include well-designed case control and cohort studies. Levels above IV are not considered rigorous enough to base practice decisions upon and include expert opinions and case studies. Table 12.2 describes various types of studies and ranks them according their level of evidence.

Once the evidence in the literature has been located through the databases, the nurse should evaluate the findings and assess the quality and generalizability of

TABLE 12.1 ONLINE EVIDENCE-BASED RESOURCES FOR HEALTH CARE PROFESSIONALS

RESOURCE	WEBSITE	TYPE OF DATA	AVAILABILITY
CINAHL: Cumulative Index of Nursing and Allied Health Literature (1982–present)	www.cinahl.com	Studies in nursing, allied health, and biomedicine	Currently owned by EBSCO publishing and requires a subscription from libraries
Medline (1966–present)	http://www.nlm.nih.gov/bsd/pmresources.html	The U.S. National Library of Medicine's (NLM) database of journal articles related to biomedicine. The NLM is a component of the National Institutes of Health	FREE for individuals
EMBASE (1947–present)	http://www.embase.com	Biomedical database that covers biomedical research and includes all Medline data plus an additional 5 million records	Requires a subscription, no individual subscriptions available
PsycINFO (1887–present)	http://www.apa.org/pubs/databases/psycinfo/index.aspx	Database with more than 3 million records devoted to peer-reviewed literature in the behavioral sciences and mental health	Institutional subscriptions as well as individual subscriptions can be purchased annually or on an as-needed basis
Cochrane Database of Systematic Reviews (CDSR) Established in 1972	http://www.cochrane.org	Full text versions of regularly updated systematic reviews	Institutional subscriptions as well as individual subscriptions can be purchased annually or on an as-needed basis
National Guidelines Clearinghouse (NGC)	http://www.guideline.gov	An initiative of the Agency for Healthcare Research and Quality (AHRQ) that provides objective, detailed information on clinical practice guidelines	FREE
Clinical Evidence	http://clinicalevidence.bmj.com/ceweb/index.jsp	An international resource for systematic reviews	Institutional subscriptions as well as individual subscriptions that can be purchased annually or on an as-needed basis
Evidence-based Nursing	http://ebn.bmj.com	An online quarterly publication of best nursing practice	Institutional and group subscriptions available
Evidence-Based Mental Health	http://ebmh.bmj.com	An online publication that provides an assessment of the clinical relevance of studies pertaining to mental health issues	Institutional and group subscriptions available

Resource	URL	Description	Cost
PubMed database	http://www.ncbi.nlm.nih.gov/pubmed	The National Center for Biotechnology Information resource of biomedical literature from Medline, life science journals, and online books	FREE
Registered Nurses' Association of Ontario	www.rnao.org	Provides links to nursing best practice guidelines	FREE
Joanna Briggs Institute	http://www.joannabriggs.edu.au	An international organization based at the University of Adelaide in South Australia that promotes synthesis, transfer, and utilization of evidence	FREE
Sarah Cole Hirsh Institute	http://fpb.case.edu/Centers/Hirsh/index.shtm	Established at the Frances Payne Bolton School of Nursing at Case Western Reserve University; it promotes the integration of best evidence into practice and offers assistance to individuals, nurses, and organizations	FREE
Center for Evidence-Based Medicine at the University of Oxford	http://www.cebm.net	Aims to develop, teach, and promote evidence-based health care and provide support and resources to health care professionals	FREE
Knowledge Translation Clearinghouse	http://ktclearinghouse.ca	Funded by the Canadian Institute of Health Research (CIHR), this serves as a repository of evidence and provides access to tools that facilitate EBP	FREE
Sigma Theta Tau International	http://www.nursinglibrary.org/vhl	Sigma Theta Tau's Virginia Henderson International Nursing Library offers nurses access to reliable nursing research and evidence-based knowledge	FREE
Academic Center for Evidence-Based Nursing (ACE)	http://www.acestar.uthscsa.edu	Based at the University of Texas Health Science Center at San Antonio, ACE is dedicated to bridging research into practice with the ultimate goal of improving care, patient outcomes, and patient safety	FREE
McGill University Health Centre	http://muhc-ebn.mcgill.ca	Provides research and clinical resources for evidence-based nursing	FREE
National Institute for Health and Clinical Excellence (NICE)	http://www.nice.org.uk	Based in the United Kingdom, NICE provides evidence-based care guidelines	FREE
Oncology Nursing Society (ONS)	www.ons.org	Provides evidence-based guidelines related to a variety of symptoms	FREE
Google Scholar	http://scholar.google.com	Allows search across many disciplines and sources: articles, theses, books, abstracts, and court opinions from academic publishers, professional societies, online repositories, universities, and other websites	FREE

TABLE 12.2 AN OVERVIEW OF TYPES OF STUDIES AND LEVELS OF EVIDENCE

LEVEL OF EVIDENCE	TYPE OF STUDY	DEFINITION
I (strongest)	Meta-analysis	A method for systematically combining pertinent qualitative and quantitative study data from several selected studies to develop a single conclusion that has greater statistical power. This conclusion is statistically stronger than the analysis of any single study, due to increased numbers of subjects, greater diversity among subjects, or accumulated effects and results.
	Systematic review	A comprehensive review of all relevant clinical studies on a particular subject. The review is created after reviewing and combining all the information from published and unpublished studies into a summary of findings.
	Practice guidelines	A statement produced by a panel of experts outlining current best practice. The statement is produced after an extensive review of available literature.
II	Randomized control study	A study design that randomly assigns participants into an experimental group or a control group. The only expected difference between the control group and the experimental group is the outcome variable being studied.
III	Well-controlled studies without randomization	A study design that similar to a randomized control study with the exception that randomization does not occur. This type of study is weaker than those with randomization; however, the variable under study may not lend itself safely to randomization.
IV (weakest)	Cohort study	A study design where one or more groups (called cohorts) are followed prospectively and subsequent status evaluations with respect to a disease or outcome are conducted to determine which initial participants exposure characteristics (risk factors) are associated with it. As the study is conducted, outcome from participants in each cohort is measured and relationships with specific characteristics determined.
	Case-control study	A study that compares patients who have a disease or outcome of interest (cases) with patients who do not have the disease or outcome (controls) and looks back retrospectively to compare how frequently the exposure to a risk factor is present in each group to determine the relationship between the risk factor and the disease.

the information. In other words, is the available research strong enough, or rigorous enough, to support a change in patient care protocols? Also, can the generated evidence be applied in the nurse's clinical setting? Is the nurse's individual institution willing to adopt change based on their unique situation, availability of resources, and climate of change?

Tools to Evaluate Evidence From the Literature

Appraising research for strength and appropriateness can be intimidating, particularly to the new-to-practice nurse. However, tools exist to aid the interprofessional team in their goal toward EBP. Specifically, several web resources are available to assist the nurse in evaluating evidence from the literature.

The Appraisal of Guidelines for Research and Evaluation (AGREE) II Instrument

The AGREE II Instrument provides a framework to evaluate clinical guidelines (The Agree Next Steps Consortium, 2009). The AGREE II is both valid and reliable and comprises 23 items organized into six quality domains:

- Scope and purpose
- Stakeholder involvement
- Rigor of development
- Clarity of presentation
- Applicability
- Editorial independence (The AGREE II Next Steps Consortium, 2009)

Each of the 23 items targets various aspects of practice guideline quality. The AGREE II also includes two final overall assessment items that requires the appraiser to make overall judgments of the practice guideline as well as consider how they would rate the 23 items. For the purposes of the nurse evaluating clinical guidelines for the implementation of EBP, the AGREE II framework for assessing guidelines provides a valuable, easy-to-use tool. The framework is free of cost and can be accessed on the web at http://www.agreetrust.org. A tutorial is included with the tool.

Critical Thinking 12.2

You are a new graduate nurse working on a medical–surgical unit delivering care to patients. You notice that the IV team nurse makes rounds daily and changes all IV catheters that were placed 3 days ago. When you ask her why this is done, she states, "This has been the policy since I started 3 years ago."

1. What action would be appropriate for the new nurse at this time?
2. How will the new nurse accomplish this?
3. Who might be a good resource for the new nurse?

The Critical Appraisal Skills Program

The Critical Appraisal Skills Program (CASP, 2010) is another available free resource that provides the nurse with tools to interpret research evidence. CASP provides checklists specific to various types of research including randomized control trials, systematic reviews, cohort studies, case-control studies, and qualitative studies (see Table 12.3). The utilization of the checklists provides a framework to determine the strength and reliability of research documents. The CASP tools can be located on the web at http://www.casp-uk.net. The website also provides tutorials for new users.

TABLE 12.3 RESEARCH TERMINOLOGY

TERM	DEFINITION
Case-control study	A study comparing certain characteristics of two study participants in order to identify causes of what makes them different. For example, a case-control study might compare two nursing home patients, one with recurrent urinary tract infections (UTIs) and one who never had a UTI in order to identify aspects that might predict the condition in others—for example, incontinence, immobility.
Clinical practice guidelines (or practice guidelines)	Statements with recommendations to assist health care professionals regarding most appropriate treatment for specific clinical situations. Evidence-based clinical practice guidelines provide the strongest level of evidence to guide practice which is based on systematic reviews of randomized clinical trials or the best evidence on the specific clinical circumstance or situation.
Cohort study	A prospective study of two groups conducted over time in order to collect and analyze data in comparison to one another. For example, a cohort study might examine a group of inner city elementary children through age 18 compared to a similar group in a rural setting.
Integrative review	An analysis of the literature on a specific topic or concept leading to implications for practice.
Meta-analysis	A comprehensive synthesis of studies on a specific topic or concept leading to inferences or conclusions about that area of focus.
Nonexperimental research	A study in which the researcher simply collects and analyzes data based on what is observed about a phenomenon versus what might occur after implementing an intervention.
Outcomes research	A study conducted to measure the effectiveness of an intervention. For example, hospitals frequently conduct outcomes research to document the effectiveness of their services by measuring the end results of patient care for example, infection rates, rates of readmission.
Prospective study	A nonexperimental study that begins with an examination of assumed causes (e.g., high-fat diet) which then goes forward in time to the presumed effect (e.g., obesity).
Qualitative research	A study that examines a phenomenon with words and descriptions rather than statistics or numbers in order to determine underlying elements and patterns within relationships.

(continued)

TABLE 12.3 RESEARCH TERMINOLOGY (*continued*)

TERM	DEFINITION
Quantitative research	A study that examines a phenomenon with numeric data and statistics rather than words in order to determine the magnitude and reliability of relationships between variables or concepts.
Randomized clinical trial (RCT)	A study that uses a true experimental design (research that provides an intervention or treatment to research participants who have been randomly chosen to experimental group or control group where they receive no treatment or intervention).
Systematic review of the literature	A study that examines, critically examines, and summarizes all evidence on a specific topic or concept.

Compiled with information from Melnyk and Fineout-Overholt (2011) and Dicenso et al. (2005).

EVALUATION OF A SYSTEMATIC REVIEW UTILIZING THE CASP TOOL

Locate the following article to be reviewed: Bernard, M. S., Hunter, K. F., & Moore, K. N. (2012). A review of strategies to decrease indwelling urethral catheters and potentially reduce the incidence of catheter-associated urinary tract infections. *Urologic Nursing, 32*(1), 29–37.

Be sure to read the article completely and make sure you understand the purpose of the study. Focus on purpose, methodology, and results. Be sure to determine what type of study this article is discussing (i.e., Randomized control trial, systematic review, cohort study, qualitative study, etc.). Do this *before* you start the evaluation of the study.

Access the appropriate evaluation tool from the CASP website, located at http://www.casp-uk.net. From the CASP homepage, there are links for various checklists based on the type of study to be evaluated. In this example, the study to be evaluated is a systematic review. Click on the appropriate link to access the systematic review evaluation tool. The evaluation tool consists of 10 questions divided into three sections that address whether the results are valid (Section A), what the results are (Section B), and if the results will help with the population of interest to the reviewer (Section C).

Section A

Question 1: Does the review address a clearly focused question?

YES—The article aims to address a very specific question. The authors are investigating a population of hospitalized patients requiring indwelling urethral catheters. The stated purpose is to reduce the incidence of catheter-associated urinary tract infections (CAUTIs). The authors do a thorough job of discussing why this is an important, relevant, and timely topic.

Question 2: Did the authors look for the appropriate sort of papers?

YES—The authors utilized several electronic databases including CINAHL, Medline, Cochrane Database, Google, and Google Scholar to locate potentially appropriate articles. Relevant search terms were used to locate applicable studies.

(continued)

The results of questions one and two indicate that the systematic review should yield valid data.

Section B

Question 3: Do you think the important, relevant studies were included?

YES—A review of 53 abstracts occurred and 44 articles were discarded because they did not address the topic of interest. The remaining nine articles were evaluated. Optimally, the included studies would be randomized clinical trials. However, there are ethical limitations to implementing randomization of interventions to hospitalized patients as potential harm may occur. Therefore, the majority of studies included in the systematic review were quasi-experimental and nonrandomized. This is most likely the best type of data that could be reviewed for the particular topic of interest. Included studies were published from 2003 to 2009, indicating that timely information was utilized. Authors also utilized grey literature to identify abstracts from conferences and presentations that were not published. One potential weakness in this area exists. There is no discussion of consultation with topic experts related to findings.

Question 4: Did the review's authors do enough to assess the quality of the included studies?

YES—There were some inherent weaknesses in the overall systematic review as well as in some of the individual studies that were included. The authors do a nice job of exposing and discussing these weaknesses. First, there were only a total of nine applicable studies to evaluate. Only one of the nine included studies was a randomized controlled study. Six studies did not include confidence intervals (CIs) within their study, making it difficult to evaluate their rigor. The authors point out that the studies took place in four different countries and in a variety of clinical settings. It is unclear whether this enhances or hinders the generalizability of the review. Another potential weakness is a lack of consistency in the definition of short-term catheterization.

All of the studies demonstrated a reduction in the duration of catheterizations. Seven of the nine studies showed a significant reduction in CAUTIs. This finding enhances the validity of the review.

Question 5: If the results of the review have been combined, was it reasonable to do so?

YES—The authors of the systematic review separated the included studies into two categories; nurse-led interventions and informatics-led interventions. This was clearly delineated and discussed in the review. As discussed above, findings within each category and between categories were similar.

Question 6: What are the overall results of the review?

Nurse-led interventions that were effective in reducing the duration of catheterizations and CAUTIs included utilizing various nursing staff to assess, at set intervals, if indwelling urinary catheters were still indicated for patients. The nurse then works collaboratively with the physician to determine if catheter use might be discontinued.

(continued)

Informatics-led interventions were also effective in reducing the duration of catheterizations and CAUTIs. These interventions utilized technology to automatically prompt health care personnel to review and act on individual patients with indwelling catheters.

Question 7: How precise are the results?

Five nurse-led intervention studies were evaluated, all of which demonstrated a decrease in duration of catheterization. CIs were not given for any of the studies. Only four of the studies looked at rates of CAUTIs. All five demonstrated a reduction in CAUTIs, CIs were not reported in any of the studies.

Four informatics-led interventions were evaluated, and results were not as clear as the nurse-led interventions. Three of the four studies demonstrated a reduction in the duration of catheterizations with no CI reported. The fourth study did not evaluate catheterization duration, but instead demonstrated a decrease in inappropriate catheter utilization at a 95% CI. Two of the four informatics-led interventions demonstrated a reduction in CAUTIs while the other two studies found no significant reduction in CAUTIs. No CIs were available.

In statistics, a CI is a measurement of how good, or how accurate a certain parameter is. The high number of included studies without reported CIs weakens the rigor of this systematic review.

Section C

Question 8: Can the results be applied to the local population you are interested in?

The answer to this question is highly variable depending on your specific population of interest. It is impossible to answer this for everyone in this explanation. However, you should take some time to ponder how this systematic review could apply to the health care setting where you work or are performing clinical rotations. Be sure to consider ways this review is appropriate to your particular setting. Also, make sure you consider how this review is not applicable to your health care setting.

Question 9: Were all important outcomes considered?

The studies that were located and included in the systematic review were categorized into nurse-led and informatics-led interventions. The relative low number of studies included indicates that further interventions and appropriate outcomes should be explored. The review met its stated purpose, but additional issues of patient satisfaction, quality of life, cost, and other indices were not included, again indicating areas for future study.

Question 10: Are the benefits worth the harms and costs?

Absolutely none of the included studies demonstrated any harm to patients. Most demonstrated improved outcomes. The few interventions that did not demonstrate improved outcomes also did not demonstrate worse outcomes. This indicates minimal risk for patients.

(continued)

The review did not examine the inherent costs of implementing and monitoring the investigated interventions. The cost would vary at different health care institutions related to unique organizational structures and resources.

Overall, the systematic review was comprehensive and well organized. Limitations to the review primarily stem from limitations in the available research. Potential harms to patients from incorporating any of the suggestions appear to be minimal. For these reasons, these findings, augmented with other research findings, are appropriate to consider when considering a policy change to decrease CAUTIs.

The Health On the Net (HON) Foundation

The Internet allows the nurse, other HCP, or health care consumer to obtain vast amounts of information with relative ease. Unfortunately, it is not always easy to determine which sites and information are accurate and of high quality. The HON Foundation (2012) is a nonprofit, nongovernmental organization dedicated to assisting patients, health care professionals, and web publishers in disseminating and locating high-quality health information. HON offers links to health topics, access to trusted health websites, a HON code certification that identifies high-quality websites as well as other tools. The HON resources can be accessed at http://www.hon.ch.

IMPLEMENTATION MODELS FOR EBP

There are several models for EBP including Titler's (2001) Iowa Model of EBP to Promote Quality Care, the ACE model (Stevens, 2004) with its focus on primary care; and Stetler's (2001) model of Research Utilization. Titler's model of EBP; is most useful in acute care settings where the majority of nurses currently practice (see Figure 12.2).

TITLER'S IOWA MODEL OF EBP

Utilizing Titler's model as a guide, nurses look for knowledge-focused triggers and problem-focused triggers from the external professional environment and the internal health care organization. **Knowledge-focused triggers** are triggers that stem from the research literature, a new philosophy of care, new national standards, or from professional guidelines. **Problem-focused triggers** are triggers that stem from internal identification of a clinical problem. For example, performance improvement and quality data as well as internal and external benchmarking can lead to identification of clinical performance problems. New procedures and treatments driven by technology, as well as by outside regulators can also contribute to the identification of clinical issues. Often these clinical issues are identified at the point of care delivery on patient care units. They are then brought to the unit practice committee and then to the organization-wide practice and quality care committees to be addressed. In conclusion, once a quality trigger is identified, there are five steps nurses can use to implement Titler's Iowa Model of EBP to Promote Quality Care (see Table 12.4).

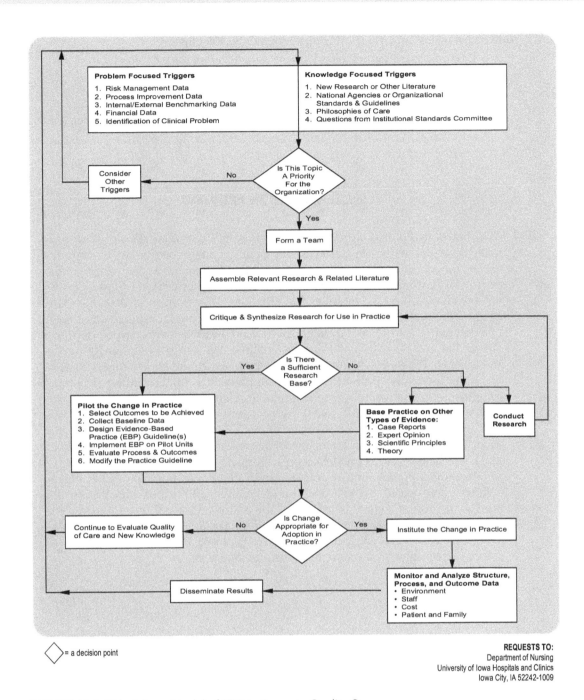

FIGURE 12.2 Titler's Iowa Model of EBP to Promote Quality Care.

Reprinted with permission from Marita G. Titler, PhD, RN, FAAN, and the University of Iowa Hospitals and Clinics, Copyright 1998. For permission to use or reproduce the model, please contact the University of Iowa Hospitals and Clinics at 319-384-9098.

TABLE 12.4 APPLICATION OF TITLER'S IOWA MODEL OF EBP

Step 1: Narrow the focus into a researchable question using the PICO format.
Step 2: Search the literature for what is known about this issue.
Step 3: Critically appraise the evidence.
Step 4: Conduct a pilot project.
Step 5: Evaluate the practice decision and outcomes of the pilot project; determine if the change is to be implemented throughout the entire organization.

REAL-WORLD INTERVIEW

Our shared governance structure includes the EBP committee. This committee is made up of staff nurses and, more recently, clinical nurse specialists. This committee has functioned since the initial days of our shared governance structure in the early 1990s. Currently, the committee meets six times a year where all participants have ready access to the Internet. The EBP committee is supported by the management team with the provision of meals and compensation for the day. Each EBP committee is structured differently based on the unit size and structure. Maria Titler's Iowa Model of EBP to Promote Quality Care, serves as a guide for nurses and other HCPs to use evidence to improve patient care and patient care processes. The Titler model has been incorporated into Bassett's EBP committee structures using evidence that includes internal data. Problems come to the attention of the EBP committee. Problems are generated by continuous performance improvement data, safety and quality issues, regulatory changes, advances in the profession, and science. Internal and external benchmarking with similar practice units in regional acute care facilities act as problem-focused triggers for process improvements.

Anytime a process improvement is indicated, those involved as key stakeholders interested in the process should be engaged and/or educated in the process. If process change is indicated, the interprofessional team explores the change, gathers, and evaluates the relevant data and determines the need to pilot the change or conduct further research of the problem. Evaluation of any change occurs to determine if the change had its intended goal.

Maureen Murray, MS, RN, NE-BC, and Jeanne-Marie Havener, PhD, RN
Bassett Healthcare
Cooperstown, New York

Application of Titler's Iowa Model of EBP

Bassett Healthcare, a Magnet™-designated facility in Cooperstown, New York, utilizes Titler's Iowa Model of EBP to Promote Quality Care to identify and implement EBPs. Bassett Healthcare's Council for the Advancement of Research and EBP is the main vehicle through which nursing standards of practice are developed and updated. Bassett's Council for the Advancement of Research and EBP is an interprofessional council that includes representatives from nursing, the library, the Institutional Review Board (IRB), and a representative of the performance improvement department as standing members. The performance improvement department representative acts as a liaison to other institutional interprofessional teams focused on creating and updating standards of practice based on new evidence. Once a quality trigger is identified, there are five steps nurses can use to implement Titler's Iowa Model of EBP to Promote Quality Care.

Step 1: Narrow the focus into a researchable question using the PICO format (Melnyk & Fineout-Overholt, 2011) described in Chapter 11. PICO is an acronym that stands for population, intervention, compare, and outcome(s). Acronyms help us remember steps in a process and can, thus, enhance quality and safety of patient care. Following PICO, the first steps are to determine the *Population* that you are focusing on and the *Intervention(s)* that you want to find evidence and best practice recommendations about. For example, the nurse in the opening scenario of this chapter may focus on a population of postoperative patients, not including C-sections, with UTIs. The nurse may wish to look at those patients with and without the intervention of an indwelling catheter.

Step 2: Search the literature for what is known about this issue. Review the evidence and compare how one recommended intervention compared to another intervention affects patient outcome(s). The nurses at the nursing practice committee may be interested in comparing which postoperative patients get more UTIs, those with or without indwelling catheters. The nurses may also wish to know if there are more infections when certain brands of catheters are used rather than others. Searching the literature in conjunction with the reference librarian often results in discovering what the state of the science and/or best practice(s) are regarding interventions.

Step 3: Critically appraise the evidence. Using the levels of evidence as described earlier and either the AGREE II or CASP tools, determine the validity and reliability of the results of the research study(s) discovered from your literature search. Then compare what is known from the literature with what the current standard of practice is at your organization. Does the current organizational practice standard incorporate results and recommendations from the literature? If not, evaluate whether or not this recommended evidence should be used by your institution to change policy and the standard of practice. Will

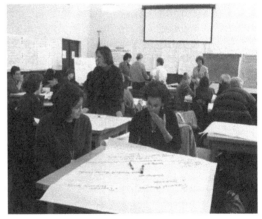

Working as a team to design a pilot study for EBP.

implementing a change improve patient care? If so, in what practice areas should the practice change be implemented?

If there is a difference determined between current organizational practice and what is recommended in the gathered evidence from the literature, an interprofessional team is assembled and a pilot project is often developed to implement and evaluate the implemented change.

Step 4: Conduct a pilot project. Pilot projects are important prior to making a decision to implement a full organizational practice change. Some practices recommended in the research literature will not be appropriate for the entire organization. Pilot projects will tell you the applicability and feasibility of potential changes in specific practice areas (Titler et al., 2001). For example, implementing a new standard of practice for indwelling catheters for postsurgical patients will most likely impact the flow of work on a general surgical unit where a nurse may be caring for six to eight patients differently than it impacts the flow of work in a critical care area where the nurse may be caring for one to two patients. A pilot project discovers what does and does not work. It allows changes to be made prior to implementing the new practice throughout the entire organization. Pilot projects allow staff to celebrate when a new EBP change works and improves patient care and to make course corrections as the implementation occurs. Outcomes discovered in the evaluation of a pilot project can prevent unintended organizational upheaval, thus enhancing the speed of adoption of the change.

Step 5: Evaluate the practice decision and outcomes of the pilot project; determine if the change is to be implemented throughout the entire organization. Determine if the outcomes you desired were achieved. Again, using the indwelling catheter example, we would want to know if there was a decrease in UTIs. Did the new EBP protocol decrease or increase the costs of care? What are other outcomes you might have specified to evaluate the pilot project?

Utilizing Titler's Iowa Model of EBP to Promote Quality Care to guide the pilot project and subsequent implementation process, the team

- Selects outcomes to be achieved from the pilot project, that is, decrease hospital-acquired UTIs.
- Gathers baseline data, that is, the incidence of UTIs in postoperative patients, not including post C-sections, over the past calendar year.
- Designs EBP guidelines, that is, designs a new EBP guideline with supporting references.
- Implements the new EBP on select pilot units for a defined period of time, not to exceed 1 year.
- Evaluates the process and outcomes using formative and summative evaluation.
- Modifies the newly developed practice guideline (Taylor, Lillis, LeMone, & Lynn, 2011).

Through this EBP implementation process, the interprofessional practice team determines whether the practice change is appropriate to implement throughout the entire organization, and/or where modifications need to be made in practice prior to implementation throughout the organization.

REAL-WORLD INTERVIEW

I feel that EBP is not implemented nearly as much as it should be in my facility. Lack of use of EBP in my care area could be due to several factors. Many of the nurses have associate degrees and may have never been educated regarding EBP and its importance. Those who have been educated may be limited by lack of access to good health care resources, lack of time, or even lack of interest. There are times where I see use of EBP being encouraged. A notebook is kept at my nurse's station where articles on various health care topics, often of recent research, are filed for us to read. We are also required to complete a number of PeriFACTS tests along with their accompanying readings each month. The PeriFACTS tests present current findings on issues pertaining to pregnancy and childbirth, therefore providing us with information to implement EBP. We also have yearly Mosby skill competencies to perform, which often include updated information relating to health care practice. These competencies are often outlined and adapted as part of hospital policy, which then reinforces the use of EBP. EBP may also be enforced by requiring documentation of specific EBP interventions, ensuring

(continued)

that they are performed. I would also like to mention how shocked I was to recently have read that the gap between the publishing of research evidence and its translation into practice to improve patient care often takes 17 years (Melnyk & Fineout-Overholt, 2011, p. 9). At this rate, when EBP is finally implemented, the research on which it is based is probably outdated! I understand that there can be many hurdles to leap before many practices can be implemented, but perhaps if we were all more proactive about learning the latest EBP recommendations and less reluctant to change our ways, this timeline could be decreased.

Sarah Stiller, RN
Staff Nurse, St. James Hospital
Hornell, New York

Barriers to the Implementation of EBP

Along the route to full implementation of EBP, additional barriers to change may be encountered due to a lack of resources, including time. There are also people barriers to be aware of such as a lack of trust, fear of the unanticipated consequences of the change, comfort with the status quo, and lack of knowledge about a new practice.

EVIDENCE FROM THE LITERATURE

Citation

Forsman, H., Rudman A., Gustavsson P., Ehrenberg A., & Wallin l. (2010) Use of research by nurses during their first two years after graduating. *Journal of Advanced Nursing*, 66(4), 878–890.

Discussion

To deliver the highest levels of patient safety and quality of care, nurses are expected to develop and utilize evidence-based patient care guidelines. As new-to-practice nurses acclimate to the realities of providing care in hospitals and other health care settings, it is important to discover how research is integrated and applied. As this study reveals, use of research within the first 2 years of graduation remained overall low at only 59%. Interesting, "low users" tended to remain infrequent users of research over the two year long, longitudinal study.

Implications for Practice

The findings of this study show discrepancy between the goal for EBP and the realities of clinical practice. More research is needed to discover better ways to develop appreciation for EBP in nursing education curricula as well as individual and organizational factors that might be modified to increase nurses' use of research.

ROGERS'S (2003) DIFFUSION OF INNOVATION FRAMEWORK

Rogers's (2003) Diffusion of Innovation framework states that new innovations and changes are social phenomena. Rogers states that if a third of any given group adopts a new practice change based on new evidence, then the rest of the group will follow, considering the practice change the norm. There are five steps in Rogers' Diffusion of Innovation framework (Table 12.5).

Nurses can use Rogers's Diffusion of Innovation framework to guide full implementation and adoption of a new EBP. To do this, nurses can first work with staff who are known innovators and early adopters of change. According to Schmidt and Brown (2009), **innovators** are people within an organization who are flexible about change, curious with a sense of inquiry, have good communication skills, and have an awareness of self and the practice unit. Once the innovators are on board, they then appeal to the majority. The early majority will soon adopt the change and the laggards

TABLE 12.5 ROGERS'S DIFFUSION OF INNOVATION FRAMEWORK

STEPS	EXPLANATION	APPLICATION
Knowledge	The change/innovation is described to the decision-making unit (individual, team, or organization) who develops a beginning understanding of the suggested change.	CDC guidelines indicate that urinary tract infections in hospitalized patients are decreased when urinary catheters are inserted only when absolutely necessary and left in for no longer than 48 hours.
Persuasion	The change agent(s) work to develop favorable attitudes toward the innovation/change.	An interprofessional Performance Improvement team provides in-service education to all staff members at initiation of trial of a new evidence-based clinical practice for 6 months on the surgical unit. The Performance team meets with staff every 2 weeks to answer questions and provide support.
Decision	A decision is made to adopt or reject the innovation/change.	Results indicate that over this 6-month period, the number of new CAUTIs on this surgical unit decreased by 50%.
Implementation/trial	The innovation is put in place. Reinvention or alterations may occur.	The new urinary catheter protocol is implemented on all hospital units.
Confirmation	The individual or decision-making unit seeks reinforcement that the decision made was correct, or a decision that was previously made may be reversed.	Over the next 6 months, the rate of CAUTIs decreases by 35%. The new protocol has become the accepted standard of practice.

CAUTI, catheter-associated urinary tract infections; CDC, Centers for Disease Control.

will eventually come along. Some will even turn out to be the greatest proponents of the new practice. Therefore, in conducting a pilot, it is smart to approach a unit with known innovators to start the project. Staff on the practice committee may be able to identify these known innovators.

Plan-Do-Check Model

The Diffusion of Innovation framework is very similar to the nursing process of assessment, planning, implementation, and evaluation (Yura & Walsh, 1988). The Joint Commission on health care organizations describes the decision-making process in a similar but different way. The Joint Commission has adopted Ransom, Joshi, and Nash's (2005) four-step model for the implementation of change. This model is called Plan-Do-Check-Act (**PDCA**), which is a systematic plan to monitor the structures, processes, and outcomes of interdependent systems that affect patient care and patient care delivery. PDCA is a simple and effective framework to use as a guide to monitor the pilot project of the practice change based on current evidence and to guide full implementation of the change in each practice area.

Relying on the PDCA framework, the EBP committee with administration's support develops a *plan* to conduct a pilot project of the EBP change on a unit(s) with known innovators. Then in the *do* phase, the pilot project is implemented. Moving to the *check* phase, the pilot project is checked and evaluated. Then the committee determines the next *action*. This PDCA cycle continues until the practice change is completely implemented in all appropriate areas. For example, the PDCA framework could be utilized to implement a new admissions policy. The hospital may choose to implement the policy on the medicine floor first to evaluate its feasibility before implementing the policy hospital wide.

All nurses can facilitate the implementation of EBP changes. A nurse's willingness to accept a new change is impacted by the nurse's previous experience with change, the nurse's educational preparation, and the length of time and experience the nurse has on the unit where the EBP change will occur. Innovators embracing change stemming from evidence, will find it important to educate nurses regarding the science behind any change, encourage them to let go of their old ideas related to delivering patient care, even if a practice is one that has always been done this way. It is also important to include all interprofessional stakeholders in planning the innovation and value their perspectives.

Nurses can promote a positive attitude regarding innovation and embrace the opportunity to assist in the implementation of EBPs, serving as mentors to others and encouraging inquisitiveness regarding best practices. Enlightened users of EBP can provide encouragement to others as they incorporate innovative change.

Critical Thinking 12.3

As a nurse with 6 months experience on a pediatric inpatient unit, you have developed an interest in how pain control is addressed for pediatric patients. You feel that improvements could be made to provide improved comfort and decreased anxiety for patients and their parents.

1. How will you explore this issue?
2. Who will need to be involved in a discussion related to the issue?
3. Who could help facilitate the discussion?

Practicing in the information age, clinicians are privileged to have the results of scientific evidence at their fingertips through a variety of devices. When considering a change in practice, the issues that arise include:

- Giving up old ways of doing and practicing
- Identifying the best evidence from the many EBP studies reviewed
- Determining the best evidence to use for the patient population in a specific practice setting
- Implementing many new practice changes in an efficient, organized manner.

Titler's Iowa Model of EBP to Promote Quality Care and other EBP frameworks referred to in this chapter are effective guides for professional nurses who choose to take on the challenge of creating an EBP culture with their interprofessional colleagues, promoting safety and quality that lead to excellence in patient care.

KEY CONCEPTS

1. EBP promotes the delivery of optimal health care through the integration of best current evidence, clinical expertise, and patient/family values (QSEN, 2012).
2. Utilizing the Internet as a search tool affords the nurse researcher the ability to obtain vast amounts of current data with relative ease.
3. Collaborating with reference librarians ensures high-quality research-based evidence.
4. A framework for assessing EBP guidelines, such as AGREE II and CASP, provides a valuable, easy to use tool for the nurse evaluating these guidelines.
5. Models such as Titler's Iowa Model of EBP to Promote Quality Care and the ACE model exist to guide the EBP implementation process.
6. PICO is an acronym that stands for population, intervention, compare, and outcome(s) and is used to focus a topic to investigate the literature.
7. Comparing what is known from the literature with what the current standard of practice is at your institution is an important component of EBP. If there is a difference, piloting a change in practice is a needed step.
8. Evaluation of the practice decision and outcomes of a pilot project assist in determining if the change is to be implemented throughout the entire organization.
9. Rogers's Diffusion of Innovation model explains how innovators are key to gaining momentum for a practice change and overcoming resistance to a new standard.

KEY TERMS

EBP	Levels of evidence
Innovators	PDCA
Knowledge-focused triggers	Problem-focused triggers

DISCUSSION OF OPENING SCENARIO

1. How would you find out?

    Narrow the Focus Through a PICO Statement: Following PICO, the first step is to determine the *Population* that you are focusing on and the *Intervention*(s) or practice(s) that you want to find evidence for, and best practice recommendations about. For example, the nurse in the opening scenario may wish to focus on a population of postoperative patients, not including C-sections, with UTIs. She or he may wish to look at those with and without the intervention of an indwelling catheter.

2. What would you do if there was a difference between your organization's practice and the evidence?

    Search the Literature: The nurse at the practice committee may be interested in comparing which postoperative patients get more UTIs, those with or without indwelling catheters. She or he may also wish to know if there are more infections when certain catheters are used than others.

    Appraise the Evidence: Does the evidence indicate that a change in procedure might be beneficial?

    Implementation: Utilizing Titler's model to guide the pilot and subsequent implementation process, the team

   1. Selects outcomes to be achieved from the pilot, that is, decreased hospital-acquired UTIs.
   2. Gathers baseline data, that is, incidence of UTIs in postoperative patients not including post-C sections over the past calendar year.
   3. Designs EBP guidelines, that is, a new practice policy/procedure with supporting references.
   4. Implements the new EBP on select pilot units for a defined period of time not to exceed 1 year.
   5. Evaluates the process and outcomes using formative and summative evaluation.
   6. Modifies the newly developed practice guideline (Taylor et al., 2011).

    Evaluation: The nurse would want to know if there was a decrease in UTIs and did the new protocol decrease or increase the costs of care. What are other outcomes you might have specified to evaluate the pilot?

CRITICAL THINKING ANSWERS

Critical Thinking 12.1

1. How will you, as a new nurse, begin to promote EBP?

    Be inquisitive, observant, and ask questions, seek clarification as to why certain care practices exist in the institution where you work. Be aware of safety issues and outcomes. When you become aware of a potential patient safety or outcome issue, be proactive. Explore the issue. Ask for advice from senior nurses your unit or the nurse educator.

    Explore what options are available to work with the quality improvement groups that exist in your institution. Ask for opportunities to collaborate with more experienced colleagues and participate in the process of exploring and implementing EBP in your place of employment.

2. What contributions can you make to EBP?

Be observant regarding areas of practice that need improvement. Be an innovator and advocate for change. Assist with the development of new procedures within your area of practice. As you become more experienced, be a mentor for newer nurses. Learn to perform literature and evaluate the quality of research effectively.

3. How can nurses help overcome potential resistance to EBP?

Nurses can promote a positive attitude regarding change and embrace the opportunity to assist in the implementation of EBPs. Nurses can serve as mentors to others and encourage inquisitiveness regarding best practices. Nurses can provide encouragement to others as they incorporate change.

Critical Thinking 12.2

1. What action would be appropriate for the new nurse at this time?

The new nurse should search further for the reason behind the protocol.

2. How will the new nurse accomplish this?

Further investigation may include looking at the written protocol, identifying the last revision date, what references were utilized, and their date of publication. You can also identify key personnel who developed the protocol. The nurse could also explore what the current literature shows related to this topic to ensure that the protocol is EBP.

3. Who might be a good resource for the new nurse?

Nurse mentor, nurse educator, nurse manager of the floor.

Critical Thinking 12.3

1. How will you explore this issue?

Examine current literature related to this topic.

2. Who will need to be involved in a discussion related to the issue?

Nurse manager, nurse educator, physicians, pharmacists—this is a multidisciplinary issue and as such requires input from all involved parties.

3. Who could help facilitate the discussion?

Nurse manager or nurse educator.

CASE STUDY ANSWERS

Case Study 12.1

1. Is it appropriate to tell the patient that he needs to do what the physician ordered because dialysis can extend life expectancy?

No

2. Why or why not?

Part of ensuring high-quality care is the use of EBP. Hemodialysis may be the best treatment option to for the patient's condition; however, if the treatment is in opposition to the patient's value system a discussion needs to occur. EBP incorporates not only the latest research and treatments but also the values and desires of the patient.

3. What would be the most appropriate action to take?

Clarify with the patient that he understands the risks and benefits of initiating hemodialysis as well as the consequences of not initiating hemodialysis. Initiate a conversation with the physician responsible for the patient and encourage dialogue between the patient and physician.

Case Study 12.2

1. Since this change is evidence based, do you just keep utilizing the new method despite concerns?

No

2. Why or why not?

The goal of EBP is to improve patient safety and outcomes. If a new procedure is providing questionable outcomes then it needs to be reevaluated.

3. What would be the most appropriate action to take?

Document all concerns that you have noticed and contact your head nurse or person in charge of implementing the new change. Together evaluation of the situation can occur and appropriate adjustments be made as needed to ensure that patient safety and optimal outcomes are obtained.

Case Study 12.3

1. What key factor has most likely hampered your ability to locate relevant information?

Inexperience with literature searches.

2. What is your next step?

Ask for assistance.

3. Who can help you with this?

Institutional librarian, nurse manager, nurse educator, nurse mentor.

REVIEW QUESTIONS

Please see Appendix D for answers to Review Questions.

1. The nurse cares for patients in the surgical unit and has noted that there have been an increased number of nosocomial UTIs for patients on the unit during the past 2 months. The nurse proposes research on comparing postoperative patients with three or more inpatient days and indwelling catheters versus patients with shorter stays and without indwelling catheters. The nurse knows that the next step in formulating the research is which of the following?

A. Outcome
B. Compare
C. Population
D. Intervention

2. The nurse manager is notified that a trauma patient is arriving at the ED with polytrauma sustained in a high-speed rollover accident. The nurse manager utilizes the Benner novice to expert continuum to assign an expert nurse to care for this patient. Which of the following nurses is most likely to be assigned?

A. An RN with a bachelor's degree in nursing and 18 months of clinical experience in the ED
B. A nurse practitioner with a master's degree in nursing and 9 months of clinical experience in the ED
C. An RN with an associate's degree in nursing and 8 years of clinical experience in the ED
D. An RN working on their PhD in nursing with 3 years of nursing research experience on ED outcomes for trauma patients and 1 year of clinical experience in the ED

3. The nurse is giving a presentation to coworkers regarding the patient benefits of adopting policies based on EBP. The nurse includes which of the following in the presentation? Select all that apply.

A. Improved quality of care
B. Improved cost savings
C. Decreased patient satisfaction
D. Decreased lengths of stay
E. Improved patient outcomes
F. Decreased cost savings

4. The nurse cares for a patient who has been diagnosed with reoccurring lung cancer. The oncology unit has a nurse-led support group for improving quality of life for cancer patients. The patient declines participation, stating that he is a private person and is not interested in participating in a group. Which of the following is the best response by the nurse?

A. "The grieving process will bring you through many phases. Many patients experience denial initially. If you change your mind at a later date, let me know."
B. "This program is based on research that found support groups help cancer patients cope with their disease. I think you should come to the next meeting anyway."
C. "I will bring over another patient who says the program has been life-changing so you can make an informed decision."
D. "What types of support have you found helpful in dealing with trying situations in the past?"

5. The nurse is gathering rigorous evidence to study improving outcomes for patients who are at high risk for falls. Which of the following should the nurse *not* use?

A. Clinical practice guidelines

    B. Meta-analyses of randomized, controlled trials

    C. Case studies

    D. Well-controlled trials not utilizing randomization

6. The nurse is involved in a task force to design patient care plans using EBP. Which of the following statements is true regarding EBP?

    A. All patients should receive the same care based on evidence.

    B. Level IV evidence does not have adequate rigor to impact patient care decisions.

    C. Patient values are a key component of EBP.

    D. Given the ease of access to scientific data, EBP can be quickly incorporated into care plan design.

7. The nurse wants to implement EBP in the care of patients on the unit. Order the following actions for appropriate implementation of EBP.

    1. Critically appraise the current evidence.

    2. Narrow the focus of interest into a PICO question.

    3. Implement a pilot project.

    4. Implement a search of the literature.

8. The nurse on the telemetry unit has initiated a pilot project to provide early intervention for arrhythmias by using a dedicated RN for cardiac monitoring in an effort to decrease adverse patient incidents. A nurse from the surgical ICU is interested in adopting this program. What is the best response initially by the telemetry unit RN?

    A. "The program outcomes have not been evaluated yet. We will share the results of the study with your unit when ready."

    B. "The initial results have been fantastic. I will give you the materials so you can share it with your nurse manager."

    C. "You will need to wait until the hospital administrators are satisfied with the cost savings benefits of this program."

    D. "I am not sure that this program is beneficial, and I may prove that change is not needed."

9. The ED nurse reads an article that states that patient morbidity and mortality are increased when patients are given plasma volume expanders in the initial treatment of hypovolemic shock. The nurse is concerned about patient outcomes in the ED as plasma volume expanders are prescribed. What is the best action by the nurse?

    A. Narrow the issue to develop a researchable PICO question.

    B. Give the article to the unit's nurse manager.

    C. Contact the chief of emergency medicine to share concerns about current ED practice.

    D. Propose a pilot program.

10. The nurse performs health screening at the community center. The nurse notes that several of the patients do not use age-appropriate child restraint systems (CRS) to transport their children in an automobile. The nurse knows that the best way to approach this issue is which of the following?

A. The nurse must take into account the individual cultural backgrounds, socio-economic issues, and support structures at play to realize that CRS usage is not always a viable option.

B. Caring is the essence of nursing, and it is the nurse's responsibility to advocate and educate parents regarding correct CRS usage.

C. The nurse should work collaboratively with the patient, other HCPs, and community resources to maximize patient health.

D. The nurse should collaborate with the hospital librarian to locate specific information regarding successful programs aimed at increasing CRS compliance.

REVIEW ACTIVITIES

Please see Appendix E for answers to Review Activities.

1. As a nurse on the medical–surgical inpatient floor, you have noticed several patients have experienced phlebitis at the site of insertion for IV catheters. You start to wonder if there are EBP changes that could be made to decrease the incidence of phlebitis. Develop an appropriate PICO statement for this issue. Choose one of the database resources listed in the chapter and locate a research article that applies to your PICO statement. Analyze the research article that you located and determine its level of evidence.

2. Consider a patient from your own clinical laboratory experience and think of interventions provided for his or her care. What level of evidence supported the care given? Were there clinical pathways or policies in place based on evidence from research? If so, what were they?

EXPLORING THE WEB

1. The Cochrane Collection (http://www. cochrane.org) produces systematic reviews and other types of evidence reports. Holdings can be searched by topic or key word.

2. The Joanna Briggs Institute (http://www. Joannabriggs.edu.au) produces systematic reviews, evidence summaries, and best practice series that tend to be nursing focused. Holdings can be searched by topic or key word.

3. Access a few of the resources outlined in Table 12.1. What terminology is consistently used by multiple resources?

4. Go to the following website to further develop your knowledge of evidence-based health care: EBM Education Center of Excellence, North Carolina: http://library. ncahec.net.

REFERENCES

The AGREE II Next Steps Consortium. (2009). *Appraisal of guidelines for research and evaluation II instrument*. The AGREE Research Trust. Retrieved from http://www.agreetrust.org

Balas, E. (2001). Information systems can prevent errors and improve quality. *Journal of the American Medical Informatics Association, 8*(4), 398–399.

Benner, P. (1984). *From novice to expert: Excellence and power in clinical nursing practice*. Menlo Park, CA: Addison-Wesley.

Burnett, F. H. (1911). *The secret garden*. New York, NY: Simon & Brown.

Critical Appraisal Skills Program (CASP). (2010). Checklists. Retrieved from http://www.casp-uk.net

Dicenso, A., Guyatt, G., & Ciliska, D. (2005). *Evidence-based nursing: A guide to clinical practice*. St. Louis, MO: Elsevier Mosby.

Forsman, H., Rudman A., Gustavsson, P., Ehrenberg A., & Wallin, L. (2010). Use of research by nurses during their first two years after graduating. *Journal of Advanced Nursing, 66*(4), 878–890.

Gallup, Inc. (2010). *Nurses top honesty and ethics list for 11th year*. Retrieved from http://www.gallup.com/poll/145043/Nurses-Top-Honesty-Ethics-List-11-Year.aspx

Health On the Network (HON) Foundation. (2012). *HONtools for medical professionals*. Retrieved from http://www.hon.ch

Leininger, M., & McFarland, M. (2006). *Culture care diversity and universality: A worldwide nursing theory* (2nd ed.). Sudbury, MA: Jones and Bartlett Publishers.

Melnyk, B., Fineout-Overholt, E., Stillwell, S., & Williamson, K. (2009). Igniting a spirit of inquiry: An essential foundation for evidence-based practice. *American Journal of Nursing, 109*(11), 49–52.

Melnyk, B. M., & Fineout-Overholt, E. (2011). *Evidence-based practice in nursing & health care. A guide to best practice*. Philadelphia, PA: Lippincott, Williams & Wilkins.

Olsen, L., Aisner, D., & McGinnis, J. M. (Eds.). (2007). *The learning health care system: Workshop summary (IOM roundtable on evidence-based medicine)*. Washington, DC: The National Academies Press.

Quality and Safety Education for Nurses (QSEN). (2012). *Evidence-based practice*. Retrieved from http://www.qsen.org/definition.php?id=3

Ransom, S. B., Joshi, M. S., & Nash, D. B. (2005). *The health care quality book: Vision, strategy, and tools*. Chicago, IL: Health Administration Press.

Rogers, E. M. (2003). *Diffusion of innovation* (5th ed.). New York, NY: Free Press.

Stetler, C. B. (2001). Updating the Stetler model of research utilization to facilitate evidencebased practice. *Nursing Outlook, 49*, 272–279.

Stevens, K. R. (2004). *ACE star model of EBP: Knowledge transformation*. Academic Center for Evidence-based Practice. The University of Texas Health Science Center at San Antonio. Retrieved from http://www.acestar.uthscsa.edu/acestar-model.asp

Taylor, C. R., Lillis, C., LeMone, P., & Lynn, P. (2011). *Fundamentals of nursing*. Philadelphia, PA: Lippincott, Williams & Wilkins.

Titler, M. G., Kleiber, C., Steelman, V. J., Rakel, B. A. Budreau, G., Everett, L. Q., . . . Goode, C. (2001). The IOWA model of evidence-based practice to promote quality care. *Critical Care Nursing Clinics of North America, 13*(4), 497–509.

Yura, H., & Walsh, M. B. (1988). *The nursing process: Assessing, planning, implementing, evaluating*. Norwalk, CT: Appleton & Lange.

SUGGESTED READING

Carter, M. J. (2010). Evidence-based medicine: An overview of key concepts. *Ostomy Wound Management, 56*(4), 68–85.

Fineout-Overholt, E. (2008). Synthesizing evidence: How far can your confidence meter take you? *AACN Advanced Critical Care, 19*(3), 335–339.

Gerrish, K., McDonnell, A, Nolan, M., Guillaum, Y., Kirshbaum, M., & Tod, A. (2011). The role of advanced practice nurses in knowledge brokering as a means of promoting evidence-based practice among clinical nurses. *Journal of Advanced Nursing, 67*(9), 2004–2014.

Lamb, J., & Zavinskis, I. (2008). Kangaroo care: Making the leap to an evidence-based practice. *American Nurse Today, 3*(3), 13–15.

McNett, S. (2012). Teaching nursing psychomotor skills in a fundamentals laboratory: A literature review. *Nursing Education Perspectives, 33*(5), 328–333.

Militello, L. K., Kelly, S. A., & Melnyk, B. M. (2012). Systematic review of text-messaging interventions to promote healthy behaviors in pediatric and adolescent populations: Implications for clinical practice and research. *Worldviews on Evidenced-Based Nursing, 9*(2), 66–77. doi:10.1111/j.1741–6786.201100239.x

Rauen, C., Vollman, K., Arbour, R., & Chulary, M. (2008). Challenging nursing's sacred cows. *American Nurse Today, 3*(4), 23–26.

Van Achterberg, T. Schoonhoven, L., & Grol, R. (2008). Nursing implementation science: How evidence-based nursing requires evidence-based implementation. *Journal of Nursing Scholarship, 40*(4), 302–310.

Wishin, J., Gallagher, T. J., & McCann, E. (2008). Emerging options for the management of fecal incontinence in hospitalized patients. *JWOCN, 35*(1), 104–110.

13

THE FUTURE ROLE OF THE REGISTERED NURSE IN PATIENT SAFETY AND QUALITY

Jerry A. Mansfield

If we only improve care as much in the next decade as we have in the last, we are failing the American public. (Sebelius, 2011)

Upon completion of this chapter, the reader should be able to

1. Discuss movement toward the future of health care
2. Describe the future transformational leadership role of the nurse
3. Explore leadership commitment to listening to the voice of the nurse
4. Discuss quality improvement (QI) and patient safety in the future
5. Discuss patient-centered care (PCC) in the future
6. Review evidence-based practice (EBP) in the future
7. Support the role of the registered nurse (RN) as a full member of the interprofessional team in the delivery of high-quality and safe patient care in the future
8. Review the importance of informatics use by the health care team of the future
9. Discuss advances in implementing *The Future of Nursing: Leading Change, Advancing Health* and the Future of Nursing/Campaign for Action
10. Identify health care strategies for getting from here to the future

You recently accepted a job as a medical–surgical nurse in a 350-bed community-based hospital about 200 miles from where you graduated from nursing school. In your nursing leadership course, you learned a great deal about how current health reform would impact future health care delivery in the United States. Now that you have started your new nursing position, you are curious as to how your hospital is preparing for the future in this era of health reform.

- *Who could you talk to or what resources could you review to learn more about how your hospital is preparing for health care reform and potential changes in future patient care delivery?*
- *How does your hospital compare with other hospitals in your geographical area in the areas of quality and safety in patient care?*
- *How satisfied are patients who receive treatment at your facility?*
- *What actions could you take to facilitate future change in patient care delivery within your own nursing unit?*

The current nursing workforce (2,824,641 RNs and 690,038 licensed practical nurses [LPNs]) is large (Health Resources and Services Administration [HRSA], 2013). Based on nurses' regular contact with patients and their families and their proximity to patients across the continuum of patient care, the RN is a unique partner with other health professionals in creating a preferred future for health care in the United States (Institute of Medicine [IOM], 2011c).

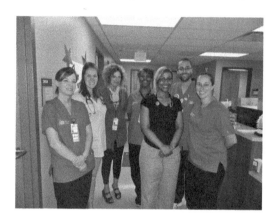

Patient-centered Medical Home interprofessional team at The Ohio State University Wexner Medical Center.

Health care as an industry continues to evolve through many changes and these changes will affect nursing and nursing education in the future, for example, patient demographic changes and increased diversity of patient populations, continuing technological and informatics explosion, globalization of the economy and society, the educated consumer-driven era, population-based care, increased cost of health care and managed care challenges, influence of health policy and regulation, need for interprofessional collaboration and education, need for workforce development and the nursing shortage, and advances in nursing and health care science and research. The eyes, ears, and voice of over 2.5 million RNs are well positioned to improve the quality and safety of patient care in the midst of all this change. Nurses, transformational nursing leadership, and the interprofessional team are evolving toward the future of ever improving patient care using concepts of PCC, teamwork, informatics, EBP, safety, and quality.

This chapter discusses the movement toward future health care and the role of transformational leadership in transitioning nursing and the health care team toward a preferred future. It explores leadership commitment to listening to the voice of the nurse and discusses QI, patient safety, PCC, and EBP in the future. The chapter reviews the role of the RN as a full member of the interprofessional team in the delivery of high-quality and safe patient care in the future and the importance of informatics use by the health care team. Finally, the chapter discusses *The Future of Nursing: Leading Change, Advancing Health* and the Future of Nursing/Campaign for Action and identifies health care strategies for getting from here to the future.

MOVEMENT TOWARD FUTURE HEALTH CARE

Americans have grown up in a health care system that operates largely within a controlled economic system, rather than a free market. A **free market** is a market where the price of a good or service is mutually determined by at least two people or groups of people; people agree to pay a price for either a commodity or service. The transaction is mutually agreed to by both parties rather than by governmental regulation (Rothbard, 2008). In a free market, if an individual consumer wants a service, they will shop for that service based on price, quality, and availability. This does not happen in a controlled economic system like health care. Payment for health care in this controlled economic system has stemmed primarily from multiple third-party payers, for example, the government, insurance companies, and so on. Health care services have been provided to the patient (first party) by health care clinicians and hospitals, and so on (second party). These clinicians and hospitals (second party) have billed their services to multiple third-party payers (Figure 13.1). This controlled economic system has led in the past to high-administrative costs in the U.S. system and decreased patient involvement in the search for cost-effective price, quality, and availability.

Americans are becoming more aware than ever of what happens in our health care institutions. Patients are beginning to hold all health care providers more accountable for the care they individually and collectively provide as a health care team. Governmental payers and insurers are increasingly demanding reimbursement

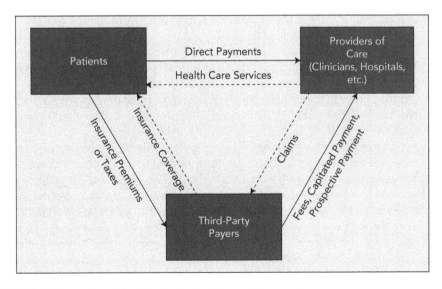

FIGURE 13.1 Economic relationships in the health care delivery system.
Source: Jonsson (1989).

changes based on measureable clinical outcomes. Also, the following free market forces are beginning to push for changes in health care payment (Binder, 2012):

- Consumer-driven health plans (CDHPs): Employees in these health plans with very high deductibles, often in the thousands of dollars, are being advised to navigate the health system to get the best prices and quality (Binder, 2012).
- Reference pricing: Employers have begun stating a price they will pay for certain health care services and letting employees pay the difference if they choose a higher cost provider. Currently, it is not uncommon for the price of a particular health care service to vary sixfold or more, depending on who delivers it, with little or no difference in quality to explain the price difference (Binder, 2012).
- National and global shopping for health services: Employers are offering employees options to travel within the United States or even abroad for services such as heart bypass surgery, transplants, and other complex procedures (Binder, 2012).
- Hospital Value-Based Purchasing Program (HVBPP): The Centers for Medicare and Medicaid Services (CMS) will make value-based incentive payments to acute care hospitals based on how well hospitals perform on certain quality measures such as care provided to patients discharged from acute care with acute myocardial infarction (AMI), community-acquired pneumonia (PN), and heart failure (HF; Binder, 2012).
- In addition, hospitals may receive incentive payments for results from patient satisfaction scores (e.g., Hospital Consumer Assessment of Healthcare Providers and Systems [HCAHPS]; CMS, Retrieved from http://www.cms.gov/apps/media/press/factsheet.asp?Counter=3947) .

Nurses in the future can expect to see more incentive-based payment programs from CMS as additional health care conditions, processes of patient care and outcomes become part of the value-based purchasing program. Other insurance providers are also beginning to add their own incentive-based programs much like the federal government. By preventing hospital-acquired conditions such as patient injury due to falls and hospital-acquired pressure ulcers (HAPUs) or enhancing the patient's experience of the hospital stay, nurses can help the hospital improve its overall performance and enhance the ability of the organization to avoid losing money in value-based purchasing arrangements (Binder, 2012).

More and more patients and consumers are accessing information on the Internet to help them make informed decisions about where they want to receive their health care. Information about quality and all of these payment changes increases consumer power to make their own decisions on price and quality, which in turn drives the health care market in a different direction than a controlled economic health care system.

Currently, there are gaps between what patients should receive in the delivery of care and the care they actually do receive. In a review of health care data, the Agency for Healthcare Research and Quality (AHRQ) identified 18 potentially preventable adverse events and complications—for example, central line–related bloodstream infections, deep vein thrombosis, pressure ulcers, and so on—that patients may experience through contact with the health care system (Zrelak et al., 2011). Nurses, in many cases, are the patient's last line of defense against these adverse events and broken care delivery work processes. For example, many patients in hospitals today are at risk of developing HAPUs. These HAPUs, if not documented as "present-on-admission" (i.e., the patient's pressure ulcer was identified by the nurse during the admission assessment and acknowledged by the physician) will be noted as a complication of the hospitalization. Even though the care of a patient with a pressure ulcer costs more to treat as compared with patients without pressure ulcers, the hospital does not receive a higher payment for such a condition as HAPUs. Nurses and interprofessional teams can put health care processes in place to ensure that patients who are at high risk do not develop skin breakdown (e.g., frequent turning schedules, ensuring adequate nutrition, frequent assessment, and accurate documentation of skin integrity, etc.). Nurses with knowledge of HAPU prevention are in an excellent position to recommend changes to improve the quality of care.

FUTURE TRANSFORMATIONAL LEADERSHIP ROLE OF THE NURSE

Porter-O'Grady and Malloch (2011) identify tomorrow's transformational nursing leaders as leaders who "create a new and improved system that allows individuals to contribute to their fullest potential to deliver the most effective health care possible" (p. 375). Transformational nursing leaders in the future will facilitate the development of highly reliable organizations and a culture of safety. They will further develop skills of improved communication, rapport, dialogue, conflict resolution, and consensus building to positively change the patient care delivery process of the future and ensure that all six Quality and Safety Education for Nurses (QSEN) elements of quality and safety, that is, QI, safety, informatics, PCC, teamwork and collaboration, and EBP (QSEN, 2012), are delivered (Table 13.1).

Health care leaders in the future are nurses, administrators, physicians, pharmacists, dieticians, respiratory therapists, rehabilitation specialists, and so on. All have a personal responsibility to work together as a team to ensure quality and safety of patient care. As mentioned earlier, the frequency and proximity of nurses in the delivery of patient care across the continuum positions nurses and nursing leadership to use firsthand knowledge and experience gained from observing active errors or mistakes and unsafe conditions or potential errors at the unit or department level to improve patient safety. However, knowledge and experience alone will not provide the greatest improvement in patient safety. It is only by changing patient care work processes and monitoring outcomes of patient care that nurses and other members of the health care team will impact today's complex health care environment. Nurses at all levels of an organization, for example, nurse leaders and managers, staff nurses, and so on, must be actively involved, not only in providing and monitoring the daily delivery of patient care, but also in sharing information to set up an environment for high-quality care delivery and prevent errors from occurring beyond their home unit or department. This information can be shared at the local, state, and national level. Shared governance, nursing practice councils, and involvement at upper levels of management in decision making, all work to create a high-level nursing presence (Sieg, 2009). Errors that happen in one clinical unit along with the steps implemented to reduce future occurrences may be useful information to share with other units in a hospital or clinic. Failure to share best practices and lessons learned across all clinical care areas may reduce the possibility of catching or preventing a repeat error. This results in patient harm that could have been prevented.

THE VOICE OF THE NURSE

The voice of the nurse is critically important in current health care practice to inform health care changes that will prevent errors in the future. Aiken (2012) states, "Organizational sociology proposes that a really good way to understand organizations is not so much to ask the people at the top what goes on, such as the elites in the

TABLE 13.1 FUTURE TRANSFORMATIONAL NURSING LEADERSHIP ROLE IN SUPPORTING QSEN QUALITY AND SAFETY ELEMENTS

QSEN QUALITY AND SAFETY ELEMENT	FUTURE TRANSFORMATIONAL LEADERSHIP ROLE
Quality improvement (QI)	• Monitor clinical, patient satisfaction, financial, and other outcomes to improve quality • Review health care rating systems. Strive to be number 1! • Benchmark with other high-performing health care organizations to improve patient care • Transfer knowledge and best practices from internal patient care departments that have shown positive health outcomes for patients and families to other patient care departments
Safety	• Structure the design of work and the health care work space to reduce error • Create and sustain health care processes to develop a culture of safety • Build flexibility into staffing models to ensure that appropriate care providers are on hand to respond quickly to an unscheduled event • Accept that errors do occur and shift from a culture of blame to a just culture in which error is perceived as an opportunity for improvement by both individuals and the total health care system • Monitor patient and staff outcomes
Patient-centered care (PCC)	• Develop policy to enhance transparency in patient care delivery • Develop more opportunities to involve patients in their care, that is, more education programs, patient satisfaction surveys, bedside hand-offs/rounds, mutual goal setting, and so on. • Reframe the work of health care to enhance partnerships between patients, families, and providers • Encourage all staff and patients to manage their own health effectively • Monitor patient outcomes for satisfaction, safety, respect, access, clinical outcomes, and so on.
Evidence-based practice (EBP)	• Support EBP • Adopt evidence-based management and leadership practices • Review evidence-based practice guidelines from professional organizations
Teamwork and collaboration	• Develop rapport with all team members and maximize the capability of the interprofessional team • Adopt TeamSTEPPS; Crew Resource Management (CRM); and/or situation, background, assessment, and response (SBAR) practices to build interprofessional teamwork • Utilize safe patient handoff communication
Informatics	• Create an environment for informatics and EBP that includes increased access to computers, librarians, continuing education programs, QI and safety information, and so on • Utilize electronic health records and other computer tools to improve documentation, monitor patient outcomes, and improve clinical decision making

Developed with information from Porter-O'Grady and Malloch (2011) and Institute of Medicine (2004).

organization, but to ask the people who really work in the main part of the organization, the people who come in contact with everyone, and use them as informants about the organization. What better informants are there, particularly in hospitals but also in health care in general, than nurses, because they are in close proximity with patients and families and with doctors?" The voice of the nurse, heard when nurses participate in patient care, hospital committees, and hospital structures, as well as when nurses monitor and improve care based on data about patients and their outcomes, will guide future patient care. Accurate assessment of patients by a RN and other health care providers along with accurate and timely data entry into electronic health records (EHRs) will help establish the evidence of what works to improve patient care delivery and patient outcomes. Ensuring that nursing assessment, patient data/findings are documented timely and accurately are foundational steps in preparing future clinical decision making as technology continues to advance in hospitals and clinics. The IOM has set a goal that by 2020, 90% of clinical decisions will be supported by accurate, timely, up-to-date information and will reflect the best available evidence (IOM, 2011a).

EVIDENCE FROM THE LITERATURE

Citation

Russell, D., Rosati, R., Rosenfeld, P., & Marren, J. (2011). Continuity in home health care: Is consistency in nursing personnel associated with better patient outcomes? *Journal for Healthcare Quality: Promoting Excellence in Healthcare*, 33(6), 33–39.

Discussion

A growing body of evidence suggests that patients who receive coordinated and uninterrupted health care services have better outcomes, more efficient resource utilization, and lower costs of health care. This study examined the relationship between consistency in nursing personnel and three patient outcomes: hospitalization, emergent care, and improvement in activities of daily living. After analyzing data from a large population of home health patients ($N = 59,854$), this study found that having the same staff care for patients on regular follow-up visits decreased the probability of patient hospitalization and emergent care and increased the likelihood of improved patient functioning in activities of daily living between admission and discharge from home health care.

Implications for Practice

This study provides an example of how data is collected and analyzed. The data shows enhanced outcomes when patients are cared for by consistent caregivers. This is an example of how data informs future practice and highlights that nurse leaders must work to ensure that patient care assignments are made in such a way as to ensure that the same staff work with the same patients as much as possible.

QI IN THE FUTURE

While all nurses have a professional obligation today to develop and improve the delivery of care in their practice, the future demands it! Nurses must develop rapport and partner with interprofessional team members and take responsibility for setting up a quality nursing care environment for patients with appropriate health care structures (environment), processes (guidelines, staffing), and monitoring of patient outcomes. Nurses of the future must work as members of an interprofessional team and identify problems in the delivery of patient care, use new QI tools to improve care, generate ideas to improve the patient care process, implement the necessary steps, track changes over time and make the necessary adjustments to ensure improvement and sustainability. Interprofessional teams are effective in improving quality of care. QI initiatives are more likely to result in sustained improvements if teams remain intact and if the teams continue to review and analyze data from the project (Hulscher, Schouten, Grol, & Buchan, 2012). All forms of QI projects can serve to support change in patient care delivery. Most of these projects involve health care teams who identify clinical problems, design innovative solutions, conduct small-scale tests of change, reflect on the outcomes achieved, and guide further action. For today's RN, participation and leadership in such projects is the form of action taken (Berwick, 2011, p. 326).

REAL-WORLD INTERVIEW

Florence Nightingale reminded us that "no system can endure that does not march. In today's health care environment, are we marching toward the future or retreating to the past? For us who Nurse, our Nursing is a thing, which, unless in it we are making progress every year, every month, every week, take my word for it, we are going back" (McDonald, 2004). For more than 100 years, the science and discipline of nursing has continued to be shaped by our efforts to continuously improve our practice. Now, more than ever, improving our practice is critical to improving health outcomes for the patients and families we serve. Nursing's focus on illness prevention and maintenance of health and its oversight in the continuum of care uniquely positions us to make a great impact on patient care quality and safety. Nurses detect and describe potential safety issues inherent in everyday work and are actively involved in creating and testing interventions to prevent patient harm. Specific nurse-sensitive indicators continue to emerge, highlighting how the practice of nursing directly correlates with patient outcomes. The impact of nursing care on the prevention of injury related to falls and pressure ulcers cannot be denied. The impact of nursing continues to grow and the growing public interest in reporting quality and safety measures will make the impact of nursing care even more visible to the society we serve.

Margaret M. Calarco, PhD, RN
Senior Associate Director for Patient Care Service and Chief of Nursing Services,
The University of Michigan Health System
Adjunct Professor, University of Michigan School of Nursing
Ann Arbor, Michigan

Critical Thinking 13.1

You have been asked to participate on a QI team in your work setting. You decide to seek out the latest information regarding how to be an active committee member. Go to the following AHRQ website: http://teamstepps.ahrq.gov. Note the discussion of TeamSTEPPS (AHRQ, 2012a).

1. Click on About TeamSTEPPS to explore the three phases of TeamSTEPPS at the website. Are you ready for TeamSTEPPS?
2. How would you know if your organization is ready to implement Team-STEPPS?

PATIENT SAFETY IN THE FUTURE

As discussed in Chapter 3, health care organizations are becoming highly reliable organizations that are working to become blame free, just cultures of safety for patient care. Clancy (2011) states, "An organization's patient safety culture exerts a powerful influence on many endeavors, including its efforts to identify behaviors, assumptions, or omissions that can lead to medical errors" (p. 193). Health care organizations are developing error detection systems that contribute to organizational learning. Organizational learning best occurs when health care team members work together to understand how patient care is delivered and what can be done to improve the process and thus enhance patient safety and quality. Organizational learning starts with systems thinking, realizing that a change in one part of the system affects other parts of the system. Organizational learning shares a vision for high-quality and safe patient care and encourages collaboration to improve patient care. When science, informatics, incentives, and culture are aligned for continuous improvement and innovation—with best practices embedded in the care delivery process and new knowledge gained as a by-product of the care delivery experience—the organization is learning (IOM, 2011a)!

By gaining new insights into change processes about how care is delivered and the outcomes produced by that care, interprofessional team members can help a health care system prevent future errors and ensure systemic changes that alter the basic circumstances in which the original error occurred. When individuals report honest mistakes, they must not be blamed for those mistakes. An organization can benefit more by learning from mistakes than they can benefit from blaming people who make errors. Clinicians currently may not report health care errors due to a fear of the unknown or due to a lack of faith that something meaningful will happen if they do report an error (Dekker, 2007, p. 41). The following example illustrates that errors can be reduced and performance improved when teams work together:

Abington Memorial Hospital, Abington, Pennsylvania
- Fewer adverse events and deaths: A 27% decline in inpatient adverse events and a 30% decline in hospital mortality rate.
- Proactive rescue of at-risk patients: Codes (i.e., code blue) called outside of critical care decreased suggesting that unit staff members improved their ability to recognize and communicate early warning signs of respiratory failure and cardiac arrest.
- Better hand hygiene: Hand hygiene compliance rates increased to 80% in 2010 from 41% in 2007.

- Improved staff perceptions of teamwork and communication: Nurse surveys conducted before and after implementation of TeamSTEPPS education found that the average score on questions related to teamwork, communication, leadership, responsibility for patient safety, support, and trust rose from roughly 3 to 4 points (on a 5-point Likert-type scale) across all units (Mimm, 2013).

REAL-WORLD INTERVIEW

Pharmacists and nurses collaborate to achieve drug therapy outcome goals that include:

- Administering the right drug and the right dose at the prescribed time
- Assuring proper quality controls for medications
- Accurately recording patient medication lists
- Providing appropriate education on risky medications to prevent side-effects or possible complications that lead to harm

Pharmacists and nurses also collaborate to assure that medications are dispensed correctly, often using unit-based medication cabinets or automated dispensing devices (ADDs) that store common medications. Other medication administration collaborative activities between pharmacy and nursing include developing policies and procedures for safe administration of medications and narcotics in ADDs. Policies and procedures on proper and safe administration of IV preparations are also often developed by a pharmacy/nursing team.

Many hospitals use bar-code medication administration (BCMA). Pharmacists and nurses develop safe medication administration processes to make sure that all medications are scanned for correctness and that BCMA alerts are correctly interpreted. Pharmacy and nursing also collaborate on making sure that patients' medication lists are accurate and that patients understand the use and side effects of their medications. This involves a collaborative team of pharmacists and nurses to observe and map out the medication workflow process and coordinate efforts to get a patient's medication history along with assuring that patients have access to medications at discharge. Pharmacists and nurses also participate in follow-up discharge phone calls to patients that help to reinforce valuable information about medications and prevent an adverse drug event.

Robert J. Weber, PharmD, MS, BCPS, FASHP, FNAP
Senior Director, Pharmaceutical Services
The Ohio State University Medical Center
Columbus, Ohio

PCC IN THE FUTURE

PCC is built on the principle that the individual patient should be the ultimate decision maker when it comes to what type of treatment and care they receive (IOM, 2011c). Individualizing the patient's plan of care to coordinate goals, interventions, and outcome measurements that are shared by all members of the interprofessional team can enhance the achievement of outcomes.

PCC in the future will increasingly be delivered in a growing number of nonhospital settings such as patient-centered medical homes, home care, telehealth, hospice, and other ambulatory settings. There will be expanding roles for nurses who help patients and their families navigate the health care system and coordinate their care across a variety of settings. Complexity in patient care will grow with advances in biotechnology, human genome mapping, and an ever-increasing capacity to predict disease and prevent illness.

Predictive, Preventive, Personalized, and Participatory Medicine (P4 Medicine)

P4 Medicine (i.e., medicine that is predictive, preventive, personalized, and participatory) is emerging out of the convergence of systems biology, the increasing activation of networked consumers, and the digital revolution in communications and information technology (IT; P4 Medicine Institute, 2012). For example, "predictive" medicine may include using the results from a genetic test to determine the risk a patient may have for a particular health problem. "Preventive" medicine could include encouraging patients and families to get an annual influenza vaccination during flu season. Hood, Balling, and Auffray (2012) envision a future where each patient will be associated with a virtual data cloud of billions of data points (e.g., height, weight, medications, diseases, lab values, hospitalizations, vital signs, etc.). As a result, examining the patients' "personalized" needs and patterns compared with others can generate hypotheses about health and/or disease for each individual patient. While care coordination has always been a part of nursing practice, the complexity of patient care in the future will increasingly require the RN to solicit patient "participation"; the nurse should assertively manage the coordination of the patient's care and serve as a patient/family advocate. In the future, the nurse will have access to much more data and information about each individual patient, which will ultimately enhance the continuity of care and communication among the interprofessional team.

Future Marketing and Nursing

Future nurses can contribute to PCC by reflecting on their unique contribution to the patient's experience. Consider if you, as a hospitalized patient, were to personally pay each day for direct nursing care, what would you "value"? Do patients want what nurses offer? Do patients really know what nurses offer in the provision of high-quality, safe nursing care? Do nurses know what patients want and need? How can nurses more effectively market themselves or their nursing services? Product, placement, promotion, and price are four classic elements of marketing (The Times 100, 1995–2013). Upon introducing oneself to a patient, a nurse shares with the patient that the nurse will monitor the patient's vital signs, listen to his lungs, check circulation in his legs and arms, watch for any unexpected complications, and ensure the highest level of quality and safe care for the next 8, 10, or 12 hours (product). This will help the patient recover from a surgical procedure on a medical–surgical floor (placement). Through this introduction, and answering the patient's questions and concerns, the nurse is "promoting" the service being provided to the patient. The price is the amount the patient pays for the product. Currently, the "price" in many hospitals is part of the room charge billed to patients. In the hospital of the future, as well as in some nurses' practices, this may change. Nurses of the future will consider, does each nursing unit or department address the product needs of a different market or group of patients? What do nurses know about their patients (i.e., customers) regarding demographics, conditions, or responses to actual or potential health problems? Consider how should nursing and health care services be paid for by patients? Answers to these and other questions will expand nursing in the future (Table 13.2).

The Health of the RN in the Future

The health of the RN in the future is also very important in PCC. The choices that nurses make, related to both personal health and professional health, impact the costs of health care and the quality of nurses' lives and the lives of their patients. For example, nurses can stop smoking and help patients stop smoking. Nurses can play an important role in helping patients and themselves live healthier lifestyles. A recent meta-analysis showed that adults with four or more healthy behaviors, compared with people who have an unhealthy lifestyle (e.g., smoking, excessive alcohol consumption, no physical exercise, unhealthy diet, obesity) have a 66% lower risk of death (Loef & Walach, 2012). In public polls, nurses are rated as having the highest honesty and ethical standards compared to other professions (Gallup, 2012a). However, another recent poll regarding healthy lifestyles of nurses is less positive! According to Gallup (2012b), physicians are in better health and have better health habits than nurses and the employed adult population. In the poll, a higher percentage of nurses had high blood pressure, depression, smoked, were obese, and had diabetes (Gallup, 2012b). So there is work to do in improving the health status of nurses in America. Nurses could help reduce overall health care costs and enhance their own health and well-being if they promoted healthy lifestyles (Table 13.3), both for themselves and for the patients to whom they provide nursing care.

EBP IN THE FUTURE

As more research is conducted, the amount of information available for development and implementation of evidence-based clinical care guidelines and protocols to ensure high-quality patient care in every setting increases. Balas (2001) noted that it takes an average of 17 years for clinical research to be fully integrated into everyday practice. The health care system of the future must do better than this. The interprofessional team of clinicians must review the literature and together develop clinical practices to ensure that patients receive the most current and safe care possible.

The nurse of the future may encounter barriers in practicing evidence-based care, for example, resistance from colleagues, nurse leaders and managers, and others (Melnyk, Fineout-Overholt, Gallaher-Ford, & Kaplan, 2012). Belonging to professional organizations that support EBP—for example, ongoing education, resources and guidelines to support EBP, continuing formal education at the undergraduate and/ or graduate level, supportive cultures that promote informed clinical practice, and so on—is useful. The Oncology Nursing Society (http://www.ons.org) is one source of resources and tools to help the nurse, for example, online EBP resources and links to national and international sources for systematic reviews/meta-analyses and guidelines; online courses on how to critique nursing research articles; and topics for putting evidence into practice, for example, anorexia, fatigue, sleep–wake disturbances, and so on (Mallory, 2010).

TABLE 13.2 EXPANDED ROLES AND IMPLICATIONS FOR FUTURE NURSES

FUTURE GROWTH	IMPLICATIONS FOR FUTURE NURSING
Telehealth and ambulatory settings	• Telehealth: Expanded roles for the registered nurse in helping patients manage chronic illnesses in their home setting via telemedicine. Telemedicine is also used by hospitals without specialty services (e.g., evaluation of patients with a stroke or psychiatric needs, etc.) and allows access to health care specialists in remote locations. Nurses in the future need to ensure that they are familiar with how to work with this technology and assure quality for their patients and families. • Ambulatory settings: There is a growing need to increase the number of registered nurses who work in clinics, community health and wellness programs, serving as care coordinators or navigators, and helping patients and families access acute care, and other community services to meet their health and illness needs.
Biotechnology	• Registered nurses in expanded roles are needed for biotechnology research in treating debilitating and/or rare diseases. Nurses are needed to provide care to patients undergoing clinical trials for new medical devices, equipment, pharmaceuticals, and so on.
Human genome mapping	• Nurses need to be experts at obtaining comprehensive family histories in order to facilitate the identification of family members at risk of developing disease, reduce the potential for genomic influenced drug reactions, helping patients understanding genetic tests and results as well as referring patients and families to experts in genetics for assessment, treatment, or follow-up.

TABLE 13.3 HEALTH AND WELLNESS TOPICS FOR REGISTERED NURSES

Diet	Dietary Guidelines for Americans, 2010, http://www.health.gov/dietaryguidelines/2010.asp Read the latest evidence regarding food groups, Nutrition Evidence Library, 2013, http://www.nel.gov
Exercise	Physical Activity Guidelines for Americans, 2008, http://www.health.gov/paguidelines/default.aspx
Body mass indicator (BMI) calculator	http://www.cdc.gov/healthyweight/assessing/bmi/adult_bmi/english_bmi_calculator/bmi_calculator.html
Sleep	Sleep guidelines, http://www.cdc.gov/sleep/about_sleep/how_much_sleep.htm
Tanning beds	Avoid tanning beds, http://www.ncbi.nlm.nih.gov/pmc/articles/PMC3004589
Smoking	How to quit smoking, http://www.cdc.gov/tobacco/quit_smoking/how_to_quit/index.htm Smoking cessation materials, http://www.cdc.gov/tobacco/quit_smoking/cessation/index.htm
Drugs and alcohol	Alcohol, http://www.cdc.gov/alcohol/index.htm Persons who use drugs, http://www.cdc.gov/pwud

Compiled with information from Health Information for Individuals and Families. (2013). Retrieved from http://www.health.gov/; http://www.cdc.gov/HealthyLiving/, and other websites identified in table above.

There are also excellent resources on the Internet to support EBP. The AHRQ website has a variety of resources including nursing research findings to support the translation of science into practice on such topics as the following:

- How EHRs improve nursing care
- Coordination and patient safety
- Drug–drug interactions, responding to call lights, end of life skills, and so on (see AHRQ, 2013; Nursing Research, Research Findings, http://www.ahrq.gov/professionals/clinicians-providers/resources/nursing/ahrq/ra/index.html

THE INTERPROFESSIONAL TEAM IN THE FUTURE

The nurse of the future must establish positive working relationships within interprofessional health care teams and ensure the coordination of care for each patient and the patient's family. In addition, the RN can educate members of the public on the role of the RN in patient quality and safety, patient comfort, assessing and treating patient responses to actual or potential health problems, and prevention of errors, and poor care decisions.

Hassmiller describes how Florence Nightingale, with her commitment to evidence and education for nurses, worked with others to achieve change, that is, "she used her existing relationships with influential people. She worked through respected colleagues in the military, business and even the monarchy. She was friends with the Queen of England. It was through these relationships that Nightingale advanced her cause for better data, quality care, an improved health care system, and the nursing profession" (Adams, 2011, p. 395).

REAL-WORLD INTERVIEW

As the chief quality and patient safety officer for an academic medical center of over 1,100 beds, 1,100 physicians, and 3,000 nurses, engaging the team is truly essential. While this sounds as if it is easy to do, it is not. One of the biggest misconceptions is that the word "team," renders a team whole. Contrary to popular belief, a team is a dynamic concept that must come together voluntarily. Fundamental to this team dynamic is that they must have a common concept or goal that unites them.

Nurses and doctors working together as a team to continuously improve PCC is a perfect example of a very powerful but potentially fragile team. There are a few ground rules that are absolutely essential for this often-underappreciated team to be successful. First, the team must have a common purpose and establish clear rules and expectations. This is often difficult in the ever present hierarchy of medicine and nursing. This hierarchy is one which we must work on together to break down to work in a more horizontal fashion. Second, there must always be a leader of the team. The leader of a team must be receptive to ideas and truly a facilitator in his or her role. Dictatorship is not acceptable for a truly

(continued)

successful leader. Third, a team must have a process to execute their goal, that is, a playbook by which to implement change and this must be explicit, not implied. Fourth, solid relationships are necessary. Not everyone should think alike; this is not the way to make change and continuously improve. Solid relationships make new ideas acceptable and worthy of consideration. Lastly, a team is only as good as the communication that exists. Nurses and physicians communicate differently. Recognition of this will only strengthen the relationships that are the key to the team being successful.

Susan D. Moffatt-Bruce, MD, PhD, FACS
Chief Quality and Patient Safety Officer
Associate Professor of Surgery
The Ohio State University
Columbus, Ohio

CASE STUDY 13.1

John is a nurse on a cardiovascular unit in a large academic health care center working on a team that cares for patients with congestive heart failure (CHF). John heard in a staff meeting that the readmission rate for CHF patients at the hospital was higher than the national benchmark. An interprofessional team is to be formed to examine the care of previously discharged patients with CHF from the hospital who were readmitted within 30 days of discharge posthospitalization.

1. *What is the role of the nurse in participating on an interprofessional team to reduce readmissions for patients with CHF?*
2. *What other interprofessional team members could be involved in the work group?*

INFORMATICS IN THE FUTURE

Increasingly, health care systems are investing in informatics including EHR and clinical intelligence decision-making tools to promote safer patient care. As more hospitals and providers use EHRs, the ability to access and share information quickly and accurately across care settings can promote high-quality and timely care. In the future, IT will provide reminders to nurses and other providers of important health care interventions. For example, reminders for preventive services such as mammograms, vaccines, and colonoscopies can be electronically triggered by a patient's age, gender, or preexisting risk factors for certain illnesses (Table 13.4).

EHR documentation communicates patient status and outcomes to the entire health care team. Accurate patient assessment and documentation of those assessment findings promotes effective and efficient team collaboration and development

TABLE 13.4 WAYS IN WHICH INFORMATICS PROMOTE SAFE PATIENT CARE

- Provides documentation systems that reflect actual patient care work processes
- Supports clinician assessment and work organization
- Integrates provider order entry, medication administration, and documentation
- Includes a professional practice framework that helps clinicians handle large amounts of data, thus increasing clinical intelligence and promoting decision making in complex clinical situations
- Integrates standards-based organizing frameworks such as Nursing Interventions (NIC), Nursing Outcomes (NOC), and North American Nursing Diagnosis Association (NANDA; Müller-Staub, 2009)
- Develops complex and comprehensive database for patient and health care research
- Includes "alerts," "pop-ups," evidence-based "clinical practice guidelines," and "protocols" to guide caregivers in clinical intelligence decision making and documentation

Compiled with information from Benner, Malloch, and Sheets (2010).

(Zrelak et al., 2011). In a retrospective review of malpractice claims between 2008 and 2010 involving nurses, 61% of individual nurse errors were determined to be failure to assess or monitor (Painter, Dudjak, Kidwell, Simmons, & Kidwell, 2011). It is important that nurses accurately document assessment findings and monitor patient outcomes and response to health care interventions.

Clinical Intelligence

EHRs provide a way for all health care providers to document patient care in automated data entry fields and contribute to clinical intelligence that becomes a resource for changing future care delivery. Clinical intelligence is the electronic aggregation of accurate, relevant, and timely clinical data into meaningful information and actionable knowledge (Harrington, 2011). Cinical intelligence data provides an opportunity to analyze the data from all patients, all treatments, and all variations of treatments, along with all variables of care and all patient outcomes. This data analysis process can help develop new patient standards of care and improve patient decision making and outcomes. For example, some patients who are discharged from the hospital are at risk for readmission. The CMS are evaluating hospital readmission patterns for a growing number of conditions (e.g., CHF, AMI, hip and knee replacement, chronic obstructive pulmonary disease). EHRs collect patient information about treatment of patients with these conditions or surgeries. Statisticians are developing algorithms that electronically scan patient information (e.g., How many medications does the patient take? Does the patient live alone? What is the patient's age and socioeconomic status?) in the EHR database and alert clinicians which patients may be at risk for readmission to the hospital. Once the health care team knows which patients are at risk for readmission, the team can implement targeted health care interventions to prevent unnecessary readmissions after discharge. Examples of interventions to prevent patient readmissions include patient education about medications, signs and symptoms to watch for, timely follow-up appointments with health care providers postdischarge, and thoroughly answering all questions that patients and families may have about the treatment plan and follow-up.

Using Clinical Intelligence

Data about the care provided to patients, pain scores, heart and lung sounds, skin integrity, and clinical outcomes can be electronically documented in an EHR by an RN or other member of the health care team. This data, when captured electronically in the EHR, is available for clinical intelligence retrieval to support better clinical decisions for research, clinical outcomes, and resource and supply planning. An interprofessional team can analyze this clinical intelligence data to investigate how to improve patient care for a group of patients. The team could also extract data information on a wider population of patients and then examine the data for patterns and trends. The data can be aggregated or grouped together and analyzed to improve the delivery of care.

Effect of EHRs on Patient Safety

EHRs that capture data entered by clinicians do not automatically guarantee patient safety or health care staff efficiency. As an example, poor human–computer interactions or loss of data, errors in medication dosing, failure to detect life-threatening illnesses, and delays in treatment have led to serious injury and death (IOM, 2011b). The IOM has recommended that the Department of Health and Human Services (DHHS), which is responsible for coordinating the development and promoting the use of national Health IT, establish a mechanism that both EHR vendors and users can use to report deaths, serious injuries, or unsafe conditions that result from using technology systems (IOM, 2011b). To improve the overall quality and safety of EHRs, the Office of the National Coordinator (ONC) for Health IT recently released the Health IT Patient Safety Action and Surveillance Plan. The key objectives of the plan are to (a) use Health IT to make patient care safer and (b) continuously improve the safety of health IT (DHHS, 2013). It is believed that patient safety and quality care can be improved if there are consistent ways in which hospitals and health care systems document and report errors through the use of electronic records.

Other New Technologies

The future will also provide other new technologies with which nurses can help patients better manage their own health. For example, Moss (2011) recently outlined advances in IT, biology, and engineering, such as the "inconspicuous wireless sensors worn on your body and placed in your home… to monitor your vital signs and track daily activities that affect your health, counting the number of steps you take and the quantity and quality of food you eat… to measure your levels of arousal, attention, and anxiety… your bathroom mirror will calculate your heart rate, blood pressure, and oxygen level" (Moss, 2011). RNs today can explore various applications (apps) on their iPhones (e.g., Nexercise [www.nexercise.com]), remind ME Health & Fitness [www.appbrain.com], Cardiograph [https://itunes.apple.com/us/app/cardiograph-heart-rate-pulse/id441079429?mt=8], etc.). These apps provide ongoing monitoring of personal key health indicators. Nurses of the future should be prepared to help patients use available technologies while ensuring that the online tools or apps used provide accurate and timely information that is useful to patients and families and not harmful.

These new technologies will promote the movement of health care outside traditional settings such as hospitals and clinics and into everyday lives. In the past century, such technological advances may have seemed like something out of a space-related television program, but not anymore. The nurse of the future will work within health care environments that develop and test new technologies constantly.

THE FUTURE OF NURSING: LEADING CHANGE, ADVANCING HEALTH AND THE FUTURE OF NURSING/CAMPAIGN FOR ACTION

The Robert Wood Johnson Foundation (RWJF)/IOM report, *The Future of Nursing: Leading Change, Advancing Health* (IOM, 2011c), clearly articulates what should be done to improve the health of the U.S. population specifically through nurse-led efforts in daily practice. It outlines a path for the nursing profession and asks that all nurses participate to create a preferred future for American health care.

The report states:

- Nurses should practice to the full extent of their education and training.
- Nurses should achieve higher levels of education and training through an improved education system that promotes seamless academic progression.
- Nurses should be full partners, with physicians and other health professionals, in redesigning health care in the United States.
- Effective workforce planning and policy making require better data collection and an improved information infrastructure.

The Future of Nursing/Campaign for Action

The Future of Nursing/Campaign for Action launched in November 2010, shortly after release of the IOM Report, *The Future of Nursing: Leading Change, Advancing Health*. The Future of Nursing/Campaign for Action is working to transform health care through nursing by mobilizing coalitions representing nurses, other health providers, consumers, educators, and businesses. Backed by the RWJF and AARP, the Campaign for Action is driven by evidence-based recommendations from the IOM. Nurses can help create the future by reviewing and joining statewide initiatives at the Campaign for Action (Initiative on the Future of Nursing, 2011). Nurses can view the Campaign for Action initiatives on the website in four main areas: practice, education, leadership, and workforce. Examples of contemporary evidence on the Initiative on the Future of Nursing website includes the quality of care provided by advanced practice registered nurses, the value of nursing education and residency programs, success stories in community health, and information about the expansion of retail health clinics.

HEALTH CARE STRATEGIES FOR GETTING FROM HERE TO THE FUTURE

The cost of health care in the United States has risen to unprecedented levels while unfortunately our health outcomes do not exceed those of other developed countries who spend much less (The Commonwealth Fund, 2011; Davis, Schoen, & Stremikis, 2010; Truffer et al., 2010). The United States is now focused on comprehensive health care reform. The momentum that is building nationally to change the delivery of health care as outlined in the IOM *Future of Nursing* report provides a great way for nurses to get involved (IOM, 2011c). The beginning nurse should watch for opportunities to learn more and get involved within their own hospitals and health care settings with team-based care, implementation, and evaluation of health IT, QI/cost control, prevention of hospital-acquired conditions (e.g., central line–associated bloodstream infections, patient falls with injury, wrong site surgery, etc.), and efforts to improve communication, coordination, and collaboration among patients, families, and other health care providers. All of these areas are critical to improving the delivery of care to patients in this era of national health reform.

The Patient Protection and Affordable Care Act (PPACA)

The PPACA provides for a variety of new changes to facilitate health care reform to gain a better handle on costs of health care delivery and outcomes of care. Health care reform changes include

- Ensuring that more Americans have access to quality affordable health care
- Prohibiting denials of health care coverage based on preexisting health care conditions
- Helping young adults by requiring insurers to permit coverage of dependents until the age of 26
- Expanding Medicaid to millions of low-income Americans
- Investing in preventive care

To make these health care reform changes, the federal government is requiring health care organizations to enhance the delivery of health care services and will reward organizations with additional money for significant QIs when compared to other health care organizations for similar care. Many of these changes and reforms in health care provide opportunities for nurses (Table 13.5).

HVBPP

One of the newer ways the federal government intends to enhance the quality of care in the future is called HVBPP. The HVBPP intends to revamp the federal payment system that historically rewarded hospitals based primarily on volume of patient services, rather than quality performance of services. Formerly, hospitals were paid by governmental payers on either a "fee-for-service" or fixed payment model (i.e., Diagnosis-Related Groups [DRGs]). In the future, HVBPP will reward hospitals that deliver high-quality care. In 2013, HVBPP will distribute money to hospitals based on their overall performance on a set of quality measures linked to improved clinical processes of care and patient satisfaction (HealthCare.gov, 2012). As quality performance measurement and pay-for-performance (P4P) efforts become an integral part of the fabric of health care, data and information will be used increasingly to leverage performance improvement and accountability (VanBuren, 2012). Hospital performance measures such as Core Measures, for example, AMI, PN, and HF, are already publicly reported on the Internet (http://www.hospitalcompare.hhs.gov). The importance of nurses taking an active role to improve the care of patients with the health care conditions that are currently monitored will grow as the number of conditions that hospitals are required to monitor grows. For example, outcome measures proposed for monitoring in 2014 may include 30-day mortality rates for AMI, PN, and HF (Park & Hiller, 2011). In addition, errors and treatment of errors that occur with hospitalized patients, for example, falls that result in severe injury, HAPUs, and

TABLE 13.5 SELECTED HEALTH CARE REFORM OPPORTUNITIES FOR NURSING

PPACA HEALTH REFORM	DESCRIPTION	NURSING OPPORTUNITY
Pay-for-performance	Performance on 42 core quality measures is linked to annual hospital bonus payment	Ensure that hospitalized patients receive all the excellent care they should receive for conditions such as acute myocardial infarction, community-acquired pneumonia and heart failure.
Patient hospital readmission penalty	Portion of Medicare Severity Diagnosis-Related Group payment is withheld from hospitals with higher than average patient hospital readmission rates	• Screen patients for risk of hospital readmission, for example, patients who are older, have a higher number of medications, live alone, and so on. • Work with nurses, case managers, social workers and the community to ensure quality patient care postdischarge.
Bundled payments	Medicare payments are combined into a single lump sum shared by hospitals, inpatient physicians, and post-acute care providers. One payment is made by the government for all pre, intra, and posthospitalization care.	• Nurses should work with the interprofessional team to reduce duplication of unnecessary tests and procedures and eliminate waste in the delivery of care to patients to reduce the overall costs of care.
Accountable care organizations	Group of health care providers create a formal structure to deliver health care to a patient population and collectively share in the achieved cost savings	• Participate in discussions in the organization around accountable care. • Help manage diseases in the lowest cost settings. • Redesign how patient care is delivered in various settings. • Develop new systems for patient care delivery. • Explore new ways to deliver preventive services. • Develop ways to live healthy lifestyle for self and patients.

Compiled with information from Advisory Board Company (2010).

catheter-associated urinary tract infections (CAUTIs), and so on, will not be reimbursed by the CMS. Nurses can make a difference by ensuring that patients get all of the care that they should receive so that the CMS audits of patient care demonstrate that patient care was delivered as promised and that patient care given is documented in the health care record. In addition to documenting patient care, nurses must work with other interprofessional team members and provide interventions for patients at risk for hospital-acquired conditions and work to prevent harm to patients while they are hospitalized. In the future, the RN can expect more and more patient conditions to be monitored with resultant reimbursement impacts under these HVBPP strategies. Greater transparency in care with more information being shared with patients plus increased reimbursement to hospitals that "outperform" their peers will help ensure future resources to enhance the quality of patient care.

Critical Thinking 13.2

To increase your knowledge of future legislation affecting nursing, go to the Library of Congress site, http://thomas.loc.gov/home/thomas.php. Review the site and then enter the word "nursing" in the Search Bill Summary and Status box. Choose one of the bills and read either the Text of Legislation or the Congressional Research Service Summary.

1. Are you in favor of the bill?
2. Will it improve patient care?

Accountable Care Organizations (ACOs)

Any nurse who will work in future health care should become familiar with concepts such as an ACO. An **ACO** is a formal network of doctors, hospitals, and health care providers that will share the responsibility of providing health care to all the patients enrolled with the ACO (Advisory Board Company, 2010). By law, the ACO must manage the care of at least 5,000 Medicare beneficiaries for a 3-year term. What does that mean for nursing? The most significant opportunity for nurses in future ACOs will be to proactively and effectively coordinate the care of patients across all levels and types of services (Jones, 2011). Nurses work in a variety of health care organizations (e.g., hospitals, health care insurers, practitioner offices, community health organizations, clinics, surgery centers, etc.) and are often in a good position to improve patient care delivery across these various settings. Opportunities for nurses in communities or health systems that are developing strategies to become or participate in an ACO are likely to grow in the following areas:

• Care coordinator/case manager
• Disease manager
• Health coach
• Community outreach coordinator
• Data analyst
• Discharge/transition planner (Jones, 2011).

The ACO will ultimately reward patients who access preventive care services, reduce unnecessary use of emergency rooms, and reduce unhealthy behaviors, for example, smoking, alcohol, lack of exercise, and so on. Nurses in the future have an opportunity to lead these health care efforts because of their education and experience in helping patients respond to health and illness.

The beginning nurse should look for a career in hospitals and other health care settings that provide strong clinical leadership, allow the nurse to participate in developing an achievable vision of the future, take risks, and innovate to improve quality and efficiency of how care is delivered. By actively participating in organizations with the characteristics described above, a nurse and the overall nursing profession is more likely to contribute to health reform that benefits patients and families into the future (Buerhaus et al., 2012).

Nurses in Various Settings

In the ambulatory setting, RNs "are uniquely qualified, autonomous providers of patient/family-centered care that is ethical, evidence-based, safe, expert, innovative, healing, compassionate, and universally accessible" (AAACN, 2011, p. 96). In rural settings, the safeguarding work of RNs includes "anticipating problems and emergencies and being prepared; careful watching, surveillance, and vigilance; negotiating safety; being able to act in emergency situations; and mobilizing emergency transport systems" (MacKinnon, 2011, p. 119).

By actively participating in all settings in every organization to improve quality, enhance safety, provide PCC, use the best available evidence, work through excellent teamwork and collaboration, and utilize informatics, nurses will facilitate change. By facilitating change, nurses will also use lessons learned in the process to enhance future improvements in health care delivery. By experiencing these changes firsthand, nurses will advocate for better health care, not only within their organizations and health systems but also by sharing best practices and advocating for policy change at the local, state, and federal level. The future is developing as we speak! Seize the moment!

Critical Thinking 13.3

You are concerned with future development of your nursing practice of the QSEN competencies below.

QSEN COMPETENCY	PERSONAL FUTURE GOAL	PATIENT'S GOAL
PCC		
Safety		
Quality improvement (QI)		
EBP		
Informatics		
Teamwork and collaboration		

1. What is a personal goal for your future development in each of the six competencies?
2. What do you think your patient's goals are in each of the competencies? Ask someone who has been a patient.

KEY CONCEPTS

1. Nursing must be a part of planning and participating in health care strategies for getting from here to the future.
2. Transformational leadership helps promote quality and safety in health care delivery systems.
3. The voice of the nurse can inform health care changes that will prevent errors in the future.
4. There are multiple national initiatives geared toward improving future patient safety, PCC, EBP, teamwork and collaboration, informatics, and QI.
5. Nursing and the interprofessional team, supported by a culture of safety where all are encouraged to learn from mistakes, will be in a good position to facilitate the journey toward a future health care system.
6. Accurate patient assessment and documentation of assessment findings promotes effective and efficient team collaboration, particularly when using EHRs.
7. The RN is a full member of the interprofessional team in the delivery of high-quality and safe patient care now and in future patient-centered and accountable care initiatives.
8. The Future of Nursing/Campaign for Action is working to transform health care by mobilizing coalitions representing nurses, other health providers, consumers, educators, and businesses.
9. Backed by the RWJF and AARP, the Campaign for Action is driven by evidence-based recommendations from the IOM.
10. Health reform offers opportunities for nurses to lead efforts to transform health care and promote health care environments that provide safe, high-quality patient care.
11. Opportunities for future nurses to improve care may include strategies related to P4P, patient hospital readmission penalties, bundled payments, and ACOs.
12. Health care payment reform strategies such as HVBPP will impact how hospitals are paid in the future. Nurses should expect to see more publicly reported data on hospital patient outcomes.
13. The nurse of the future will likely perform most nursing documentation of patient care using EHRs. Such patient care data, stored in large databases and subsequently analyzed, will facilitate future evidence-based decision making, clinical practice, and research.
14. Nurses need to take advantage of future opportunities to learn about new ways to deliver preventive services in new and existing settings. Nurses should also explore opportunities to learn more about how to live healthy lifestyles, both for themselves and for their patients.
15. Nurses now must begin to set future goals for safety, PCC, EBP, teamwork and collaboration, informatics, and QI.

KEY TERMS

ACO
CI
Free market

DISCUSSION OF OPENING SCENARIO

1. Who could you talk to or what resources could you review to learn more about how your hospital is preparing for health reform and potential changes in future patient care delivery?

    As a new nurse, some of the questions/thoughts identified below could have been part of your initial interview with your new supervisor! It is important to know the mission, vision, and values of the organization and what community or population of patients they serve currently as well as plans for future patient services. Note what newspaper articles have been posted from hospital administration and/or health care providers in the local media news or newspaper regarding advances in health care to meet current and future needs of patients in the surrounding community? Does the organization have relationships with skilled nursing facilities, home care agencies, durable medical equipment companies, and so on? Does the hospital have a strategic plan that you can review and get a copy? Does the strategic plan talk about health reform and what the organization intends to do in order to meet future demands for care?

2. How does your hospital compare with other hospitals in your geographical area in the areas of quality and safety in patient care?

    To compare your hospitals performance in quality and safety patient care access Hospital Compare, http://www.medicare.gov/hospitalcompare. Select at least two hospitals for comparison. Graphs and data are available among the following categories:

    - Patient satisfaction survey results
    - Timely and effective care
    - Readmissions, complications, and death
    - Use of medical imaging devices
    - Medicare payment
    - Number of Medicare patients

3. How satisfied are patients who receive treatment at your facility?

    You can learn how satisfied patients are who receive treatment at your facility via the same website (Hospital Compare, http://www.medicare.gov/hospitalcompare) under "Patient Survey Results."

4. What actions could you take to facilitate future change in patient care delivery within your own nursing unit?

    Once you know what your hospital is doing to prepare for the future of health care delivery, you could volunteer to be a part of hospital focus groups or committees and help create solutions to current problems. By creating more efficient and effective ways to deliver nursing care and reducing waste and/or redundancy, you are helping the hospital save money and resources for investment in other patient care projects and programs. If you care for a particular patient population (e.g., patients with orthopedic problems), and you know that Medicare/Medicaid will start evaluating patient outcomes/readmissions for total hip and total knee replacements, there are several potential projects you could work with other hospital staff to prepare for. For example:

1. How well are patients prepared to take care of themselves after discharge?
2. Do patients understand their exercise, mobility restrictions, medications, diet?
3. What is the main reason patients are readmitted postdischarge from your nursing unit?
4. What changes can the interprofessional team make that facilitate patient/family participation in mutual goal setting and care planning?
5. What is the best way to provide evidence-based care to a particular patient population that reduces complications, prevents readmissions, and offers the best possible patient experience?

Get involved and help change happen!

CRITICAL THINKING ANSWERS

Critical Thinking 13.1

1. Click on About TeamSTEPPS to explore the three phases of TeamSTEPPS at the website. Are you ready for TeamSTEPPS?

   TeamSTEPPS can help QI teams to effectively address problems in patient care delivery in health care organizations. The team should include representatives from areas involved in any QI efforts and must work to understand the clinical implications of any proposed change in practice and what the consequences of any change may have on other areas or departments. Even though senior leadership may not be directly involved in the delivery of care, they do provide advice, oversight, and resources to assess, plan, implement, and evaluate any planned QI changes. It is sometimes helpful to have an "executive sponsor" from the hospital's leadership team available to the team who can facilitate the acquisition of resources. The Institute for Healthcare Improvement (IHI) website offers a variety of tools and examples to help QI teams and team members. Be sure to explore the website to learn more about QI.

   TeamSTEPPS is a three-phase process aimed at creating and sustaining a culture of safety with

   - A pretraining assessment for site readiness
   - Training for onsite trainers and health care staff
   - Implementation and sustainment

2. How would you know if your organization is ready to implement TeamSTEPPS?

   You would know if your organization is ready to implement TeamSTEPPS by reviewing the strategies of TeamSTEPPS Phase 1—Assess the Need. The goal of Phase 1 is to determine an organization's readiness for undertaking a TeamSTEPPS-based initiative. Such practice is typically referred to as a training needs analysis, which is a necessary first step to implementing a teamwork initiative. For more information about conducting a needs assessment, review Details of a Site Assessment (http://teamstepps.ahrq.gov/about-2cl_3.htm# PIAN).

Critical Thinking 13.2

1. Are you in favor of the bill?

    When you go to the site and choose one of the bills you will have access to all Library of Congress Pending Bills Summary and Status. The information found will tell you the bill name and number, the sponsor, date introduced, any co-sponsors, which congressional committees are reviewing the bill, and the latest major action on the bill. Review the bill carefully to determine if you are in favor of the bill.

2. Will it improve patient care?

    Review the bill carefully to determine if it will improve patient care.

Critical Thinking 13.3

1. What is a personal goal for your future development in each of the six competencies?

    A personal goal for future development in each of the six competencies will vary from nurse to nurse. Consider how to develop yourself in each of them.

2. What do you think your patient's goals are in each of the competencies? Ask someone who has been a patient.

    Your patient's goals in each of the six competencies will vary from patient to patient. Be sure to ask someone who has been a patient. It is critical that patients receive patient-centered, evidence-based, safe care and that the interprofessional team collaborates and uses informatics and quality improvement to help achieve this.

CASE STUDY ANSWERS

Case Study 13.1

1. What is the role of the nurse in participating on an interprofessional team to reduce readmissions for patients with CHF?

    The role of the nurse in participating on an interprofessional team to reduce readmissions for patients with CHF includes such things as developing rapport with the interprofessional team, reviewing QI data about these patients, taking appropriate actions to reduce the readmissions, and so on.

2. What other interprofessional team members could be involved in the work group?

    Other interprofessional team members that could be involved in this work group include physicians, case managers, physical therapists, dieticians, pharmacists, rehabilitation unit staff, emergency room staff, discharge unit staff, and so on.

REVIEW QUESTIONS

Please see Appendix D for answers to Review Questions.

1. Transformational leadership is an essential component to drive positive change in future health care delivery. Select the best example below of the use of transformational leadership to support safety.

    A. Discuss patient safety issues at staff meetings.

    B. Accept that errors do occur and shift from a culture of blame to a just culture in which error is perceived as an opportunity for improvement.

    C. Notify all staff members when a safety event occurs.

    D. Let the nurse manager know when you witness any staff member providing unsafe patient care.

2. In health care settings that are creating new models of PCC delivery, who should be the ultimate decision maker regarding the care of the patient?

    A. The patient

    B. The RN

    C. The physician

    D. The patient's attorney

3. RNs should take an active role in the development and implementation of evidence-based clinical practice guidelines. What resource should be used by the nurse to ensure future care is based on the best available evidence?

    A. Unit-based staff meeting minutes

    B. The Internet

    C. Professional nursing organizations (e.g., Oncology Nursing Society, American Academy of Ambulatory Care Nursing, etc.)

    D. Members of the interprofessional team

4. Health care organizations around the country are investing in EHRs. Which of the following is the best way that an EHR promotes safe patient care?

    A. Ensures all of the patient information is entered the same way by every nurse

    B. Computer-based charting is easier to read than handwritten documentation

    C. Notifies management when a nurse forgets to document patient care

    D. May include a professional practice framework that helps clinicians handle large amounts of data and promotes decision making in complex clinical situations

5. If patient data is recorded in an EHR and stored in a clinical data repository, the data can later be analyzed to improve quality and safety of care for more patients in the future. Select the best term that describes the electronic aggregation of accurate, relevant, and timely clinical data and transforms the data into meaningful information and actionable knowledge?

    A. Clinical intelligence

    B. Root cause analysis

    C. Evidence-based practice

    D. Quality improvement

6. Preventing hospital readmissions is a health care reform opportunity for future nurses. How can nurses prevent unnecessary hospital readmissions?

    A. Screen patients "at risk" for readmission (e.g., older patients, patients with a higher number of medications, etc.) and work with case managers and social workers on the discharge plan of care.

    B. Document that the patient states understanding of any discharge teaching.

    C. Provide medication information handouts to the patients' family members.

    D. Give the patient/family the nursing unit phone number so that the patient can call with any questions after discharge.

7. An example of a national initiative geared toward improving future quality and safety in patient care delivery is which of the following?

A. Patient satisfaction scores
B. HVBPP
C. EBP
D. Shared governance

8. A formal network of doctors, hospitals, and health care providers that share responsibility for providing health care to all patients enrolled within that network is known as which of the following?

A. Health care system
B. Patient-centered medical home
C. ACO
D. Academic medical center

9. Patient outcome measures proposed for quality monitoring in the year 2014 may include 30-day mortality rates for certain health care conditions. Which of the following diagnoses are included in quality monitoring by the CMS? Select all that apply.

A. Diabetes
B. AMI
C. PN
D. Asthma
E. Congestive heart failure
F. Stroke

10. The PPACA (2010) provides a variety of new changes to facilitate health reform, reduce health care costs, and improve outcomes of patient care. Which of the following health reform changes can nurses take an active role in improving the process and outcomes of patient care? Select all that apply.

A. Telling patients or families to file malpractice claims
B. P4P
C. Patient hospital readmission penalty
D. Bundled payments
E. ACOs
F. QI

REVIEW ACTIVITIES

Please see Appendix E for answers to Review Activities.

1. Explore the Centers for Disease Control website, http://www.cdc.gov/HealthyLiving, to determine what resources are available for nurses and patients to live healthier lifestyles. For example, what resources are available to help you help your patient stop smoking?
2. The RWJF/IOM report, *The Future of Nursing: Leading Change, Advancing Health* (2011), outlines a path for the nursing profession in transforming health care delivery in the United State. Explore the Future of Nursing, Campaign for Action, at,

http://thefutureofnursing.org/about. Go to the site and click on Get involved with the Campaign for Action. Scroll down to learn more about your state. Click on states, and then click again on your state. Join your online community. Who can you contact in your home state for more information?

EXPLORING THE WEB

1. Explore the AHRQ tab for Clinicians and Providers, see patient safety, http://www.ahrq.gov/qual.
2. Note the role of measurement in quality, see National Quality Forum, ABCs of Measurement, http://www.qualityforum.org/Measuring_Performance/ABCs_of_Measurement.aspxm.
3. Review the Veterans Administration, National Center for Patient Safety, tips and tools for patients, http://www.patientsafety.gov/patients.html#tools.
4. Review The Joint Commission, National Patient Safety Goals, site for standards applicable to your anticipated work environment, http://www.jointcommission.org/standards_information/npsgs.aspx.
5. Review the most recently published Joint Commission Sentinel Event Alert at http://www.jointcommission.org/standards_information/up.aspx.
6. Review the National Patient Safety Foundation website, http://www.npsf.org/for-patients-consumers/tools-and-resources-for-patients-and-consumers/what-you-can-do-to-make-healthcare-safer. Note what it tells patients to do to promote safety in their personal care.

REFERENCES

AAACN. (2011). *American Academy of Ambulatory Care Nursing—Ambulatory care nursing defined*. Retrieved from http://www.aaacn.org/cgi-bin/WebObjects/AAACNMain.woa/1/wa/viewSection?s_id=1073743905&ss_id=536873820&wosid=KGJG2pLHo6jl2ug2Ttb7ceRbaU4

Adams, J. M. (2011). Influencing the future of nursing, an interview with Sue Hassmiller. *Journal of Nursing Administration, 41*(10), 394–396.

Advisory Board Company. (2010). Optimizing accountable care clinical operations. Retrieved from http://www.advisory.com/~/media/Advisory-com/Research/HCAB/Events/Webconference/2011/Optimizing-Accountable-Care-Clinical-Operations-HCAB.pdf

Agency for Healthcare Research and Quality (AHRQ). (2012). *TeamSTEPPS*. Retrieved from http://teamstepps.ahrq.gov

Agency for Healthcare Research and Quality (AHRQ). (2013). *Research findings: Nursing research*. Retrieved from http://www.ahrq.gov/professionals/clinicians- providers/resources/nursing/ahrq/ra/index.html

Aiken, L. (2012). Improving health care outcomes through research (Part One). *Reflections on Nursing Leadership, 38*(1). Retrieved from http://www.reflectionsonnursingleadership.org/Pages/Vol38_1_Aiken_Morin.aspx

Balas, E. A., & Boren, S. A. (2000). *Managing clinical knowledge for health care improvement*. Yearbook of Medical Informatics 2000: Patient-Centered Systems, Stuttgart, Germany (pp. 65--70).

Benner, P. E., Malloch, K., & Sheets, V. (Eds.) (2010). *Nursing pathways for patient safety*. St. Louis, MO: Mosby Elsevier.

Berwick, D. M. (2011). Preparing nurses for participation in and leadership of continual improvement. *Journal of Nursing Education, 50*(6), 322–327.

Binder, L. (2012). *No matter who's in the white house: Three trends that will transform healthcare.* Forbes. Retrieved from http://www.forbes.com/sites/leahbinder/2012/10/29/no-matterwhos-in-the-white-house-three-trends-that-will-transform-healthcare

Buerhaus, P. I., DesRoches, C., Applebaum, S., Hess, R., Norman, L. D., & Donelan, K. (2012). Are nurses ready for health care reform? A decade of survey research. *Nursing Economics, 30*(6), 318–330.

Centers for Disease Control (2014). *Healthy living.* Retrieved January 7, 2014 from http://www.cdc.gov/HealthyLiving

Centers for Medicare and Medicaid Services (CMS). (2011). *CMS issues final rule for first year of hospital value-based purchasing program.* Retrieved from http://www.cms.gov/apps/media/press/factsheet.asp?Counter=3947

Clancy, C. M. (2011). New research highlights the role of patient safety culture and safer care. *Journal of Nursing Care Quality, 26*(3), 193–196, doi:10.1097/NCQ.0b013e31821d0520

The Commonwealth Fund. (2011). *Why not the best? Results from the national scorecard on U.S. health system performance.* Retrieved from http://www.commonwealthfund.org/~/media/Files/News/Nat%20Scorecard/1500_WNTB_Natl_Scorecard_2011_web.pdf

Compiled with information from Healthy Living (CDC, 2014). Centers for Disease Control (2014). *Healthy living.* Retrieved January 7, 2014 from http://www.cdc.gov/Healthy Living

Davis, K., Schoen, C., & Stremikis, K. (2010). *Mirror, mirror on the wall: How the performance of theU.S. health care system compares internationally, 2010 Update.* Retrieved from http://www.commonwealthfund.org/Publications/Fund-Reports/2010/Jun/Mirror-Mirror-Update.aspx?page=all

Dekker, S. (2007). *Just culture: Balancing safety and accountability.* Bodmin, Cornwall Great Britain: Ashgate.

Department of Health and Human Services (DHHS). (2013). *Health IT patient safety action and surveillance plan, Office of the National Coordinator (ONC) for Health Information Technology (IT).* Retrieved from http://www.healthit.gov/policy-researchers-implementers/health-it-and-patient-safety

Gallup. (2012a). *Honesty/ethics in professions.* Retrieved from http://www.gallup.com/poll/1654/honesty-ethics-professions.aspx#1

Gallup. (2012b). *U.S. physicians set good health example.* Retrieved from http://www.gallup.com/poll/157859/physicians-set-good-health-example.aspx Harrington, L. (2011). Clinical intelligence. *Journal of Nursing Administration, 41*(12), 507–509, doi:10.1097/NNA.0b013e318237eca0

HealthCare.gov. (2012). *Administration implements new health reform provision to improve care quality, lower costs.* Retrieved from http://www.healthcare.gov/news/factsheets/2011/04/valuebasedpurchasing04292011a. html

Health Resources and Services Administration (HRSA). (2013). *The U.S. nursing workforce: Trends in supply and education.* Retrieved from http://bhpr.hrsa.gov/healthworkforce/reports/nursingworkforce/nursingworkforcefullreport.pdf

Hood, L., Balling, R., & Auffray, C. (2012). Revolutionizing medicine in the 21(st) century through systems approaches. *Biotechnology Journal, 7*(8), 992–1001. doi:10.1002/biot.201100306

Hulscher, M. E., Schouten, L. M., Grol, R. P., & Buchan H. (2012). Determinants of success of quality improvement collaboratives: What does the literature show? *BMJ Quality & Safety.* doi:10.1136/bmjqs-2011–000651

Initiative on the Future of Nursing. (2011). *About the campaign.* Retrieved from http://thefutureofnursing. Org

Institute of Medicine (IOM). (2004). *Keeping patients safe: Transforming the work environment of nurses.* Washington, DC: National Academies Press.

Institute of Medicine (IOM). (2011a). *The learning health system and its innovation collaboratives.* Retrieved from http://www.iom.edu/Activities/Quality/~/media/Files/Activity%20Files/Quality/VSRT/Core%20Documents/ForEDistrib.pdf

Institute of Medicine (IOM). (2011b). *Health IT and patient safety, building safer systems for better care.* Report Brief. Retrieved from http://iom.edu/~/media/Files/Report%20Files/2011/Health-IT/HealthITandPatientSafetyreportbrieffinal_new.pdf

Institute of Medicine (IOM). (2011c). *The future of nursing: Leading change, advancing health*. Washington, DC: National Academies Press.

Jones, P. (2011). *The nurse's role in accountable care*. Milliman Healthcare Reform Briefing Paper, Retrieved from http://publications.milliman.com/publications/healthreform/pdfs/nurses-role-accountable-care.pdf

Jonsson, B. (1989, December). *What can Americans learn from Europeans?* Health Care Financing Review. Spec No: 79–93; discussion 93–110. Retrieved from http://www.cms.gov/Research-Statistics-Data-and-Systems/Research/HealthCareFinancingReview/List-of-Past-Articles-Items/CMS1191067.html?DLPage=1&DLFilter=jonsson&DLSort=1&DLSortDir=ascending (Note to publisher Jonsson ref above—All published material that appeared in HCFR is in the public domain and may be reproduced or copied without permission; however, citation to source is appreciated, http://www.cms.gov/Research-Statistics-Data-and-Systems/Research/HealthCareFinancingReview/index.html?redirect=/HealthCareFinancingReview.)

Loef, M., & Walach, H. (2012). The combined effects of healthy lifestyle behaviors on all cause mortality: A systematic review and meta-analysis. *Preventive Medicine, 55*(3), 163–170. doi:10.1016/j.ypmed.2012.06.017

MacKinnon, K. (2011). Rural nurses' safeguarding work: Reembodying patient safety. *Advances in Nursing Science, 34*(2), 119–29. doi:10.1097/ANS.0b013e3182186b86

Mallory, G. (2010). Professional nursing societies and evidence-based practice: Strategies to cross the quality chasm. *Nursing Outlook, 58*(6), 279–286. doi:10.1016/j.outlook.2010.06.00

McDonald, L. (Ed.) (2004). *Florence Nightingale on public health care* (Vol. 6). Ontario, Canada: Wilfried Laurier University Press.

Medicare (2014). *Hospital Compare*. Retrieved January 7, 2014 from http://www.medicare.gov/hospitalcompare/search.html

Melnyk, B., Fineout-Overholt, E., Gallagher-Ford, L., & Kaplan, L. (2012). The state of evidence-based practice in US Nurses: Critical implications for nurse leaders and educators. *The Journal of Nursing Administration (JONA), 42*(9), 410–417. doi:10.1097/NNA.0b013e3182664e0a

Mimm, L. (2013). *Team communication improvement initiatives enhance a hospital's culture of safety, leading to improved outcomes*. Retrieved from http://innovations.ahrq.gov/content.aspx?id=1783

Moss, F. (2011, November 9). *Our high-tech health-care future*. The New York Times, Retrieved from http://www.nytimes.com/2011/11/10/opinion/our-high-tech-health-care-future.html

Müller-Staub, M. (2009). Evaluation of the implementation of nursing diagnoses, interventions, and outcomes. *International Journal of Nursing Terminologies and Classifications, 20*(1), 9–15. doi:10.1111/j.1744–618X.2008.01108.x

Oncology Nursing Society. (2012). *Clinical practice*. Retrieved from http://www.ons.org/ClinicalResources

Oncology Nursing Society. (2014). *ONS putting evidence into practice (PEP)*. Retrieved January 7, 2014 from https://www.ons.org/practice-resources/pep.

P4 Medicine Institute. (2012). *P4Medicine*. Retrieved from http://p4mi.org/p4-medicine Painter, L. M., Dudjak, L. A., Kidwell, K. M., Simmons, R. L., & Kidwell, R. P. (2011), The nurse's role in the causation of compensable injury. *Journal of Nursing Care Quality, 26*(4), 311–319. doi: 10.1097/NCQ.ob013e31820f9576

Park, M. H., & Hiller, E. A. (2011). Medicare hospital value-based purchasing: The evolution toward linking Medicare reimbursement to health care quality continues. *Health Care Law Monthly, 2011*(2), 2–9.

Porter-O'Grady, T., & Malloch, K. (2011). *Quantum leadership: Advancing innovation, transforming health care* (3th ed.). Sudbury, MA: Jones & Bartlett Learning.

Quality and Safety Education for Nurses (QSEN). (2012). Retrieved from http://www.qsen.org

Reinhardt, U. E. (1989). Economic relationships in the health care delivery system. (Source: Adapted from "What Can Americans Learn from Europeans?") *Health Care Financing Review* (Suppl), 97–103.

Rothbard, M. N. (2008). *Free market*. Retrieved January 7, 2014 from http://www.econlib.org/library/Enc/FreeMarket.html

Russell, D., Rosati, R., Rosenfeld, P., & Marren, J. (2011). Continuity in home health care: is consistency in nursing personnel associated with better patient outcomes? *Journal for Healthcare Quality: Promoting Excellence in Healthcare, 33*(6), 33–39. doi:10.1111/j.1945–1474.2011.00131.x

Sebelius, K. G. (2011). *Keynote presentation – The Richard and Hinda Rosenthal lecture: New frontiers in patient safety.* Retrieved from http://www.nap.edu/openbook.php?record_id=13217&page=3

Sieg, D. (2011). *What nursing leaders know: Seven truths from top health care professionals.* Retrieved from http://www.reflectionsonnursingleadership.org/pages/vol35_3_sieg_nursingleaders.aspx

The Times 100. (1995–2013). *Business case studies, marketing mix (price, place, promotion, product).* Retrieved from http://businesscasestudies.co.uk/business-theory/marketing/marketing-mix-price-place-promotion-product.html#axzz2ZqHdqGJg

Truffer, C. J., Keehan, S., Smith, S., Cylus, J., Sisko, A., Poisal, J. A., . . . Clemens, M. K. (2010). Health spending projections through 2019: The recession's impact continues. *Health Affairs, 29*(3), 522–529.

U.S. Department of Health and Human Services (2014). *Key Features of the Affordable Care Act.* Retrieved January 7, 2014 from http://www.hhs.gov/healthcare/facts/timeline/index.html

VanBuren, A. (2012). *Timeline: CMS quality measures.* E-mail Communication.

Zrelak, P. A., Utter, G. H., Sadeghi, B., Cuny, J., Baron, R., & Romano, P. S. (2011). Using the Agency for Healthcare Research and Quality patient safety indicators for targeting nursing quality improvement. *Journal of Nursing Care Quality, 27*(2), 99–108. doi:10.1097/NCA.0b013e318237e0e3

SUGGESTED READING

Berwick, D., Nolan, T., & Whittington, J. (2008). The triple aim: care, health, and cost. *Health Affairs, 27*(3), 759–769. doi:10.1377/hlthaff.27.3.759

Bittner, N. P., Gravlin, G., Hansten, R., & Kalisch, B. J. (2011). Unraveling care omissions. *Journal of Nursing Administration, 41*(12), 510–512. doi:10.1097/NNA.0b013e3182378b65

Clancy, C., & Berwick, D. (2011). The science of safety improvement: Learning while doing. *Annals of Internal Medicine, 154*(10), 699–701. doi:10.1059/0003–4819-154–10-201105170–00013

Donabedian, A. (1966). Evaluating the quality of medical care. *Milbank Memorial Fund Quarterly, 44*, 166–206.

Kelly, L., McHugh, M., & Aiken, L. (2011). Nurse outcomes in Magnet® and non-magnet hospitals. *The Journal of Nursing Administration (JONA), 41*(10), 428–433. doi:10.1097/NNA.0b013e31822eddbc

Kendall-Gallagher, D., Aiken, L., Sloane, D., & Cimiotti, J. (2011). Nurse specialty certification, inpatient mortality, and failure to rescue. *Journal of Nursing Scholarship: An Official Publication of Sigma Theta Tau International Honor Society of Nursing/Sigma Theta Tau, 43*(2), 188–194. doi:10.1111/j.1547–5069.2011.01391.x

Kendall-Gallagher, D., & Blegen, M. (2010). Competence and certification of registered nurses and safety of patients in intensive care units. *The Journal of Nursing Administration (JONA), 40*(10 Suppl), S68–S77. doi:10.1097/NNA.0b013e3181f37edb

McHugh, M., & Lake, E. (2010). Understanding clinical expertise: Nurse education, experience, and the hospital context. *Research in Nursing & Health, 33*(4), 276–287. doi:10.1002/nur.20388

Needleman, J., Buerhaus, P., Pankratz, V., Leibson, C., Stevens, S., & Harris, M. (2011). Nurse staffing and inpatient hospital mortality. *New England Journal of Medicine, 364*(11), 1037–1045. doi:10.1056/NEJMsa1001025

O'Neill, S., Jones, T., Bennett, D., & Lewis, M. (2011). Nursing works, the application of lean thinking to nursing processes, *Journal of Nursing Administration, 41*(12), 546–552. doi:10.1097/NNA.0b013e3182378d37

Rees, S., Leahy-Gross, K., & Mack, V. (2011). Moving data to nursing quality excellence. *Journal of Nursing Care Quality, 26*(3), 260–264, doi:10.1097/NCQ.0b013e31820e0e8c

Schluter, J., Seaton, P., & Chaboyer, W. (2011). Understanding nursing scope of practice: A qualitative study. *International Journal of Nursing Studies, 48*(10), 1211–1222. doi:10.1016/j.ijnurstu.2011.03.004

Shekelle, P., Pronovost, P., Wachter, R., Taylor, S., Dy, S., Foy, R., ... Walshe, K. (2011). Advancing the science of patient safety. *Annals of Internal Medicine, 154*(10), 693–696. doi:10.1059/0003–4819-154–10-201105170–00011

Squires, M., Tourangeau, A., Spence Laschinger, H., & Doran, D. (2010). The link between leadership and safety outcomes in hospitals. *Journal of Nursing Management, 18*(8), 914–925. doi:10.1111/j.1365–2834.2010.01181.x

Titler, M., Shever, L., Kanak, M., Picone, D., & Qin, R. (2011). Factors associated with falls during hospitalization in an older adult population. *Research & Theory for Nursing Practice, 25*(2), 127–148.

Vogus, T., & Sutcliffe, K. (2011). The impact of safety organizing, trusted leadership, and care pathways on reported medication errors in hospital nursing units. *The Journal of Nursing Administration (JONA), 41*(7–8 Suppl.), S25–S30. doi:10.1097/NNA.0b013e318221c368

White, S. V. (2011). Interview with a quality leader: Carol Wagner on Washington State Hospital Association (WSHA) and their statewide improvement. Interview with a Quality Leader: Carol Wagner on Washington State Hospital Association (WSHA) and their Statewide Improvement. *Journal for Healthcare Quality: Promoting Excellence in Healthcare, 34*(1), 62–64. doi:10.1111/j.1945–1474.2011.00161.x

Yee, T., Needleman, J., Pearson, M., & Parkerton, P. (2011). Nurse manager perceptions of the impact of process improvements by nurses, *Journal of Nursing Care Quality, 26*(3), 226–235, doi:10.1097/NCQ.0b013e318213a607Mel

APPENDIX A

INSTITUTE OF MEDICINE (IOM) REPORTS

1st Annual Crossing the Quality Chasm Summit: A Focus on Communities. Released September 14, 2004

A Foundation for Evidence-Driven Practice: A Rapid Learning System for Cancer Care. Workshop summary released June 4, 2010

A Summary of the December 2009 Forum on the Future of Nursing: Care in the Community. Workshop summary released June 3, 2010

A Summary of the February 2010 Forum on the Future of Nursing: Education. Workshop summary released August 31, 2010

A Summary of the October 2009 Forum on the Future of Nursing: Acute Care. Workshop summary released April 14, 2010

Advancing Quality Improvement Research: Challenges and Opportunities. Workshop summary released May 23, 2007

Adverse Drug Event Reporting: The Roles of Consumers and Health Care Professionals. Workshop summary released April 12, 2007

Cancer Care for the Whole Patient: Meeting Psychosocial Health Needs. Released October 15, 2007

Certifying Personal Protective Technologies: Improving Worker Safety. Released November 11, 2010

Child and Adolescent Health and Health Care Quality: Measuring What Matters. Released April 25, 2011

Clinical Data as the Basic Staple of Health Learning. Workshop summary released February 3, 2011

Clinical Practice Guidelines We Can Trust. Released March 23, 2011

Creating a Business Case for Quality Improvement and Quality Improvement Research. Workshop summary released April 7, 2008

Crossing the Quality Chasm: A New Health System for the 21st Century. Released March 1, 2001

Digital Infrastructure for the Learning Health System: The Foundation for Continuous Improvement in Health and Health Care. Workshop series summary released May 23, 2011

Emerging Safety Science. Workshop summary released April 9, 2008

Engineering a Learning Healthcare System: A Look at the Future. Workshop summary released July 8, 2011

Evidence-Based Medicine and the Changing Nature of Healthcare. Released October 9, 2008

Finding What Works in Health Care: Standards for Systematic Reviews. Released March 23, 2011

Fostering Rapid Advances in Health Care: Learning from System Demonstrations. Released November 19, 2002

Future Directions for the National Healthcare Quality and Disparities Reports. Released April 14, 2010

Health IT and Patient Safety: Building Safer Systems for Better Care. Released November 8, 2011

Health Literacy Implications for Health Care Reform. Workshop summary released July 15, 2011

Health Professions Education: A Bridge to Quality. Released April 18, 2003

Initial National Priorities for Comparative Effectiveness Research. Released June 30, 2009

Innovations in Health Literacy Research. Workshop summary released March 10, 2011

Institute of Medicine of the National Academies, 2012. Accessed June 12, 2012.

Keeping Patients Safe: Transforming the Work Environment of Nurses. Released November 3, 2003

Key Capabilities of an Electronic Health Record System. Released July 31, 2003

Leadership by Example: Coordinating Government Roles in Improving Health Care Quality. Released October 30, 2002

Leadership Commitments to Improve Value in Healthcare: Toward Common Ground. Workshop summary released June 14, 2010

Learning What Works: Infrastructure Required for Comparative Effectiveness Research. Workshop summary released July 25, 2011

Medicare's Quality Improvement Organization Program: Maximizing Potential. Released March 9, 2006

Patient Safety: Achieving a New Standard for Care. Released November 20, 2003

Patient-Centered Cancer Treatment Planning: Improving the Quality of Oncology Care. Workshop summary released June 13, 2011

Patients Charting the Course: Citizen Engagement in the Learning Health System. Workshop summary released October 3, 2011

Performance Measurement: Accelerating Improvement. Released December 1, 2005

Preventing Medication Errors: Quality Chasm Series. Released July 20, 2006

Priority Areas for National Action: Transforming Health Care Quality. Released January 7, 2003

Public Health Effectiveness of the FDA 510(k) Clearance Process: Balancing Patient Safety and Innovation. Workshop report released October 14, 2010

Redesigning Continuing Education in the Health Professions. Released December 4, 2009

Redesigning the Clinical Effectiveness Research Paradigm: Innovation and Practice-Based Approaches. Workshop summary released December 6, 2010

Retooling for an Aging America: Building the Health Care Workforce. Released April 11, 2008

Rewarding Provider Performance: Aligning Incentives in Medicare. Released September 20, 2006

Standardizing Medication Labels: Confusing Patients Less. Workshop summary released April 22, 2008

The Future of Drug Safety: Promoting and Protecting the Health of the Public. Released September 22, 2006

The Future of Nursing: Leading Change, Advancing Health. Released October 5, 2010

The Healthcare Imperative: Lowering Costs and Improving Outcomes. Workshop series summary released February 24, 2011

The Learning Healthcare System. Released March 30, 2007

The Richard and Hinda Rosenthal Lecture 2002: Fostering Rapid Advances in Health Care. Released January 1, 2002

The Richard and Hinda Rosenthal Lecture 2003: Keeping Patients Safe. Released November 11, 2004

The Richard and Hinda Rosenthal Lecture 2005: Next Steps Toward Higher Quality Health Care. Released October 12, 2006

The Richard and Hinda Rosenthal Lecture 2011: New Frontiers in Patient Safety. Released October 5, 2011

The Richard and Hinda Rosenthal Lecture Spring 2001: Crossing the Quality Chasm. Released May 1, 2001

The Safe Use Initiative and Health Literacy. Workshop summary released December 1, 2010

The State of Quality Improvement and Implementation Research: Expert Views. Workshop summary released October 5, 2007

To Err Is Human: Building A Safer Health System. Released November 1, 1999

Value in Health Care: Accounting for Cost, Quality, Safety, Outcomes, and Innovation. Workshop summary released December 16, 2009

APPENDIX B

PRELICENSURE KNOWLEDGE, SKILLS, AND ATTITUDES (KSAs)

Listed below are the prelicensure Quality and Safety Education for Nurses (QSEN) competencies. The chapter of this textbook that has information related to the competency is also identified (see http://qsen.org/competencies/pre-licensure-ksas).

PATIENT-CENTERED CARE (PCC)

Definition: Recognize the patient or designee as the source of control and full partner in providing compassionate and coordinated care based on respect for patient's preferences, values, and needs.

KNOWLEDGE	SKILLS	ATTITUDES
Integrate understanding of multiple dimensions of PCC: patient/family/community preferences, values coordination, and integration of care information, communication, and education physical comfort, and emotional support involvement of family and friends, transition, and continuity • Chapter 1 • Chapter 2 • Chapter 5 • Chapter 6 • Chapter 13	Elicit patient values, preferences, and expressed needs as part of clinical interview, implementation of care plan, and evaluation of care • Chapter 6 Communicate patient values, preferences, and expressed needs to other members of health care team • Chapter 5 • Chapter 6	Value seeing health care situations "through patients' eyes" • Chapter 1 • Chapter 2 • Chapter 5 • Chapter 6 • Chapter 13 Respect and encourage individual expression of patient values, preferences, and expressed needs • Chapter 5 • Chapter 6

(continued)

PATIENT-CENTERED CARE (PCC) (*continued*)

KNOWLEDGE	SKILLS	ATTITUDES
Describe how diverse cultural, ethnic, and social backgrounds function as sources of patient, family, and community values • Chapter 6	Provide PCC with sensitivity and respect for the diversity of human experience • Chapter 2 • Chapter 6	Value the patient's expertise with own health and symptoms • Chapter 5 • Chapter 6 Seek learning opportunities with patients who represent all aspects of human diversity Recognize personally held attitudes about working with patients from different ethnic, cultural, and social backgrounds • Chapter 6 Willingly support PCC for individuals and groups whose values differ from own • Chapter 5 • Chapter 6 • Chapter 13
Demonstrate comprehensive understanding of the concepts of pain and suffering, including physiological models of pain and comfort. • Chapter 6	Assess presence and extent of pain and suffering Assess levels of physical and emotional comfort • Chapter 6 Elicit expectations of patient and family for relief of pain, discomfort, or suffering • Chapter 6 Initiate effective treatments to relieve pain and suffering in light of patient values, preferences, and expressed needs	Recognize personally held values and beliefs about the management of pain or suffering Appreciate the role of the nurse in relief of all types and sources of pain or suffering Recognize that patient expectations influence outcomes in management of pain or suffering • Chapter 6
Examine how the safety, quality, and cost-effectiveness of health care can be improved through the active involvement of patients and families • Chapter 5 • Chapter 6	Remove barriers to presence of families and other designated surrogates based on patient preferences Assess level of patient's decisional conflict and provide access to resources	Value active partnership with patients or designated surrogates in planning, implementation, and evaluation of care • Chapter 5 • Chapter 6

(*continued*)

PATIENT-CENTERED CARE (PCC) (*continued*)

KNOWLEDGE	SKILLS	ATTITUDES
Examine common barriers to active involvement of patients in their own health care processes • Chapter 6 Describe strategies to empower patients or families in all aspects of the health care process • Chapter 5 • Chapter 6	Engage patients or designated surrogates in active partnerships that promote health, safety and well-being, and self-care management • Chapter 5 • Chapter 6	Respect patient preferences for degree of active engagement in care process • Chapter 5 • Chapter 6 Respect patient's right to access to personal health records • Chapter 5 • Chapter 6 • Chapter 10
Explore ethical and legal implications of PCC • Chapter 1 • Chapter 6 Describe the limits and boundaries of therapeutic PCC	Recognize the boundaries of therapeutic relationships Facilitate informed patient consent for care	Acknowledge the tension that may exist between patient rights and the organizational responsibility for professional, ethical care • Chapter 5 Appreciate shared decision making with empowered patients and families, even when conflicts occur • Chapter 5 • Chapter 6
Discuss principles of effective communication • Chapter 5 • Chapter 6 Describe basic principles of consensus building and conflict resolution • Chapter 5 Examine nursing roles in assuring coordination, integration, and continuity of care • Chapter 5	Assess own level of communication skill in encounters with patients and families • Chapter 5 • Chapter 6 Participate in building consensus or resolving conflict in the context of patient care • Chapter 5 Communicate care provided and needed at each transition in care • Chapter 5 • Chapter 6	Value continuous improvement of own communication and conflict resolution skills • Chapter 5 • Chapter 6

TEAMWORK AND COLLABORATION

Definition: Function effectively within nursing and interprofessional teams, fostering open communication, mutual respect, and shared decision making to achieve quality patient care.

KNOWLEDGE	SKILLS	ATTITUDES
Describe own strengths, limitations, and values in functioning as a member of a team • Chapter 1 • Chapter 2 • Chapter 5 • Chapter 13	Demonstrate awareness of own strengths and limitations as a team member • Chapter 5 Initiate plan for self-development as a team member Act with integrity, consistency, and respect for differing views • Chapter 5 • Chapter 6	Acknowledge own potential to contribute to effective team functioning • Chapter 1 • Chapter 2 • Chapter 5 • Chapter 13 Appreciate importance of intra and interprofessional collaboration • Chapter 5 • Chapter 6
Describe scopes of practice and roles of health care team members • Chapter 5 Describe strategies for identifying and managing overlaps in team member roles and accountabilities Recognize contributions of other individuals and groups in helping patient/family achieve health goals • Chapter 5	Function competently within own scope of practice as a member of the health care team Assume role of team member or leader based on the situation Initiate requests for help when appropriate to situation Clarify roles and accountabilities under conditions of potential overlap in team member functioning Integrate the contributions of others who play a role in helping patient/family achieve health goals	Value the perspectives and expertise of all health team members • Chapter 1 • Chapter 2 • Chapter 5 • Chapter 6 • Chapter 13 Respect the centrality of the patient/family as core members of any health care team • Chapter 6 Respect the unique attributes that members bring to a team, including variations in professional orientations and accountabilities • Chapter 5
Analyze differences in communication style preferences among patients and families, nurses, and other members of the health team • Chapter 5	Communicate with team members, adapting own style of communicating to needs of the team and situation • Chapter 5 Demonstrate commitment to team goals • Chapter 5	Value teamwork and the relationships upon which it is based • Chapter 1 • Chapter 2 • Chapter 5 • Chapter 6 • Chapter 13

(continued)

TEAMWORK AND COLLABORATION (*continued*)

KNOWLEDGE	SKILLS	ATTITUDES
Describe impact of own communication style on others • Chapter 5 Discuss effective strategies for communicating and resolving conflict • Chapter 5	Solicit input from other team members to improve individual, as well as team, performance • Chapter 5 Initiate actions to resolve conflict • Chapter 5	Value different styles of communication used by patients, families, and health care providers • Chapter 5 • Chapter 6 Contribute to resolution of conflict and disagreement • Chapter 5
Describe examples of the impact of team functioning on safety and quality of care • Chapter 1 • Chapter 2 • Chapter 5 • Chapter 13 Explain how authority gradients influence teamwork and patient safety	Follow communication practices that minimize risks associated with handoffs among providers and across transitions in care • Chapter 5 Assert own position/ perspective in discussions about patient care • Chapter 5 Choose communication styles that diminish the risks associated with authority gradients among team members • Chapter 5	Appreciate the risks associated with handoffs among providers and across transitions in care • Chapter 5
Identify system barriers and facilitators of effective team functioning Examine strategies for improving systems to support team functioning	Participate in designing systems that support effective teamwork	Value the influence of system solutions in achieving effective team functioning

EVIDENCE-BASED PRACTICE (EBP)

Definition: Integrate best current evidence with clinical expertise and patient/family preferences and values for delivery of optimal health care.

KNOWLEDGE	SKILLS	ATTITUDES
Demonstrate knowledge of basic scientific methods and processes • Chapter 1 • Chapter 2 • Chapter 9 • Chapter 11 • Chapter 12 • Chapter 13	Participate effectively in appropriate data collection and other research activities • Chapter 9 • Chapter 11 • Chapter 12	Appreciate strengths and weaknesses of scientific bases for practice • Chapter 11 • Chapter 12

(*continued*)

EVIDENCE-BASED PRACTICE (EBP) (*continued*)

KNOWLEDGE	SKILLS	ATTITUDES
Describe EBP to include the components of research evidence, clinical expertise, and patient/family values • Chapter 12	Adhere to Institutional Review Board (IRB) guidelines Base individualized care plan on patient values, clinical expertise, and evidence • Chapter 5 • Chapter 6 • Chapter 12	Value the need for ethical conduct of research and quality improvement • Chapter 2 Value the concept of EBP as integral to determining best clinical practice • Chapter 12
Differentiate clinical opinion from research and evidence summaries • Chapter 7 • Chapter 12 Describe reliable sources for locating evidence reports and clinical practice guidelines • Chapter 11 • Chapter 12	Read original research and evidence reports related to area of practice • Chapter 12 Locate evidence reports related to clinical practice topics and guidelines • Chapter 11 • Chapter 12	Appreciate the importance of regularly reading relevant professional journals • Chapter 11
Explain the role of evidence in determining best clinical practice • Chapter 12 Describe how the strength and relevance of available evidence influences the choice of interventions in provision of PCC • Chapter 12	Participate in structuring the work environment to facilitate integration of new evidence into standards of practice Question rationale for routine approaches to care that result in less-than-desired outcomes or adverse events • Chapter 1 • Chapter 2 • Chapter 4 • Chapter 13	Value the need for continuous improvement in clinical practice based on new knowledge • Chapter 5 • Chapter 11 • Chapter 12 • Chapter 13
Discriminate between valid and invalid reasons for modifying evidence-based clinical practice based on clinical expertise or patient/family preferences • Chapter 12	Consult with clinical experts before deciding to deviate from evidence-based protocols	Acknowledge own limitations in knowledge and clinical expertise before determining when to deviate from evidence-based best practices

QUALITY IMPROVEMENT (QI)

Definition: Use data to monitor the outcomes of care processes and use improvement methods to design and test changes to continuously improve the quality and safety of health care systems.

KNOWLEDGE	SKILLS	ATTITUDES
Describe strategies for learning about the outcomes of care in the setting in which one is engaged in clinical practice • Chapter 1 • Chapter 2 • Chapter 3 • Chapter 5 • Chapter 8 • Chapter 9 • Chapter 10 • Chapter 12 • Chapter 13	Seek information about outcomes of care for populations served in care setting • Chapter 6 • Chapter 7 • Chapter 8 • Chapter 9 Seek information about QI projects in the care setting • Chapter 9	Appreciate that continuous QI is an essential part of the daily work of all health professionals • Chapter 1 • Chapter 2 • Chapter 3 • Chapter 4 • Chapter 5 • Chapter 7 • Chapter 8 • Chapter 9 • Chapter 12 • Chapter 13
Recognize that nursing and other health professions students are parts of systems of care and care processes that affect outcomes for patients and families • Chapter 3 • Chapter 7 • Chapter 8	Use tools (such as flow charts, cause-effect diagrams) to make processes of care explicit • Chapter 4 • Chapter 9 Participate in a root cause analysis of a sentinel event • Chapter 5 • Chapter 7	Value own and others' contributions to outcomes of care in local care settings • Chapter 3 • Chapter 4 • Chapter 5 • Chapter 6 • Chapter 7 • Chapter 12
Give examples of the tension between professional autonomy and system functioning • Chapter 3 • Chapter 7		
Explain the importance of variation and measurement in assessing quality of care • Chapter 9	Use quality measures to understand performance • Chapter 8 • Chapter 9 Use tools (such as control charts and run charts) that are helpful for understanding variation • Chapter 9 Identify gaps between local and best practice • Chapter 8	Appreciate how unwanted variation affects care • Chapter 9 • Chapter 13 Value measurement and its role in good patient care • Chapter 8 • Chapter 9

(continued)

QUALITY IMPROVEMENT (QI) (*continued*)

KNOWLEDGE	SKILLS	ATTITUDES
Describe approaches for changing processes of care • Chapter 3 • Chapter 5 • Chapter 6 • Chapter 7 • Chapter 9 • Chapter 12	Design a small test of change in daily work (using an experiential learning method such as Plan-Do-Study-Act) • Chapter 7 • Chapter 9 Practice aligning the aims, measures and changes involved in improving care • Chapter 8 • Chapter 9 Use measures to evaluate the effect of change • Chapter 8 • Chapter 9	Value local change (in individual practice or team practice on a unit) and its role in creating joy in work • Chapter 3 Appreciate the value of what individuals and teams can to do to improve care • Chapter 5 • Chapter 6 • Chapter 7 • Chapter 8 • Chapter 13

SAFETY

Definition: Minimizes risk of harm to patients and providers through both system effectiveness and individual performance.

KNOWLEDGE	SKILLS	ATTITUDES
Examine human factors and other basic safety design principles as well as commonly used unsafe practices (such as, work-arounds and dangerous abbreviations) • Chapter 1 • Chapter 2 • Chapter 3 • Chapter 4 • Chapter 5 • Chapter 13 Describe the benefits and limitations of selected safety-enhancing technologies (such as barcodes, Computer Provider Order Entry, medication pumps, and automatic alerts/alarms) • Chapter 10 Discuss effective strategies to reduce reliance on memory • Chapter 4	Demonstrate effective use of technology and standardized practices that support safety and quality • Chapter 4 • Chapter 5 • Chapter 6 • Chapter 10 Demonstrate effective use of strategies to reduce risk of harm to self or others • Chapter 5 Use appropriate strategies to reduce reliance on memory (such as forcing functions, checklists) • Chapter 4	Value the contributions of standardization/reliability to safety • Chapter 1 • Chapter 2 • Chapter 3 • Chapter 4 • Chapter 13 Appreciate the cognitive and physical limits of human performance • Chapter 3

(*continued*)

SAFETY (*continued*)

KNOWLEDGE	SKILLS	ATTITUDES
Delineate general categories of errors and hazards in care Describe factors that create a culture of safety (such as, open communication strategies and organizational error reporting systems) • Chapter 3 • Chapter 4 • Chapter 5	Communicate observations or concerns related to hazards and errors to patients, families, and the health care team • Chapter 3 • Chapter 4 Use organizational error reporting systems for near miss and error reporting • Chapter 3	Value own role in preventing errors • Chapter 3 • Chapter 4 • Chapter 5
Describe processes used in understanding causes of error and allocation of responsibility and accountability (such as, root cause analysis and failure mode effects analysis) • Chapter 4 • Chapter 5 • Chapter 7	Participate appropriately in analyzing errors and designing system improvements • Chapter 3 • Chapter 7 Engage in root cause analysis rather than blaming when errors or near misses occur • Chapter 3 • Chapter 4 • Chapter 5 • Chapter 7	Value vigilance and monitoring (even of own performance of care activities) by patients, families, and other members of the health care team • Chapter 4 • Chapter 6 • Chapter 10
Discuss potential and actual impact of national patient safety resources, initiatives, and regulations • Chapter 3 • Chapter 7	Use national patient safety resources for own professional development and to focus attention on safety in care settings • Chapter 3 • Chapter 4 • Chapter 7 • Chapter 8	Value relationship between national safety campaigns and implementation in local practices and practice settings • Chapter 3 • Chapter 4

INFORMATICS

Definition: Use information and technology to communicate, manage knowledge, mitigate error, and support decision making.

KNOWLEDGE	SKILLS	ATTITUDES
Explain why information and technology skills are essential for safe patient care • Chapter 1 • Chapter 2	Seek education about how information is managed in care settings before providing care • Chapter 10	Appreciate the necessity for all health professionals to seek lifelong, continuous learning

(*continued*)

INFORMATICS (continued)

KNOWLEDGE	SKILLS	ATTITUDES
• Chapter 5 • Chapter 6 • Chapter 10 • Chapter 11 • Chapter 12 • Chapter 13	Apply technology and information management tools to support safe processes of care • Chapter 1 • Chapter 2 • Chapter 5 • Chapter 6 • Chapter 10 • Chapter 12 • Chapter 13	of information technology skills • Chapter 1 • Chapter 2 • Chapter 10 • Chapter 13
Identify essential information that must be available in a common database to support patient care • Chapter 10 • Chapter 12 Contrast benefits and limitations of different communication technologies and their impact on safety and quality • Chapter 10	Navigate the electronic health record • Chapter 10 Document and plan patient care in an electronic health record • Chapter 10 Employ communication technologies to coordinate care for patients • Chapter 10	Value technologies that support clinical decision making, error prevention, and care coordination • Chapter 1 • Chapter 2 • Chapter 5 • Chapter 10 • Chapter 12 • Chapter 13 Protect confidentiality of protected health information in electronic health records • Chapter 10
Describe examples of how technology and information management are related to the quality and safety of patient care • Chapter 1 • Chapter 2 • Chapter 5 • Chapter 10 • Chapter 13 Recognize the time, effort, and skill required for computers, databases, and other technologies to become reliable and effective tools for patient care • Chapter 10	Respond appropriately to clinical decision making supports and alerts • Chapter 5 • Chapter 10 Use information management tools to monitor outcomes of care processes • Chapter 10 Use high-quality electronic sources of healthcare information • Chapter 10 • Chapter 12	Value nurses' involvement in design, selection, implementation, and evaluation of information technologies to support patient care • Chapter 10

Reprinted from Cronenwett, L., Sherwood, G., Barnsteiner, J. Disch, J., Johnson, J., Mitchell, P., . . . Warren, J. (2007, May–June). Quality and safety education for nurses. *Nursing Outlook,*, 55(3), 122–131, with permission from Elsevier.

APPENDIX C

CRITICAL THINKING EXTRAS WITH ANSWERS

Critical Thinking C.1

You are concerned with improvement of your nursing practice of the Quality and Safety Education for Nurses (QSEN) competencies below. Review all the competencies and knowledge, skills, and attitudes (KSAs) in Appendix B. Identify a personal goal for your development of one of them in each of the six areas. What do you think a patient's wish for quality care might be in each of the competencies? Do you think there are differences in a patient's wishes depending on the care setting? For example, would a patient have different wishes for patient-centered care (PCC) in a hospital clinic, an ambulatory surgery center, a primary care office, or an inpatient nursing unit?

QSEN COMPETENCY	PERSONAL FUTURE GOAL	PATIENT'S WISH
Patient-centered care (PCC)		
Safety		
Quality improvement (QI)		
Evidence-based practice (EBP)		
Informatics		
Teamwork and collaboration		

Answer: Your personal goals for improvement in each of the six QSEN competencies and their KSAs will reflect your personal values about each of them and their importance in future patient care quality and safety. Your patient's wishes may be different than yours. Patients in a hospital clinic, an ambulatory surgery center, a primary care office, or an inpatient nursing unit will often have different wishes for PCC. Be sure to ask the patients for their opinions. Be sure to listen to their answers well and meet their needs.

Critical Thinking C.2

You are a new nurse just out of orientation on a 30-bed medical patient care unit. Many of the patients on this unit are elderly and suffer from various cardiac and respiratory health care conditions. Staffing for the patients on this unit is usually one registered nurse (RN) to five patients. There are two nurse aides on the unit also, in addition to a charge nurse. You arrive for your evening shift and begin to plan your patient care.

- *Identify which health care structures and processes you will assess early in your shift to ensure patient safety and quality. Incorporate these into your patient care, as needed. Refer to Table 4.1 when necessary.*
- *What patient outcomes should be monitored on these patients?*
- *What criteria will you use to assess this patient staffing situation from a safety perspective?*
- *What actions will you take if you feel this is an unsafe staffing situation?*

Answer: Before beginning your shift, clarify the patient care assignments with the charge nurse and the other staff, as needed. The charge nurse will develop the unit's staffing pattern using the hospital's patient classification system to determine the correct mix of nursing staff, depending on patient acuity. Check that you are comfortable that the right type and number of staff have been identified to meet the needs of patients for the various classifications of patient acuity on your unit. Identify patient care priorities to ensure patient safety and check on the need to request additional staff as patient needs determine this. Be sure that all staff understand their assignments. Check that your unit has good working equipment, for example, suction, computer technology, monitors, side rails on beds, and so on. Identify which patients need to be fed and assign this activity. Ensure that medications and IV fluids are given on schedule. Be sure that all patient care routines have been built into the appropriate staff's shift activities, for example, regular patient rounds, priority patient physical assessments, turn, cough, and deep breathe bedfast patients every 2 hours, ambulate patients on limited activity every 4 to 6 hours, check vital signs every 4 hours, check bedfast patient's skin condition every shift, and so on.

Outcomes to be monitored on these patients include:

- Morbidity and mortality figures, for example, incidence of decubitus ulcers, pneumonia, pulmonary embolism, infection, and so on; level of patient patient satisfaction, and so on.
- To assess this patient staffing situation from a safety perspective, you will consider such elements as patient acuity; staff numbers and qualifications; safety of the environment, e.g., fall rate, presence of side rails, and so on.
- If you feel this is an unsafe staffing situation, you will notify your supervisor immediately using the chain of command. Set priorities and monitor all your patients' airway, breathing, circulation, and safety on your shift until staffing can be quickly

adjusted safely. Determine which patient care needs are critical and must always be done. Reassess patient care priorities depending on patient needs and staffing levels. Less critical patient needs may have to be met at another time if staffing is short.

Critical Thinking C.3

You have just been named to an interprofessional health care team to design a future surgical nursing patient care unit for your hospital. Identify which structure quality elements you will incorporate into the new unit for patient-centered safe care. What health care quality processes will you put in place? Which interprofessional health care team members could help on this team? What health care quality outcomes will you monitor? Be sure to identify and plan for which types of major and minor postoperative surgical patients will be cared for on this nursing unit. What is their acuity level? Review the evidence-based literature and benchmark with other organizations on length of stay and care modalities for your identified surgical patient populations (e.g., postoperative gallbladder surgery, hip surgery, total knee surgery, etc.). Consider how to include necessary interprofessional service units, for example, physical therapy, pharmacy, dietary, laboratory, housekeeping, and so on. Plan to monitor surgical infection rates for each patient population and surgeon. Refer to Table 4.1 as needed. How will you assure that the QSEN elements are built into this future unit? Give at least one example of each of the quality elements as well as one example of the QSEN elements in the table below for this future unit. We did part of the first one in each category below for you.

QUALITY ELEMENTS	EXAMPLES OF ELEMENTS	EXAMPLES OF YOUR IDEAS FOR QUALITY AND QSEN ELEMENTS FOR FUTURE PATIENT CARE UNIT
Structures	• Safe environment • Clean air • Staffing guidelines • Supervisor support • Chain of command policy • High-reliability environment • Just culture • Assignment sheets • Informatics	Side rails on beds, medication reconciliation, competency-based orientation, staff involvement in decision-making councils, and so on
Processes	• Evidence-based patient care surgical standards, guidelines, bundles, and so on. • Delegation policies and procedures • Routines for medication administration, IV monitoring, and postoperative patient care to prevent lung, leg, bowel, bladder, bleeding, and infection problems	

(continued)

Critical Thinking C.3 *(continued)*

QUALITY ELEMENTS	EXAMPLES OF ELEMENTS	EXAMPLES OF YOUR IDEAS FOR QUALITY AND QSEN ELEMENTS FOR FUTURE PATIENT CARE UNIT
Outcomes	Interprofessional team to review the following outcomes monthly • Patient-centered care (PCC) • Patient satisfaction • Patient safety • Infection rates • Morbidity and mortality rates • Staff safety	
Quality and Safety Education for Nurses (QSEN) elements		
Team and colla-boration		Include representatives from nursing, medicine, pharmacy, dietary, physical therapy, laboratory, and so on, in planning of unit
PCC		
Safety		

(continued)

QUALITY ELEMENTS	EXAMPLES OF ELEMENTS	EXAMPLES OF YOUR IDEAS FOR QUALITY AND QSEN ELEMENTS FOR FUTURE PATIENT CARE UNIT
Quality		
Informatics		
Evidence-based practice (EBP)		

Source: Patricia Kelly, unpublished manuscript.

Answer: Use the table in this question above to work with the interprofessional health care team to design a future surgical nursing unit for your hospital. Refer to Table 4.1 as needed, to design this unit. Your answer will include elements of health care structures and processes for this future unit. Consider all the interprofessional health care team members that work with patients at your hospital to include on this team. Health care quality outcomes that you will monitor include patient and staff satisfaction as well as patient morbidity and mortality. You can build the QSEN elements into this future unit by considering them for inclusion early in the planning process. Consider the anticipated acuity level of your patients as you plan the unit.

Critical Thinking C.4

You are a new nurse just out of orientation on a 30-bed surgical patient care unit. You have just arrived for your 7 a.m. to 7 p.m. shift. There are six RNs for the 30 patients. Based on the staffing classifications for patient acuity, you have been assigned five patients on this unit. There are three nurse aides on the unit. Identify how you will plan your day and the day of your fellow team members. Remember to consider, with all of this work, what requires the skills and knowledge of an RN and what could be safely delegated to another health care team member? Note the example of this patient care routine on a surgical unit. How would you alter this routine on another unit?

06:45	Arrive on unit; check assignment sheet
07:00–09:00	Receive shift handoff report. Delegate, as needed. Go over assignments with staff, as needed. Make rounds on high-priority patients, for example, patients with airway, breathing, bleeding, circulation, or safety needs
	Check IV fluids, surgical dressings. Ensure that preoperative patients are ready for the operating room (consents, labs, NPO, etc.). Serve breakfast, feed patients as needed; complete vital signs, pass medications
	Turn, cough, and deep breathe surgical patients, check bleeding, bladder, dressings, lung and bowel sounds, ambulation, and so on. Based on your patient assessments, determine the frequency needed for rounds on priority patients. Check vital signs.
09:00–11:00	Work with nurse aides to complete AM care; review new orders regularly throughout shift, consult with interprofessional team as needed. Pass medications.
	Turn, cough, and deep breathe surgical patients, ambulate new surgical patients, give fresh drinking water to patients
11:00 – 13:00	Lunch, check vital signs, pass medications
	Turn, cough, and deep breathe surgical patients, check bleeding, dressing, lung and bowel sounds, and so on
1300–1500	Check vital signs
	Turn, cough, and deep breathe surgical patients
	Patient reassessment as indicated based on patient's condition
1500 – 1700	Check vital signs, pass medications
	Turn, cough, and deep breathe surgical patients, ambulate new surgical patients
	Patient reassessment as indicated based on patient's condition
1800–1900	Check vital signs
	Turn, cough, and deep breathe surgical patients, check bleeding, dressing, lung and bowel sounds, and so on
	Prepare and give shift handoff report to oncoming staff

Answer: Identify the unit and patients for whom you are developing this patient care routine. Use another form to plan your care. Also, be sure to plan out the times to complete your patient care.

Critical Thinking C.5

Take a look at your nursing unit's policy and procedure book. Pick a policy and examine the type of evidence used as a reference for the policy. Use the pyramid of evidence sources in the evidence-based practice chapter (Chapter 12) to evaluate the types of evidence used to support the policy. Is the evidence appropriate? If possible, can you tell how the evidence was evaluated? Why is it important to evaluate the evidence used to support the policy?

Answer: This activity will help you identify the types of evidence used to support policies. There should be several references for every policy. Ideally, a policy will have a systematic review as one piece of evidence. If only a few articles are included that are expert opinion (nonresearch) articles, you should question whether or not a thorough search was conducted for evidence. Evaluating the evidence is a key step in EBP. Evaluating evidence helps identify the strength of the evidence using standardized guidelines rather than accepting the evidence at face value. Work with other members of the interprofessional team to keep all policies evidence based and current.

Critical Thinking C.6

You are a professional RN on an interprofessional team at your hospital. Sometimes you notice that nursing's input into decisions does not seem to be respected. Some of the team members are dismissive and condescending to the nursing team members.

How can you work to change this and build respect for the profession of nursing as skilled practitioners with much to bring to patient care?

Does the way you dress, introduce yourself as an RN, and communicate with patients and other members of the interprofessional team convey that you expect to be respected?

How do other members of the interprofessional team dress, communicate, and introduce themselves to patients and to you?

Answer: When team members are dismissive and condescending to the nursing team members, you can work to begin to change this and build respect for the profession of nursing as skilled practitioners with much to bring to patient care by increasing your awareness of the inappropriateness of this behavior. Seek the support of nursing, hospital, and medical leadership to change this behavior. Work to develop team training programs such as the TEAMStepps™ program (http://teamstepps.ahrq.gov)

and communication strategies such as the SBAR (situation, background, assessment, recommendation) technique (http://www.ihi.org/knowledge/Pages/Tools/SBAR-TechniqueforCommunicationASituationalBriefingModel.aspx).

The way that nurses dress, introduce themselves as an RN, and communicate with patients and other members of the interprofessional team must convey that nurses expect to be respected. When clothing, introductions, and communications are unprofessional, this may be a sign that patients' needs may not be met in a professional manner. Notice how other members of the interprofessional team dress, communicate, and introduce themselves to patients and to you. Are they professional? Does their behavior convey to patients that they will work to meet patient needs?

Critical Thinking C.7

In an effort to make health care more affordable and accountable, data are being released by the Centers for Medicare and Medicaid Services (CMS) that shows significant variation across the country in what health care providers charge for common services. See https://data.cms.gov/Medicare/Inpatient-Prospective-Payment-System-IPPS-Provider/97k6-zzx3. These data include information comparing the charges for the 100 most common inpatient services and 30 common outpatient services. Compare the average covered charges and the average total payment for a diagnostic related group (DRG) with a large number of total discharges at two of the hospitals in your state. What did you see there? Can you make some decisions about quality care using this information?

Answer: When you compare the average covered charges and the average total payment for a DRG with a large number of total discharges at two of the hospitals in your state, you will often see large variations between the two hospitals. As you begin to study this information more in the future, you may be able to make some decisions about quality care using this information. Look for more of this type of information in the future. Also look for assistance in interpreting the data as we continue to study health care information, quality, and cost in the future.

Critical Thinking C.8

Have you asked a patient, "What is PCC?" Have you considered what outcomes you should monitor to evaluate PCC? Do you get any patient feedback that allows you to examine patient satisfaction with respect, caring, timeliness of service, and so on, offered to them? Should nurses be concerned with patient satisfaction or is it enough to focus just on assuring high-quality physical outcomes?

Answer: QSEN states that PCC recognizes the patient or designee as the source of control and full partner in providing compassionate and coordinated care based on respect for patient's preferences, values, and needs. Patient needs must be considered when delivering care. Nurses must ask patients what is important to them and monitor patient outcomes related to this. Increasingly, patient's feedback is being solicited to determine patient satisfaction and these scores are affecting hospital reimbursement. Nurses should be concerned with patient satisfaction as well as high-quality physical outcomes. Patient satisfaction with respect, caring, timeliness of service, and so on, offered to them is an important outcome and must be reviewed.

Critical Thinking C.9

Look at how informatics is used at a hospital where you have a clinical experience. Has an electronic patient care record documentation system been developed? Is informatics used to improve clinical decision making, medication safety, evidence-based care, and so on? How does informatics improve patient care?

Answer: When you look at how informatics is used at a hospital where you have a clinical experience, you will probably note their electronic patient care record documentation system, as well as the use of informatics to improve clinical decision making, medication safety, evidence-based care, and so on. Informatics has the potential to improve patient care in many ways. See how many type of informatics you note at your agency.

Critical Thinking C.10

The Affordable Care Act (ACA), http://www.hhs.gov/opa/affordable-care-act/index. html, aims to increase the quality and affordability of health insurance, lower the uninsured rate by expanding public and private insurance coverage, and reduce the costs of health care for individuals and the government. It provides a number of mechanisms—including mandates, subsidies, and insurance exchanges—to increase coverage and affordability. The law also requires insurance companies to cover all applicants within new minimum standards and offer the same rates regardless of preexisting conditions or sex. Take a look at the website. What did you see? Do you think the ACA will improve patient care?

Answer: It is early to know the answer to this query. If the ACA aims of increasing the quality and affordability of health insurance, lowering the uninsured rate by expanding public and private insurance coverage, and reducing the costs of health care for individuals and the government are achieved, the ACA will improve patient care.

Critical Thinking C.11

Look at how informatics is used at a hospital where you have a clinical experience. Has an electronic patient care record documentation system been developed? Is informatics used to improve clinical decision making, medication safety, evidence-based care, and so on? Does informatics improve patient care and communication among the various health care professionals working with patients?

Answer: When you look at how informatics is used at a hospital where you have a clinical experience, you will often note that an electronic patient care record documentation system has been developed. Informatics also improves patient care in many ways such as by improving clinical decision making, medication safety, evidence-based care, and so on. Informatics does improve patient care and communication among the various health care professionals working with patients.

Critical Thinking C.12

Read through the quality improvement (QI) methodology provided by the Department of Health and Human Services at http://www.hrsa.gov/quality/toolbox/methodology/index.html. Identify a quality problem during a clinical experience. Work as a group or individually to use the steps provided in the QI methodology to address the quality problem. While working on the project, reflect on the need for nurses to be involved in the QI process.

Answer: By using the QI methodology as a guide, you can work through an actual quality problem that reflects actual QI processes in the clinical setting. This process will help you understand the depth and breadth of the QI process as well as the need for nurses to be involved in all clinical QI projects.

Critical Thinking C.13

Read through the QI measures at http://www.hrsa.gov/quality/toolbox/measures/index. html. Select one of the QI measures and read about the identification of indicators, the measurement of indicators, the development of clinical practice guidelines, and the creation of pathways to support compliance and support for sustaining improvement. Identify where nurses are affected by the measures. How do the QI measures affect interprofessional team members? How do interprofessional team members affect the measures? Why is it important to have representation from a variety of health care professions involved in the development of QI measures?

Answer: During this exercise, you will gain an understanding of the QI processes involved in developing and implementing measurements for quality initiatives, clinical practice guidelines, and pathways. An awareness of the need for the involvement of nurses and a variety of health care professionals in quality improvement will probably be evident in your responses to the questions.

Critical Thinking C.14

Complete the Institute for Healthcare Improvement (IHI) Open School courses at http:// app.ihi.org/lms/onlinelearning.aspx. You will need to register for the free courses. Once all the modules are completed, you will receive a certificate of completion. After each course, reflect on what you have learned. Think about your most recent clinical experience. Do you see any of what you have learned being used in clinical practice? Do you see opportunities to use what you have learned in clinical practice? Use the following table to document your reflections for each IHI Open School course completed.

IHI OPEN SCHOOL COURSE	CLINICAL EXPERIENCE THAT REFLECTED THE COURSE TEACHINGS	CLINICAL PRACTICE THAT DID NOT REFLECT THE COURSE TEACHINGS	OPPORTUNITIES FOR USE IN THE CLINICAL SETTING (YOUR SUGGESTIONS FOR USING THE COURSE TEACHINGS)
Patient safety			
Leadership			
Improvement capability			

(continued)

Critical Thinking C.14 (continued)

IHI OPEN SCHOOL COURSE	CLINICAL EXPERIENCE THAT REFLECTED THE COURSE TEACHINGS	CLINICAL PRACTICE THAT DID NOT REFLECT THE COURSE TEACHINGS	OPPORTUNITIES FOR USE IN THE CLINICAL SETTING (YOUR SUGGESTIONS FOR USING THE COURSE TEACHINGS)
Patient- and family-centered care			
Quality cost and value			
Triple aim for populations			
Overall thoughts:			

Answer: When you reflect on what you have learned at the IHI Open School courses, think about your most recent clinical experience. Hopefully, you will see at least some of what you have learned being used in clinical practice. There should be many opportunities to use what you have learned in clinical practice. Your documentation of your reflections for each course completed should help you recall these lessons in your future practice.

APPENDIX D

ANSWERS AND RATIONALE TO REVIEW QUESTIONS

CHAPTER 1

1. **D**

   Answers A, B, and C all are appropriate actions to take to start an improvement project. National websites such as www.hospitalcompare.org will provide the nurses with benchmark comparison information from other hospitals. Posting current hospital performance data allows for transparency of how the organization is doing specific to this core measure. Interprofessional teams will provide the best approach to addressing this core measure. It involves physicians, nurses, and EKG technicians. Answer D assumes there is someone to blame rather than reviewing how system processes can be improved. This choice would most likely not achieve consistent quality improvement (QI) results.

2. **A**

   It is best to look at reliable and professional recourses to help you determine what has already been published to make improvements. The Institute for Healthcare Improvement (IHI) is a well-established website that has published multiple QI strategies. It is important not to get distracted with unrelated websites that are focused on other diseases, for example, cancer. Drug companies do have information about new treatment options; however, these are not recognized as the best evidence-based source for overall process improvements. Google is not recommended for this search because there are unreliable sites that can be referenced there that can distract professionals from accurate information.

3. **B**

   The patient had been in the hospital for 3 days. The contents of the advance directive should have been reviewed with the family and patient care should have incorporated the patient's wishes with the family participating. The organization has an ethical and legal obligation to ensure it has the patient's advance directive and has reviewed its contents.

4. A

The Joint Commission has standards that address the inclusion of core measures, safe practices, and process improvement processes. The Joint Commission does not mandate standardized billing models.

5. A

Higher spending does not match up with better outcomes. U.S. life expectancy is lower than other Westernized countries.

6. D

The care associated with a Stage IV pressure ulcer acquired by a patient while in the hospital is not reimbursed by Centers for Medicare and Medicaid Services (CMS). That is why it is very important for nurses to document a thorough skin assessment upon admission to ensure that the patient does not have any preexisting pressure ulcers, especially Stages III or IV pressure ulcers.

7. C

Typically, communication problems between caregivers are involved when there are health care errors. It is important to ensure open and honest communication between professionals. They also need to check in with each other to make accurate clear patient report handoffs.

8. A

Quality and Safety Education for Nurses (QSEN) suggests that we can make a difference in ensuring safety and quality for our patients. This organization emphasizes that we should incorporate six key elements into our practice; QI, team work and collaboration, evidence-based practice (EBP), patient-centered care (PCC), safety, and informatics.

9. A

Public reporting of hospital data is now available on websites so that patients can make informed decisions on where they might seek care based upon quality information about different hospitals.

10. A

This answer *best* represents the top patient quality concerns as described by the HFMA value project (2011).

CHAPTER 2

1. C

PCC is defined as "recognize the patient or designee as the source of control and full partner in providing compassionate and coordinated care based on respect for patient's preferences, values, and needs." This clearly fits the scenario described in the question.

2. A, B, C, D, E, and F

After identifying a QI patient care issue while using informatics in the electronic health care record (EHR), the primary nurse used principles of QI and EBP and collaborated with another nursing team member. The consultation with the wound care nurse was effective in providing safe, PCC.

3. **A**

Teamwork and collaboration is defined as "Function effectively within nursing and interprofessional teams, fostering open communication, mutual respect, and shared decision making to achieve quality patient care." One of the skills associated with this competency is to communicate clearly to minimize risks associated with patient handoff reports during transitions of care.

4. **B**

QI requires that nurses "use data to monitor the outcomes of care processes and use improvement methods to design and test changes to continuously improve the quality and safety of health care systems." The nurse may use a root cause analysis (RCA) to ensure QI in this situation.

5. **D**

While many of the competencies are reflected in this scenario, the most appropriate answer is teamwork and collaboration. The focus of the teamwork competency is to "function effectively within nursing and interprofessional teams, fostering open communication, mutual respect, and shared decision making to achieve quality patient care." Asepsis is an important national patient safety goal and can be achieved through teamwork and hand washing.

6. **B and D**

Bar-code medication administration is an example of a safety strategy, as it standardizes recurring processes. Additionally, this is an good example of the informatics competency.

7. **C**

PCC is ensured when the nurse works with patients and the interprofessional team to ensure patient safety and quality.

8. **B**

QI requires that nurses "use data to monitor the outcomes of care processes and use improvement methods to design and test changes to continuously improve the quality and safety of health care systems." The nurse is using a unit-based control chart to help understand the variation in patient response and develop effective pain management standards.

9. **A**

The focus of the safety competency is to "minimize risk of harm to patients and providers through both system effectiveness and individual performance." One of the key knowledge aspects of safety is to examine human factors and other basic safety design principles as well as commonly used unsafe practices like the use of work-arounds and unsafe abbreviations.

10. **D**

The focus of the informatics competency is to "use information and technology to communicate, manage knowledge, mitigate error, and support decision making." The nurse uses the data within the EHR to help support decision making and ensure that the patient's progress is appropriate within the care regimen.

CHAPTER 3

1. **D**

Not only are nurses key to changing a culture, but all disciplines within an organization work together to change the culture. A, B, and C are all correct statements.

2. **C**

The opposite is true, high-reliability organizations (HROs) understand that fragmentation of tasks lead to problems and work toward standardizing the task processes. HROs use a systems thinking and process approach to health care. In addition, HROs find that small problems are indicators of a larger issue and are aware of what is going on in the organization.

3. **A**

The hospital provides time and support for a committee to look at patient outcomes and practice issues on the nursing units. This is a sign of a strong culture for quality, safety, and performance improvement. B is incorrect, as the nurses were not supported through the hospital to look at the quality issue. C is not correct since the nurse took the initiative but the director was not supporting the change. D is incorrect as no nurses were involved in the interprofessional committee that looked at nursing practice.

4. **A, B, D, and F**

Each of these are examples of simplifying the nurse's work. Color-coded scrubs help to quickly identify who is who and is valuable in critical situations when working with unknown people from across the hospital. Placing laptop computers on movable stands allows the nurse to access information at the point of care. The availability of insulin syringes where medications are withdrawn helps eliminate steps required to search for syringes. Highlighting lab abnormal lab values helps to quickly identify those readings that require additional interventions for safe patient care. C is incorrect because the information about patient satisfaction surveys is good to know but not vital for patient care. E is incorrect in that although it eliminates interruptions and distractions, it also makes it more difficult for health care providers to reach their patients.

5. **D**

The number of respondents replying with "very satisfied" on their survey is a reflection of PCC. This answer is the only one that reflects the patient's perception of care provided. The other three relate to nursing care delivery.

6. **A**

Allowing interprofessional committees the autonomy to identify health care delivery problems and make changes to patient care practices is essential for an organization with high reliability and a focus on safety. Although B, C, and D can be good for an HRO, they are not essential to an HRO culture development.

7. **A**

The quality and patient safety department is responsible for submitting data to regulatory agencies, quality, and safety reporting for public reporting, as well as database submissions for benchmarking, process improvements, clinical documentation, infection prevention, and control. The quality and patient safety department is not directly responsible for ethical delivery of care, overseeing Institutional Review Board (IRB), or the distribution of resources. Other departments and committees have responsibilities in these areas.

8. **B**

This is the only response that supports the inclusion of a person who is not from the unit involved and does not include names. A and B include telling the unit director about the incident and the people involved, which can lead to blame and punishment. D involves the charge nurse.

9. **B, C, E,** and **F**

Each of these are definitions of the four key measurement criteria as described by The Joint Commission. A and D are not included in the four key measurement criteria.

10. **D**

An indication that an HRO has enculturated quality and safety is the willingness of interprofessionals to work together and devote both time and energy to process improvements. This is done with the knowledge that changes will happen and improvements will occur. A is incorrect, although employees feel comfortable reporting, it does not mean that an HRO exists. In addition, reporting to the unit director does not mean that the error or near miss will be examined. B is incorrect, counseling employees is a form of placing blame, something that an HRO does not do. C is incorrect as the problem is handed off to different individuals in different roles rather than examined using an interprofessional team to identify bigger problems.

CHAPTER 4

1. **C**

A system approach to safety is used in a culture of safety. After reviewing the data, the committee would look at the broader picture of how the one particular unit operates in delivering patient care. For example, the committee could look at nurse staffing, the unit's environment, and available equipment. A system approach to safety does not blame people. A system approach to safety will use education after the root causes have been identified, not before.

2. **B**

By removing sharps, medications, and other means of self-harm from the patient's access area, you will be keeping the patient immediately safe. Continuous observation of the patient and alerting other team members will also strengthen the safety of the immediate environment for the patient.

3. **C**

An adverse event is when there is harm to a patient. Administration of the wrong medication falls into this category. The harm to the patient may not be immediately evident.

4. **B**

Correcting a coworker requires deft skill in any situation. When the correction needs to be done in front of a patient, it is important to integrate the corrective element in such a way as to be inobtrusive. Offering sanitizer can also help and serve as a gentle reminder to your coworker about proper hand hygiene. If the behavior does not change, it may be necessary to take stronger action in the future.

5. **C**

First, the nurse should call the physician and ask for a clarification of the medication order. After this is done, the nurse should check with pharmacy to ask about and learn more about the drug interaction alert. The alert is a safety feature that brings attention to the potential of harm if the medication is administered. The nurse should not assume that the medication can be safely administered based on how long the patient has been in the hospital.

6. **C**

First, notify the patient physician. The rapid response team (RRT) can then be called to help prevent a cardiac arrest or unexpected death. For RRTs to be effective, the ideal time to call an RRT is when the patient appears to be deteriorating to maximize the timeliness of rescue interventions.

7. **A, D, and E**

Skid-resistant floor mats, chair alarms, and bed alarms would create a safe environment for a patient who might forget to call the nurse for assistance and might fall to the floor due to orthostatic changes. The chair alarms and bed alarms alert the nurse that the patient is in motion and needs immediate attention. The skid-resistant floor mat softens any potential falls and helps reduce injuries. Lighting should be bright, not dim. Ceiling-mounted lift equipment is typically used for patients who have impaired mobility.

8. **B**

Workplace bullying is not always physical or dramatic. Repeatedly responding to a coworker in a manner that is intimidating or negative indicates an attempt to isolate and diminish the individual.

9. **A, B, D, and E**

A routine, bundle, protocol, and checklist all include standardized clinical patient care and will help reduce variation when caring for this patient. A core measure is a quality measurement, not a clinical tool.

10. **D**

Add the total nursing hours for all nurses on that day (8 × 8 = 64 nursing hours). Divide the total nursing hours by the number of patients cared for (midnight census) on the same day (64/32 = 2.0 nursing hours per patient day)

CHAPTER 5

1. **D**

When taking a telephone order, safe practice includes writing the order, then reading it back to the prescribing physician so that it can be verified as accurate. This ensures that what is written as the order is what is intended by the prescriber.

2. **A**

RRTs consist of a physician, a critical care nurse, and a respiratory therapist among other members. The RRT can be summoned to any bedside to provide immediate assistance to nurses caring for patients with deteriorating health conditions, in an effort to prevent ICU admissions or arrests.

3. **B**

SBAR (situation, background, assessment and recommendation) is an acronym for a structured communication framework used to promote safety. Using SBAR, the situation describes the patient's general information, background describes the events leading up to this moment, assessment describes the manifestations currently exhibited by the patient, and recommendations describes the suggestions for actions needed for correction.

4. **C**
De-escalation strategies for challenging communications such as when team members raise their voices include refocusing the communication on the patient's needs that prompted the communication in the first place.

5. **A**
An interprofessional team brings multiple disciplines together with varying perspectives and expertise to contemplate options and deliberate alternatives in forming a comprehensive plan to address patient's needs.

6. **A**
An RCA is an orderly process used to investigate errors or potential errors. The process works to identify the underlying problems that increase the likelihood of errors while avoiding the trap of focusing on mistakes of individuals.

7. **B**
During team huddle, those involved in the patient's care have a brief, informal review of the plan of care, and identify pertinent information regarding the patient's status.

8. **C**
The nurse assists the family to connect to the team. Empathy is conveyed with understanding of their concerns and as a member of the team, the nurse organizes a team meeting with family members address those concerns and promote communication.

9. **B**
Eliciting constructive feedback from colleagues allows the nurse to reflect on practice and make adjustments that enhance individual and team performance.

10. **C**
Sentinel events are those that cause serious harm to others. Many sentinel events are the result of communication errors or misunderstandings. Skilled communication uses strategies that promote safety and guard against misinterpretations.

CHAPTER 6

1. **D**
Nursing and interprofessional health care providers have awakened to the need for health care to keep the patient central to all services provided to patients and their families. Nursing has always professed that patients are their primary focus and see this movement as a "return to the basics."

2. **C**
Relationship-based care is a model to operationalize a patient-centered approach to care. This is accomplished through the application of reflection, professional knowledge, and knowing the patient with every encounter with the patient and family.

3. **D**
The best assessment of a patient's understanding is direct observation. Teach back techniques are used to close the gap between what is taught and what is learned. By observing the patient changing her own dressing, the nurse can determine how effective the teaching was for the patient.

4. B

Effective communication requires the congruency of verbal and nonverbal communication. Unless the nurse both demonstrates and verbalizes her availability to the patient, the patient may receive mixed messages from the nurse.

5. D

Health homes are designed to be patient-centered systems of care that provide comprehensive care management, care coordination, and health promotion, comprehensive transitional care across inpatient and outpatient settings with adequate follow-up, and individual and family support.

6. B

Significant medication errors can occur when patients transition from one level of care to another. It is important for the clinician to reconcile medications at every transition to ensure patients have a clear understanding of the medications they have been prescribed. Care providers must also have an accurate account of a patient's medication regimen to improve care and prevent errors.

7. C

A personal health record helps patients manage their own health information and serves as a tool to help record details of their care.

8. F

Patient satisfaction encompasses many components beyond the actual provision of care requiring clinicians to be sensitive to patient-centered values and incorporate those values into the care provided.

9. A

Health care providers must understand that culture will dictate the acceptance of caring behaviors. Organizations must make a commitment to ensure that clinicians have the knowledge and resources to facilitate culturally sensitive, PCC.

10. C

The Hospital Consumer Assessment of Healthcare Providers and Systems (HCAHPS) survey represents a core set of questions that allow valid comparisons of patient care experiences at hospitals locally, regionally, and nationally. This data can be used to help clinicians understand indicators of patient satisfaction in their hospital.

CHAPTER 7

1. A, C, D, E, F, and H

Each of these actions are found in the definition. B is incorrect, efficiency is not the focus of QI efforts although it can be a side product of improving care. G is incorrect, QI efforts focus on an aspect of care within a health care system, not the entire organization. I is incorrect, the definition does not prescribe when data should be reported. Quality data should be provided monthly or quarterly to the affected personnel rather than annually.

2. A

Improving patient outcomes is a primary goal of QI. Although the other three responses are outcomes from QI efforts, they are not the main goal for conducting QI project.

3. **D**

Value-based purchasing is a current quality issue and is presently shaping the quality of care provided in health care organizations. Peer reviews, outlier identification, and publicly reporting of data are all historic in that they formed where quality health care provision is today.

4. **C**

The nurses used a systematic method of reviewing and evaluating evidence on the health literacy tools available. They also considered the type of patients found on the medical–surgical units when considering the tool. A is incorrect, no new knowledge was gained and the type of design was not research. B is incorrect, although the goal was to improve care, the group intended to evaluate evidence on available tools that would identify literacy levels. No pre- or postdata collection was done. D is incorrect, the nurses performed a review of the evidence using a systematic method and evaluated each piece of evidence.

5. **B**

This answer follows the Plan-Do-Study-Act (PDSA) cycle. The other responses do not follow the PDSA cycle.

6. **A**

Lean optimizes existing processes focusing on elimination of waste and inefficiency and Six Sigma seeks to reduce variability. B is incorrect, Lean does not focus efforts over time and Six Sigma does not focus on efficiency. C is incorrect, Lean Six Sigma is frequently combined. D is incorrect, the statement reflects the opposite of what Lean and Six Sigma do as QI techniques.

7. **D**

A fishbone diagram is used to examine a process and the related factors that contribute to a problem. A is incorrect, a fishbone diagram does not determine variability. B is incorrect, a fishbone diagram does not represent the entire process from beginning to end. C is incorrect, a fishbone diagram does not identify cause and effects, only relationships.

8. **A**

Health care failure mode and effect analysis (HFMEA) is proactive whereas the RCA is reactive. B is incorrect, the definitions are opposite of the statements. C is incorrect, HFMEA is not a documentation system and RCAs are not done annually on every significant event. D is incorrect, HFMEA does not enhance the quality culture directly. RCAs are not part of every PDSA.

9. **All the answers are correct.**

All of the responses can be classified as sentinel events or near misses. For A, if a patient is considered suicidal they cannot be allowed to sign themselves out and should have a 72-hour detention in place. For B, this is a sentinel event that probably resulted in harm to the patient. For C, this is considered a "never" event, something that should never happen and a sentinel event. For D, this is a sentinel event due to the inadvertent overdose. For E, a patient fall in most hospitals is considered an event (near miss if no harm, sentinel if resulting in harm). For F, no discharged patient should return within 24 hours with the same diagnosis and this needs to be investigated.

10. **A**

New nurses can easily learn how to collect data and share with others. Responses B, C, and D require more experience and training and are better suited to an advanced practice nurse role.

CHAPTER 8

1. **B and it is a definition of benchmarking.**
   A is incorrect as benchmarking can help define the goal but it is not a key element of benchmarking. C is incorrect. Benchmarking can help identify clinical areas in need of improvement but only if the data is benchmarked against the best performers. D is incorrect. Although collaboration is important, it is not a key element in benchmarking.

2. **C**
   Internal benchmarking is used when a health care organization wants to evaluate the quality of a process and no current standardized benchmarks exist. Look at Table 8.1. A is incorrect. Benchmarking against a nationally recognized standard is considered external benchmarking against existing high performers. B is incorrect. Using internal benchmarking solely based on poor outcomes is not the best way to evaluate performance. In this case, a search of widely available and standardized benchmarks is appropriate. D is incorrect. Many of the nationally recognized databases and benchmarks provide the opportunity to select benchmarks that are size appropriate for the organization.

3. **C**
   Compliance rates are below national average making this a trigger for process improvement. A, B, and D are all examples of improvements in quality.

4. **D**
   The checklist provides specific steps that are evidence based and lead to a decreased incidence of ventilator-acquired pneumonia. The checklist is a process of care indicator, allowing measurement of each step of the process such as checking "yes" to the step. A is incorrect. The question asks about the process of care steps that are taken to minimize the incidence of the outcome, not the outcome of ventilator-acquired pneumonia itself. B is incorrect. Quality is what indicators measure but it is not an indicator in and of itself. C is incorrect. Clinical care is not an indicator.

5. **A, B, and E**
   A, B, and E are absolutely necessary to include on the team as they directly influence the transition of care from the ED to the admitting unit. C, D, and F are not absolutely necessary as they do not play a role in the transition of care to the admitting unit.

6. **A**
   Many projects fail to sustain change due to inadequate education or lack of dissemination to the right staff members. B is incorrect. Finding other problems that relate to the problem under investigation is expected and becomes part of the changes. C is incorrect. All problem assessments arise from data and include a way of measuring change. This is an essential element to QI. D is incorrect. Timetables provide a guide on when specific tasks will be done. Times can, and often do change.

7. **C**
   Participating in National Database of Nursing Quality Indicators (NDNQI) allows comparisons against benchmarks from a large database of a variety of health care organizations. A is incorrect. Only nurse-sensitive quality indicators are included. B is incorrect. The database only allows for comparison benchmarking, it does not provide information on how to fix quality problems. D is incorrect. Unless an

organization pays a subscription, they do not have access to the information. The database does not allow comparisons locally, only nationally.

8. **D**
As of 2011, the National Quality Forum endorses over 600 health care quality indicators.

9. **A**
In areas where quality indicators and benchmarks are less common, a professional organization that is directly linked to the specific health care area is appropriate.

10. **D**
If data is collected differently in other organizations then the findings cannot be compared. One hospital may collect fall rate data based on one definition where a fall is any time a person goes to the floor, even if assisted. Another hospital may collect data on only those falls that are unassisted and not count those where a patient is assisted to the floor. A is incorrect. Similar resources and measurement styles is necessary for comparisons. B is incorrect. It is expected that different health care organizations may select different benchmarks. C is incorrect. The similarity in demographics of the community only help to support benchmarking against other health care organizations.

CHAPTER 9

1. **D**
Option D meets the criteria for a special cause variation in that the data point is outside 3 standard deviations above or below the mean.

2. **B and E**
Option B and E are the only options that are based on data and relate directly to the problem.

3. **B**
One staff nurse's poor performance would not indicate a need for a quality improvement project. The problem is specific to one person. The other responses include a specific reason for a quality improvement project.

4. **B**
Option B is correct based on calculations of mean and range.

5. **B**
The run, Pareto, and control charts increase in scientific significance. A and C are incorrect as the range only shows the spread of numbers. D is incorrect because the run and Pareto charts can also show process variation.

6. **B and E**
The other three options refer to either a run or control chart.

7. **A**
Both a run and a control chart allow for statistical process control (SPC). Option B is incorrect because a run chart can provide statistical analysis. C is incorrect because SPC requires a median centerline for the run chart or the mean as the centerline for the control chart. D is incorrect because there is potential error assessing for SPC (when assessing for an outlier) because that requires some guessing if the data point is truly an outlier.

8. D

Option A refers to a mean. Option B refers to the range. Option C refers to special cause variation.

9. A

Option A is correct because a flow map helps the team to outline the process from beginning to end. A fishbone is used to identify cause and effects of a process. A scatter plot is useful to assess for the relationship between two variables. The Pareto chart depicts the frequency distribution of a variable.

10. D

Option A is referring to statistical process control. Option B is incorrect because baseline data alone may not trigger a QI project if it is not prioritized. Option C is incorrect because there is no ability to trend with one baseline piece of data.

11. B

Option A is incorrect because the dictionary may not capture a relevant health care definition. Option C and D are not incorporated into an operational definition. Option B is correct because a clear numerator and denominator are crucial when collecting data to ensure everyone is collecting the data using the same process.

CHAPTER 10

1. C

Computer-based technologies often contain point of care alerts that help the nurse to consider potential conflicts with the medications being administered. Although technology is considered an advancement in patient safety, it does not eliminate the responsibility of the nurse to double check the five rights (right patient, right medication, right dose, right route, right time), and review patient allergies.

2. D

It is the responsibility of each institution to establish local policies and guidelines for using the electronic medical record (EMR). Each provider should receive adequate training in using the locally designed EMR. Each facility must take responsibility to provide employees with education and training on the particular EMR in their institution along with contingency plans for emergency situations.

3. C

Users of EMR systems should have a voice in the design and utilization of the system. Collaborating with the nurse informaticist is the best way to design a system that is user friendly and efficient. Allowing excessive pop-ups or alerts can be dangerous as it may promote a tendency of providers to ignore them, or attempt to suppress them.

4. A

Computerized provider order entry (CPOE) provides a system in which the provider no longer has to handwrite orders, which is a contributing factor in medical errors and patient harm. CPOE requires providers to generate orders in the computer, promoting accuracy and timeliness in the orders being complete. All of these add to patient safety.

5. C

Although not fully realized at this point, the potential future of EHR is envisioned to be a complete health record for a patient. This record would contain evidence of health promotion, disease prevention, continuous list of medications and allergies, as well as medical treatments and interventions.

6. **D**
Each facility should have a designated security officer responsible for maintaining the computer security. While each health care team member is charged with maintaining standards of patient privacy and confidentiality, he or she is not responsible for breaches in system security.

7. **B**
The pop up features are provided to aid clinical decision making and to promote increased safety in providing patient care.

8. **A**
One of the benefits of information technology to provide readily available, accurate and evidence-based research. This information can be used to promote efficiency, help with decision making in bedside care, and to facilitate patient education.

9. **C**
Telehealth promotes the provision of health care across miles, saving the patient and provides expense and time in travel. Although modern technologies provide real time data feeds to computers, nurses need to remember to validate the information by first performing a patient assessment. Calling the patient to see how they feel, and to verify the placement of the pulse oximeter is the primary action the nurse should take.

10. **A**
TIGER (Technology Initiative Guiding Educational Reform) consists of a collaborative group of experts working to infuse technology information, guidelines, and best practice protocols into nursing education at various levels.

CHAPTER 11

1. **A**
Boolean commands are used in electronic databases to define relationships between relevant search terms.

2. **C**
It is necessary to determine that the literature demonstrates a cause and effect between frequent ambulation and pain control.

3. **C**
To find the greatest amount of relevant literature, it is necessary to consult at least one, and ideally more than one, specialized literature database, such as PubMed or CINAHL.

4. **B**
PICO questions are represented by the following: (P) patient/population of interest, (I) issue of interest, (C) comparison, and (O) outcome. The other choices do not include all required components.

5. **A**
A literature search could provide methods to help you design your study, making it easier to get started. It could help you to avoid duplicating previous research in your study design. In fact, a thorough search of the literature could

demonstrate that a specific model has been identified as the standard of care and further research is unnecessary. Even if a literature search does not identify a standard of care, it can help identify existing patient assignment models to study and test.

6. **A**

Before proceeding with any inquiry, it is necessary to review your hospital's current policy and practice for how best to care for tracheostomy patients. Understanding the policy will give you a sense of whether you are already utilizing the best available practice or if there is opportunity for improvement.

7. **B**

Most databases will employ a controlled subject headings vocabulary and will index articles with a single, agreed-upon subject heading whenever possible. Therefore, best result will be achieved when the words used in the search are picked from the controlled subject headings vocabulary.

8. **C**

It is generally much better to search for main concepts separately and then combine the concepts after the initial search results are retrieved. This allows for much greater flexibility in search design and eliminates the need to start over completely if your initial search efforts do not produce the desired results.

9. **B**

When searching electronic databases for evidence, especially databases employing a controlled vocabulary, it is often best to start your search more broadly and see what initial results are returned before searching for every component of a search.

10. **A**

Bibliographic databases are often the best choice when looking for evidence because they allow the user to search a wide range of relevant literature without limiting results only to articles that the user would be able to access in full text.

CHAPTER 12

1. **D**

The "P" in PICO is the first step and is the step that focuses on identifying the populations. The nurse has identified the population, so the next step is for the nurse to determine the intervention he or she would like to consider.

2. **C**

Benner (1984) stated that regardless of how much education a nurse possessed, he or she could never be an expert without actual clinical experience.

3. **A, B, D,** and **E**

EBP promotes the safety and well-being of patients and promotes optimal delivery of health care.

4. **B**

The nurse understands that his or her primary role is to help patients achieve their desired plan of care. Although research and scientific data are important, personal beliefs and values of the patient must be considered.

5. **C**

Research findings have different levels of quality. Levels up to Level IV are considered to be rigorous enough to be used to make practice-based decisions. Expert opinions are case studies above Level IV.

6. **C**

Scientific data and evidence cannot be applied to all patient situations. To optimize patient outcomes, the patient's values and individual needs must be taken into account.

7. **2, 4, 1, and 3**

The first step is to create a PICO question; next the nurse must search existing literature. The third step is to analyze the evidence gleaned from the literature to assist in the creation of step four, implementing a pilot project.

8. **A**

It is best to evaluate the effectiveness of the pilot program prior to rolling it out to prevent unintended organizational upheaval, thus enhancing the speed of adoption of the innovation.

9. **A**

Nurses in clinical practice will often identify knowledge-focused triggers, which can stem from the external professional environment. Once an issue is identified, the first step is to narrow the focus into a researchable question using the PICO format.

10. **A**

While it is important to note that application of EBP must consider the personal circumstances of the patient, the child cannot advocate for himself or herself and therefore it is the role of the nurse to act as patient advocate. This is supported by nurse theorist Madeleine Leininger.

CHAPTER 13

1. **B**

It is important and standard management practice to discuss patient safety issues at staff meetings. It is not always appropriate for staff to be notified when a safety event occurs until after a full investigation into the root cause of the event. While it's important to notify a supervisor when an event occurs, it may be more feasible to enter the facts of an event into an electronic reporting system; inability to notify leadership in a timely manner may result in another event happening due to a system problem that needs to be resolved. The best answer for the transformational leader is to accept that errors occur and create an environment that works to improve the system and reduce the likelihood of errors occurring in the future.

2. **A**

The registered nurse (RN) and physician should facilitate patient-centered decision making. Always notify your manager or hospital risk management department before talking to any attorney representing a patient. The best decision-maker for the patient's care is the patient.

3. C

Evidence-based clinical practice guidelines include a review of the recent litera-ture about a patient care problem and outline the preferred interventions to assist the patient in reaching the best possible outcome. Staff meetings may be a good place to let people know about new policies and procedures—but evidence-based resources are the best source for the development and implementation of guide-lines. The Internet may be used for help, but use caution when accessing informa-tion from unreliable sources. Other members of the interprofessional team may provide good input, but active involvement requires the nurse to review the evi-dence. Professional nursing organizations are great resources for EBP and include reference lists for further study by the nurse.

4. D

While computers may assist in the consistency of data collection by nurses, not every nurse interprets and documents patient assessment findings exactly the same. Some electronic health system records may notify a nurse that documenta-tion is missing—but this practice does not automatically ensure safe patient care. Computer-based charting is certainly easier to "read" by the interprofessional team rather than handwritten documents; again, it does not always ensure safety. The best way to ensure safe patient care is to help clinicians' record data and sup-port decision making in patient care situations that are complex.

5. A

RCA is a tool used in QI efforts to help uncover the reason for an error or a poten-tial error in the delivery of patient care. EBP is clinical practice by any interpro-fessional health care provider based on experts, published research, and so on that should promote high-quality, effective patient care. Clinical intelligence is the transformation of many individual data elements about patients in the medical record and through analysis, it becomes meaningful and useful.

6. A

Screening patients on admission for "high risk" for readmission is the best way to identify patient problems and concerns so that care is delivered that minimizes the chance for readmission after the patient goes home. Documenting that the patient understands teaching at discharge may not prevent readmission; patient education should occur throughout the patient's stay. A telephone number for the patient to call with any questions may be helpful—but cannot ensure prevention of readmission.

7. B

Patient satisfaction scores are publicly reported, but reflect the patients' experience with their hospitalization; however, this has not been shown to improve patient safety. EBP is clinical practice by any interprofessional health care provider based on experts, published research, and so on, that should promote high-quality, effec-tive patient care. Shared governance is being implemented in hospitals to enhance the RNs' ability to impact decisions that impact clinical practice and day-to-day decision making. HVBPP is a national program that will distribute money to hos-pitals based on their overall performance on a set of quality measures linked to improved clinical processes of care and patient satisfaction

8. C

An accountable care organization (ACO) is a formal network of doctors, hospitals and health care providers that will share the responsibility of providing health care to all the patients enrolled with the ACO. A health care system is a grouping of hospitals and/or other outpatient centers (both for-profit and nonprofit) that provide illness care and health care in a particular community. A patient-centered medical home is an outpatient clinic or physician office that provides interprofessional care to patients who come for illness/wellness services. An academic medical center is a hospital or health system with a tri-part mission of teaching, research, and patient care.

9. **B, C,** and **E**

Diabetes, asthma, and stroke are medical conditions, but they are not currently included in publicly reported clinical conditions monitored by CMS.

10. **B, C, D,** and **E**

Telling patients or families to file malpractice claims is unrelated to health reform recommendations or actions. There is no evidence that malpractice claims reduce health care costs or improve patient care outcomes. QI is a methodology to improve structure, process, and outcome of clinical patient care delivery. While QI in health care is important, it is not a specific health reform change.

APPENDIX E
ANSWERS TO REVIEW ACTIVITIES

CHAPTER 1

1. You may see some clinical dashboards or other evidence of quality improvement (QI) activities around your agency. They reveal information about patient access, cost, quality, patient satisfaction, and so forth. Are the scores improving? Which areas need improvement?
2. Nurses and other members of the interprofessional team are usually involved in various safety projects to improve the quality of patient care. Information about patient quality is being gathered and used to improve patient care. This information is being gathered also for The Joint Commission and other accreditation bodies.
3. The QSEN Institute website has many resources to identify prelicensure and graduate quality and safety competencies and teaching strategies to achieve them.

CHAPTER 2

1. When you read your local paper, you may find various articles that examine health care quality or safety issues. Your discussions with your classmates and instructor will probably be very interesting and informative.
2. When you interview three nurses where you are currently doing a clinical rotation about the most pressing patient safety issue on the unit, you will probably get many different answers. The discussion of these patient safety issues with your classmates and instructor in postconference may highlight beginning strategies to improve patient care safety.

CHAPTER 3

1. Discussion: In a high-reliability organization that has a just culture, the nurse should be able to respond to the question and describe the process. If no repercussions, such as punishment, occur from reporting an error then the process is blame free. This includes policies that focus on fixing the problem, rather than punishment

for committing an error. A clear process that includes how an error is reported, who it is reported to, what happens once the error is reported, and how nurses are involved in examining the process should be clear.

2. Correlations should occur with preoccupied with failure, reluctance to simplify, sensitivity to operations, resilience, and deference to expertise. Probing questions to ask would be: Is there a methodology to report near misses and how are those reports utilized? Are investigations completed when an event occurs and ask for an investigation analysis? Are safeguards in place to minimize distractions? What steps are taken to minimize the risk of harm when an event occurs? Do staff feel safe speaking up prior to a procedure to ensure a time out step is completed?

3. Mindfulness of the complexity of the processes, how easily a failure may occur even when support processes are in place mitigates harm. Aviation tools like the checklist, double checks, entire team engagement for process checks are steps that are put into place recognizing the complexity of health care processes. Each team member brings his or her professional expertise and it is essential the team benefits from that knowledge. Being able to speak up mitigates harm because other team members can often see things that nurses take for granted because it becomes routine or a work-around may have occurred. Being able to speak up holds each team member accountable for the safety outcome of the patient.

4. Transparency and the sharing of information allow the consumer to make choices for their health care. It becomes imperative for the organization to have process improvements and excellent outcomes to be able to meet our mission to the community. Communication and coordination across the continuum of care is essential to prevent further harm to the patient. Transitions of care are highly vulnerable for error. Coordination allows the patient to receive care at a lower cost setting and keeps the entire health care team knowledgeable of patient health care needs and preferences. Effective medication management and patient understanding of his or her disease process are key to preventing readmissions, decreasing the length of stay, and improving the overall health of the patient.

   The Joint Commission used the Donabedian conceptual framework to revise the core ORYX measurement. They identified key criteria for a measure to be an accountability measure. There has to be evidence that the intervention has a direct impact on the quality outcome for the patient. It needs to be measurable as to whether the care occurred and had to closely align with the outcome and with minimal unintended consequences.

   In a Magnet™-designated hospital, the chief nursing officer (CNO) is an active leader in creating a high-reliability organization (HRO) by establishing strategic goals in conjunction with the hospital's executive team for quality and safety. These goals support the organization's commitment to zero major quality failures. Transformational leadership and structural empowerment require the active engagement of nurses. For example, nurses serve on committees at the unit, department, and organizational levels. Nurses also participate on QI teams to find innovative solutions to move health care into the future. Exemplary professional nursing practice with evidence-based new knowledge, innovation, and improvements provide the framework to sustain improvements.

CHAPTER 4

1. The nursing hours per patient day calculation will probably vary on different days from two different weeks at your assigned clinical unit, depending on staffing and

patient census. Reaching out to a safety leader in your agency will facilitate your understanding of its culture of safety and related QI efforts. You will also gain an appreciation of how the way in which nurse staffing and the way you perform patient care contributes to patient and personal safety.

2. A clinical tool is only as good as the people who are using it. Shortcuts, work-arounds, or a climate of disregard for clinical tools and patient safety undermines safety tool effectiveness. Patient and/or staff are placed at risk for injury when this occurs. Discussions about safety heighten awareness and understanding about possible consequences of not adhering to safe clinical practices that have predictable and safe outcomes.

3. Using a safe work practice such as the SBARR format during your provision of patient care is one of the best ways to evaluate and assure patient safety. Standardizing the format for report handoffs reduces variation and moves toward increasing the predictability of a safe quality environment for patients. The main difference in the process between use of the SBARR format compared to other report handoffs is the standardization of the SBARR process. Standardization tends to contribute to an environment for safety.

CHAPTER 5

1. *Situation:* I am calling about Mrs. Smith. She is your patient admitted yesterday for pulmonary edema.
   Background: We have been treating her with 4 L via nasal cannula and 40 mg Lasix every 12 hours. She received the last dose 6 hours ago.
   Assessment: She is now complaining of shortness of breath. Her respiratory rate is 30. Her pulse oximetry reading is 91%. I auscultated crackles half way up her back.
   Recommendation: I think she needs her Lasix adjusted.

2. The nurse would implement the CUS (concerned, uncomfortable, safety) strategy.
   The nurse would implement it by stating: I *concerned* about giving this medication. I'm *uncomfortable* with the dose being so high. I don't think it is *safe*.

3. The nurse would implement the read-back strategy. In doing so, the nurse would record the lab value and then repeat back the patient's name and the lab value to the caller so it could be verified for accuracy.

CHAPTER 6

1. Holding the patient's hand too firmly may convey restraint. There is an art and gentleness with hand holding that is documented and shows comforting reassurance and support.
   When one shows caring attention through hand holding a sense of trust is encouraged and exchanged through this simple act.
   Patients often times convey anxiousness through a variety of nonverbal expressions. Some of these may be fidgeting, frowned brow, grimaced face, wide eyes, tightness of facial muscles, stiffened body, staring without expression.
   When the nurse is in a position whereby hand holding is not possible, eye contact, a nod, touch to the cheek, or rested hand on the shoulder could all convey reassurance and support to the patient.

2. Collaboration and effective communication across the health care team is critical to promote positive patient outcomes. Collaborative strategies include consulting with each other on the information gathered from chart reviews, documented sources related to his condition, and assessment of the patient.

   Both students could interview the patient together with spontaneously asking questions in a conversation type approach as opposed to a rigid interview of questions.

   Communication barriers could be self-intimidation and insecurity when rounding with experts on the health care team. Others may be competiveness with peer as opposed to collectively working together for the benefit of the patient, not self-gratification.

   Communication enhancers could be the confidence one experiences when the student partners begin to see beyond a few notes taken during chart review and really begin to discover the patient's perspective of health. Rounding as a member of the interprofessional team within a collaborative relationship fosters inquiry and openness to learn as opposed to feeling being called upon with expectation will need to know everything about the patient.

   There is no "I" in a team; all work together and collaboratively when on a team. Communication can be enhanced through self-reflection exercises, such as journaling, creating tool kits, utilizing shared standard clinical communications, such as SBAR (situation, background, assessment, recommendations); communication enhancers through email, electronic devices in the workplace for learning about patient care options, drug therapies, definitions, lab values, and so on.

3. Communicating between the academic and service settings are very important so all parties have a common understanding of the purpose and goals for the clinical arrangement as a learning environment within a work environment. Together they will develop as a collaborative team at the administrative level as well as among the mentor–mentee partnership. Formalizing a mentor–mentee program requires selecting the correct mentor who is willing to work with students. The partnerships between the academic environment and the hospitals will lead to greater outcomes when formal processes such as support from both settings agree to make this work. The staff mentor would need to be willing and possess the interpersonal skill and patience needed for interacting and guiding student nurses.

   Opposition usually occurs as staff workloads have increased over time and patient safety is always the primary concern of the nurse. The staff and team in service may argue there is little time to allow students learning opportunities as there are crises, busy schedules to meet with caring for six to eight acute care patients, and little time to explain what needs to get done. Some argue "it is faster if I just do it myself."

   Champions of the seamless example with the paired assignment can explain a paired, shared assignment helps the students to learn how to effectively communicate together. They also learn how to collaborate with each other as they review materials related to the patient's history, and learn from each other as would experience in a health care team approach, such as rounding.

CHAPTER 7

1. Students should complete the course and provide evidence by printing off the certificate of completion.

2. Students can work in teams or individually to conduct the HFMEA on a clinical process. This activity provides students with an understanding of how an HFMEA works and what the outcome should be for the activity. Complete one as a class to familiarize students with the process.

3. This activity is designed to enable students to self-evaluate their readiness for change. The results can be used to foster a discussion on what it means to be ready for change and to develop a plan to increase readiness for change.

4. This activity is designed to help the student understand aspects of readiness for QI from the perspective of a practicing nurse. The real-world implications of an organization's preparedness for QI affects the success or failure of quality initiatives.

CHAPTER 8

1. The website provides a repository of information about quality health care, including benchmarks and databases. The student should understand the depth and breadth of reporting mechanisms by reviewing the contents of the site.

2. This activity is designed to illustrate variances in health care outcomes from different geographical locations using a scorecard format. The student can understand how a scorecard helps to represent data in an easy to understand format, facilitates actionable data, and can be understood by a variety of health care professions.

3. This activity demonstrates the outcomes of care based on publicly reportable quality measures for hospitals and providers. It is designed to have students become aware of variances in outcomes among health care organizations and providers.

4. This activity helps students understand the evidence-based guidelines and the variances between what should be done in the clinical setting and what is currently done. Students can examine how the data collected on the outcomes of care from the inappropriate use of guidelines can affect the health care organizations outcomes.

5. Students should at minimum, identify the need for consistent, evidence-based guidelines that reflect best practices in the clinical setting. The ability to freely access guidelines helps the smaller hospitals that do not have access to a library, access evidence-based guidelines for care. Free access to clinical guidelines can help improve the outcomes from health care delivery.

6. Under or overreporting falls occurs due to the variances in the definition of falls. Falls can be related to intrinsic or extrinsic factors, can be a facilitated descent, or may be a partial fall. Problems also arise among hospitals as the definition of falls is interpreted differently in hospitals.

   Falls can be decreased or minimized when the organization identifies those at risk early and implements fall prevention strategies. Having a standardized fall risk scale, assessing risk for falls upon admission, and implementing guidelines to minimize the risk for falls consistently are essential steps for fall prevention.

   Other disciplines have an impact on fall rates. Pharmacy should examine patient medication lists for polypharmacy implications that increase the risk for falls. Physicians should be included as a co-coordinator of care with nurses through medication adjustments and ordering necessary lab work or treatments. Physical therapists can evaluate a patient's activity level and provide assistive devices that can minimize the risk for falls. Nursing assistants spend the most time with the patient and can provide invaluable information about the patient's status.

7. The student should provide specific criteria that can be measured to determine compliance. The guideline provides specific steps that can be measured using a checklist format. The person responsible for the collecting the data can be a person from the quality department or a nurse working with the data. The data should be reported through a central department within the hospital to ensure consistency in reporting.

8. The improvement stories are updated continuously and can be used to demonstrate how benchmarking supports quality performance. Students can work in groups or individually to report back on the issue under investigation.

9. This activity is designed to help students understand that not all indicators can be measured or affected by one discipline. It takes a variety of health care professionals working together to make an improvement to the delivery of health care.

CHAPTER 9

1. Students should identify patient engagement, reducing racial and ethnic differences, and creating a national reform in the delivery of health care. The students should examine how this program has evolved over time to create and sustain change.

2. Students should identify a recent sentinel event alert and the data that supports the problem. In addition, students should be able to provide information about the prevalence of the problem for health care organizations. Guide students to develop a QI plan to address the problem.

3. Students can present their findings about cases from the frontlines to the class. Have the students compare the findings from the case study to their current clinical experiences. Discuss how the improvement might be implemented in the clinical setting. Because the case studies are frequently updated, have students share knowledge gained from the readings and how it might be implemented in another clinical setting.

CHAPTER 10

Activity A: Matching

1. d
2. a
3. e
4. b
5. c

Activity B: Fill in the Blank

1. HITECH
2. CPOE system
3. Quality Chasm
4. Department of Veterans Affairs

Activity C: Short Answer

1. Some of the issues noted include:

   - Missing or incomplete charts
   - Lost charts
   - Illegible handwriting
   - Misinterpreted orders
   - Lack of available current patient information
   - Inability to track patient interactions with multiple providers
   - Incomplete recording of test results, leading to duplicate testing

2. Point of care decision prompts are designed to aid providers in patient care and promote patient safety. Some of the prompts are alerts, such as medication conflicts, allergies, or potential adverse reactions. Other prompts may offer references to local policies and procedures. Still others may assist with patient education by providing readily available, up-to-date information.

3. Some advantages of EHR use include:

   - Time-saving features with documentation
   - Easy access to up-to-date, evidence-based literature to enhance patient care
   - Real-time access to patient information such as allergies, lab results, and updated orders
   - Interprofessional interaction with the patient information, with all members having access to the most current patient information
   - Increased patient safety related to reduced errors from poorly written orders
   - Reduction of errors related to poorly transcribed orders
   - Automated systems that promote timeliness in care provision and medication administration
   - Information database systems that promote increase patient education

4. Confidentiality is described as a responsibility of providers to keep patient health information protected and maintain the patient's privacy. This contrasts with a system approach to protect patient information.

   Security is defined as protection features that are designed into the computer. These security measures are meant to protect the patient's privacy by blocking unauthorized access to the database. Generally this is the responsibility of the information security manager within a facility.

5. VISTA—an acronym for Veterans Health Information Systems Technology Architecture, provides an array of features in managing patient health information. Some of these features include:

   - A summary screen—providing a concise overview of key health issues, medication, allergies, vital signs history, and lab results
   - Built-in navigation tools alert providers to critical information
   - Clinical reminders promote timeliness of care by alerting providers of due dates for follow-up tests, routine exams, and prescription refills
   - Vista promotes patient involvement and enhanced self-care by providing patients with web-based access to aspects of their health information.

CHAPTER 11

1. You will probably find that searching in Medline, for example, using the subject headings *myocardial infarction* and *aspirin* produces a highly relevant data set that is easy to focus even further using the limit commands. Limiting the search to articles published in English, articles published in the past 5 years, and meta-analyses should produce a small but highly relevant data set.

   You probably found that searching for literature regarding how the involvement of a patient's family impacts outcomes is a bit harder. Using key words like *family involvement* and *outcomes* in CINAHL can lead to relevant articles. At this point, you can use the "pearl growing" technique to find more evidence. Pearl growing is a technique for refining a literature search through examining the complete record of one highly relevant article to see which subject headings have been attached to it, thus finding clues for how to search the literature for other relevant articles.

2. At the time of publication, a Medline search for keywords "myocardial infarction AND aspirin" yielded 6,160 results, and a search using the subject headings "myocardial infarction" and "aspirin" using the search builder function yielded 2,744 results. Search limits can be used to increase the relevancy of both data sets, but initial results are more relevant when the search is conducted using subject headings.

3. This is an example of why it is sometimes best to initially conduct a broad search for literature and then narrow your focus if necessary. You will likely find that searching for literature regarding patient-to-staff ratios in NICUs produces a small data set, and that adding in the criteria of charge nurses and night shift leads to zero results. Had you begun by searching for all four criteria at once, it would have appeared as though no relevant data on this topic existed.

CHAPTER 12

1. P—The population of interest is patients on a medical–surgical inpatient unit with IV catheters

   I—The intervention would be a new evidence-based IV catheter protocol
   C—The comparison would be the current IV catheter care policy
   O—The outcome of interest would be the incidence of phlebitis

   Therefore, in a complete sentence the PICO statement is as follows:
   For patients on a medical–surgical unit with IV catheters, what is the impact of a new evidence-based IV catheter care protocol, compared to the current IV catheter protocol, on the incidence of phlebitis?
   It is important to note that PICO statements should never be able to be answered with a "yes" or "no" answer.
   Learning to locate articles and data within databases is a learned process, and each database has its unique qualities. The data is within the system, but the nurse must utilize proper methods of extraction to obtain the data. This is a process that takes time and practice. Practice locating articles. If you have difficulty, ask for assistance from a school or institution librarian or nurse educator.
   Read the article that you have located and determine the level of evidence that the article represents. Refer to Figure 12.2 as you critically examine the article. If

you are unclear about determining levels of evidence seek out the assistance of a nurse educator or a librarian.

2. When considering interventions for patient care, first consider policies and procedures established by the health care institution you work in. Ideally, a policy will list the source of evidence from which it was established. In reading the policy, consider the level of evidence it provides. Keep in mind, a clinical pathway is ideally based on research providing evidence of superior safety and quality of care.

CHAPTER 13

1. The Centers for Disease Control website offers a wide variety of resources to help nurses and the general public live healthier lifestyles such as exercise, smoking cessation, better nutrition, and so on. After "clicking" on a particular topic, note that each section includes health information for the general public as well as sections specifically for health professionals.

2. The Robert Wood Johnson/Institute of Medicine report, *The Future of Nursing: Leading Change, Advancing Health* (2011 website, http://thefutureofnursing.org), offers resources to help RNs find out what activities are being conducted to promote the Campaign for Action. The Campaign for Action is a collaborative effort to implement solutions to the challenges facing the nursing profession, and to build upon nurse-based approaches to improving quality and transforming the way Americans receive health care. The website discusses the campaign as well as the names and telephone numbers of individuals who are leading efforts in each state. The website also offers quick facts, information about upcoming events, individual state action coalitions, facebook, and so on. When you click on the site for your state, you will find information about your state's leadership, contacts, education, Facebook, and so on.

GLOSSARY

Accountable care organization (ACO) is a formal network of doctors, hospitals, and health care providers that will share the responsibility of providing health care to all the patients enrolled with the ACO (Advisory Board Company, 2010).

Accredited hospital is one that demonstrates that the hospital meets the minimal standards for quality developed by The Joint Commission (TJC) or another accrediting agency; this includes monitoring of standards such as infection control standards, medication management standards, and emergency management standards, and so on, as well as measurement of core measures, safe practice measures, and process improvement.

Adverse event is an undesired or intended consequence of the care provided (The Joint Commission, 2012).

Bar-code medication administration (BCMA) uses bar codes printed on the patient's wristband and the medication packet to determine if the medication is intended for the correct patient.

Benchmarking is "the continual and collaborative discipline of measuring and comparing the results of key work processes with those of the best performers in evaluating organizational performance" (Hughes, 2008).

Bibliographic databases, such as Medline, provide a basic record, or citation, for an article and often provide an abstract or brief summary, of the article; they do not necessarily contain the complete text of the article itself (Rosenberg & Donald, 1995).

Boolean commands are terms such as AND, OR, or NOT that are used to either expand or limit your literature search results when searching the literature in most electronic databases.

Clinical intelligence is the electronic aggregation of accurate, relevant, and timely clinical data into meaningful information and actionable knowledge (Harrington, 2011).

Collaboration is an interpersonal personal process characterized by health care professionals from multiple disciplines with shared objectives, decision making, responsibility, and power, working together to solve patient care problems (Petri, 2010).

Computerized provider order entry (CPOE) allows health care providers to enter orders directly into a computer system.

Core accountability measures are standardized performance indicators that allow for comparison of quality measures between organizations.

Critical appraisal guide to the literature is essentially a checklist containing questions to ask about key aspects of a study (Melnyk & Fineout-Overholt, 2011).

Cross-monitoring is the process of monitoring the actions of other team members for the purpose of sharing the workload and reducing or avoiding errors (Agency for Healthcare Research and Quality [AHRQ] TeamSTEPPS. n.d.).

Culture of safety refers to the extent to which individuals and groups will commit to personal responsibility for safety; act to preserve, enhance, and communicate safety concerns; strive to actively learn, adapt, and modify both individual and organizational behavior based on lessons learned from mistakes; strive to be honored in association with these values (von Thaden & Gibbons, 2008).

Dashboard is a tool to display quality data in a systematic manner from a specific point in time that allows users to quickly extract the meaning. Dashboards can include color graphics and highlights to help users see the data, identify trends or patterns, extract meaning, and clarify implications.

Debriefing is recounting key events and analyzing why they occurred; include what worked, what didn't work, leading to a discussion of lessons learned, and how they will alter the plan next time (AHRQ TeamSTEPPS, n.d.)

De-escalation strategies in health care, actions that decrease aggressive behaviors during challenging communications, which include refocusing attention on the patient (Altmiller, 2011).

Electronic health record (EHR) is a lifelong record of an individual's medical encounters, health screenings, and preventive health care. The record is in digital form and it can be exchanged between different computer systems.

Empathetic communication is a process by which we seek to appreciate or understand the perspective of the person first and then convey meaning in an attempt to create a shared understanding.

E-patient is a health care consumer who is equipped, enabled, empowered, and engaged in his or her health and health care decisions.

Error was defined as "any event in a patient's medical care that did not go as intended and either harmed or could have harmed the patient" (Plews-Ogan, Nadkarni, Forren et al., 2004).

Evidence-based practice (EBP) is a process that promotes the delivery of optimal health care through the integration of best current evidence, clinical expertise, and patient/family values (QSEN, 2012).

External benchmarking provides a way to measure quality with another health care organization or with professional standards, and compare what you are doing against what others are doing (Hughes, 2008).

Failure to rescue occurs when clinicians fail to notice patient symptoms or they fail to respond adequately or quickly enough to clinical signs that may indicate that a patient is dying of preventable complications in a hospital.

Fair and just culture is the demonstration of an open, free, and nonpunitive environment, which readily admits its weaknesses and commits to learning from its mistakes (Hughes, 2008).

Free market is a market where the price of a good or service is mutually determined by at least two people or groups of people; people agree to pay a price for either a commodity or service. The transaction is mutually agreed to by both parties rather than by governmental regulation (Rothbard, 2008).

Full-text databases provide the complete text of an article as well as the article citation.

Handoff is the process of one health care professional updating another on the status of one or more patients for the purpose of taking over their care (AHRQ Glossary of Terms, n.d.).

Health care quality is the degree to which health services for individuals and populations increases the likelihood of desired health outcomes and are consistent with current professional knowledge (IOM, 2013, para 3).

Health care transparency has been defined by the Institute of Medicine (IOM, 2001) as making available to the public, in a reliable and understandable manner, information on the health care system's quality, efficiency and consumer experience with care, which includes price and quality data, so as to influence the behavior of patients, providers, payers and others to achieve better outcomes (quality and cost of care).

Health care failure mode and effect analysis (HFMEA) is a proactive approach to mitigate harm that involves a comprehensive risk assessment of a select high-risk process that the organization has identified. The goal of the team is to improve the high-risk processes before an adverse event occurs.

Health literacy is the degree to which individuals have the capacity to obtain, process, and understand basic health information and services they need to make health decisions.

High-reliability organization (HRO) are those organizations that establish and maintain high-quality and safety expectations for patient care delivery and keep rates of quality and safety failures near zero (Weick & Sutcliffe, 2007).

HIPAA is an acronym for Health Insurance Portability and Accountability Act (1996). Enacted safeguards for the privacy and security of individually identifiable health information.

HITECH is an acronym for Health Information Technology for Economic and Clinical Health Act (2009). Provided funding for development of EHRs.

Hospital quality initiative (HQI), a voluntary program where hospitals report their performance on a set of core quality measures to a public website, www.hospitalcompare.hhs.gov.

Hospital Value-Based Purchasing Program (HVBPP), incentive payments will be made by CMS to hospitals who either demonstrate improvement in performance of quality measures from a baseline period, or by how well benchmarks are achieved (Centers for Medicaid and Medicare Services, 2012).

Human factors engineering is the discipline concerned with understanding human characteristics and applying that knowledge to the design of systems that are reliable, safe, efficient, and comfortable to use (Gosbee & Gosbee, 2012).

Innovators are individuals who exhibit characteristics such as being flexible about change, curious with a sense of inquiry, have good communications skills, and have an awareness of self and the practice unit (Schmidt & Brown, 2009).

Internal benchmarking "is used to identify best practices within an organization, to compare best practices within the organization, and to compare current practice over time" (Hughes, 2008, para. 6)

Key word is a self-identified literature search term that uses your own personal natural language to search the literature.

Knowledge-focus triggers are those situations that stem from the research literature, a new philosophy of care, new national standards or professional guidelines.

Lateral violence is an aggressive, destructive behavior of nurses against each other (Woelfle & McCaffrey, 2007).

Lean thinking, originating from the Toyota Motor Corporation, that strives to eliminate forms of waste within a process to increase efficiency while enhancing effectiveness. There are eight identified sources of waste in organizations that include unused human potential, waiting, transportation, defects, inventory, motion, overproduction, and processing.

Lean Six Sigma is a combination of Lean thinking (to reduce waste) and Six Sigma methodologies (reduce variation) within an improvement process.

Levels of evidence is a hierarchy of information that allows practitioners to temper their clinical decisions with more or less certainty; provides some degree of strength to the practice recommendations.

Literature search is "a systematic and explicit approach to the identification, retrieval, and bibliographic management of independent studies (usually drawn from published sources) for the purpose of locating information on a topic, synthesizing conclusions, identifying areas for future study, and developing guidelines for clinical practice" (Auston, Cahn, & Selden, 1998).

Literature search limit commands will edit your literature search results to only include results that meet your limiting criteria, for example, articles published in the last 5 years.

Medical identity theft is posing as another person and using that person's health insurance to illegally obtain free medical care.

Mindfulness is staying focused with the ability to see the significance of early and weak signals and to take strong and decisive action to prevent harm (Weick & Sutcliff, 2001).

Misuse of health care services is when incorrect diagnoses, medical errors, and avoidable health care complications occur.

MyHealtheVet is a patient portal for the Department of Veterans Affairs Veterans Health Information Systems and Technology Architecture (VISTA) system.

Near miss is an event or situation that did not produce a patient injury but only because of chance; considered a close call (AHRQ Glossary of Terms, n.d.).

Never events are health care situations that arise that are serious, often preventable, and not expected to occur in a hospital, such as a patient acquiring a new Stage IV pressure ulcer.

Nurse informaticist is a person who practices nursing informatics and who may have a professional certification in that area.

Nursing research is a process of inquiry that is systematic, adheres to rigorous guidelines, and, at the most significant level, produces unbiased answers to questions of nursing practice (Houser, 2008).

Outcome indicators include the end result from the delivery of care, such as the presence of falls, pressure ulcers, hospital-acquired infections, patient satisfaction, or readmission to the hospital (AHRQ, 2011).

Outcomes refer to the "changes (desirable or undesirable) in individuals and populations that can be attributed to health care" such as patient satisfaction results or outcomes of care (Donabedian, 2003, p. 46).

Overuse of health care services is when a health care service is provided even though it is not justified by the patient's health care needs.

Participatory medicine is a model of care that supports a cooperative approach by all members of the health care team across the full continuum of care.

Patient acuity refers to the degree of health care service complexity needed by a patient related to their physical or mental status.

Patient advocacy are actions directed at decision makers to support and promote patients' health care rights, enhance community health and policy initiatives, and focus on the availability, safety, and quality of care.

Patient handoff is the transfer of responsibility for a patient from one clinician to another and involves sharing current information that is pertinent to the patient's care with time allowed for discussion, questions, and clarification.

Pearl growing is a technique for refining a literature search through examining the complete record of one highly relevant article to see which subject headings have been attached to it, thus finding clues for how to search the literature for other relevant articles.

Performance gaps describe the difference between current practice and the recommended standard of care (AHRQ, 2010).

Person approach to safety in which we only blame the person at the end of the long chain of errors for making an error that caused an adverse event from overuse, underuse, or misuse of health care services.

Plan-Do-Check-Act (PDCA) is a decision-making framework to monitor the structures, processes, and outcomes of interdependent systems that affect patient care and patient care delivery; a simple and effective framework to guide and monitor full implementation of a practice change.

Plan-Do-Study-Act (PDSA) incorporates knowledge of engineering, operations, and management with the goal of improving accuracy, reducing costs, increasing efficiency and safety, and is composed of four parts: (a) appreciation for a system, (b) understanding process variation, (c) applying theory of knowledge, and (d) using psychology.

Population-focused health care is care based on the health status and needs assessment of a target group of individuals who have one or more personal or environmental characteristics in common.

Practice change involves changing a standard of care/pattern of action from what it was due to new scientific evidence.

Problem-focus triggers are situations identified within the organization and include risk management data, internal and external performance improvement data, financial data, and indications of a clinical problem.

Process refers to "the activities that constitute health care" such as health care policies and standards of care (Donabedian, 2003, p. 46).

Process of care indicators include the evidence-based steps (interventions, actions, or tasks) that when performed help to meet desired outcomes (AHRQ, 2011).